T0136794

Low Protein Cookery

for

Phenylketonuria

LOW PROTEIN COOKERY

for

PHENYLKETONURIA

Virginia E. Schuett

THIRD EDITION

The University of Wisconsin Press

The University of Wisconsin Press
1930 Monroe Street
Madison, Wisconsin 53711

3 Henrietta Street
London WC2E 8LU, England

9   10

Printed in the United States of America

All illustrations are by Virginia E. Schuett.

Library of Congress Cataloging-in-Publication Data
Schuett, Virginia E., 1947–
Low protein cookery for phenylketonuria /
Virginia E. Schuett.—3rd. ed.
570 pp.   cm.
Includes index.
ISBN 0-299-15384-3 (pbk.)
1. Phenylketonuria—Diet therapy—Recipes. 2. Low-phenylalanine
diet—Recipes. 3. Low—protein diet—Recipes. I. Title.
RJ399.P5S38   1997
641.5′638—dc21   97-5931

ISBN-13: 978-0-299-15384-7 (pbk: alk. paper)

Contents

Helpful Hints

Everyday Tips

Foreword

This book was written on behalf of children and others with phenylketonuria (PKU). Since parents play such a fundamental role in managing treatment in the early years of life, I would like to relate some of the history of PKU and emphasize the importance that parents have had over the years. With their interest and energy, we have now come to the point where this book of recipes and ideas can help in preventing the mental retardation formerly associated with PKU.

The initial discovery of PKU in 1933 was prompted by the desperate attempt of one mother with two mentally retarded children to find someone who could help them, according to a story related to me by Dr. George Jervis (who is credited with first describing the enzyme defect in PKU). Several physicians in Europe failed in their attempts to provide assistance. In fact, one of the doctors referred her to a psychiatrist to help with her "delusion" when she described the penetrating and peculiar odor of her children's urine. Finally, Dr. Asbjørn Følling of Norway was impressed with her story, verified the presence of the unusual urine odor, and was able to identify it as coming from a chemical compound called phenylpyruvic acid, from which PKU gets its name. Thus, identification of PKU was stimulated by the persistence of one mother. Dr. Følling later went on to test hundreds of mentally retarded children and adults with the simple chemical urine test he had used initially. By this method he determined that PKU was in fact an inherited condition that can happen when both parents are carriers of the disease.

The next major development in the history of PKU was identification and preparation of a treatment. Again a parent of a child with PKU was highly influential. In the early 1950s, Dr. Horst Bickel, a German physician working in England, set up a new screening method for testing urine in children with suspected "metabolic diseases" such as PKU. The story he told me is that almost immediately after he began his screening, he confirmed a diagnosis of PKU in a two-year-old girl who was hyperactive and severely retarded. When the mother was told that there was no treatment available, she refused to accept this. Her persistence and devotion to her child had an important influence on Dr. Bickel's decision to embark on the research that led to the development of the special formula that would provide a basis for treatment. With the aid of a biochemist colleague, Dr. Bickel prepared a phenylalanine-free mixture of amino acids to replace normal food protein (which is high in phenylalanine) in the child's diet. After the child had consumed this mixture for several days, her blood phenylalanine level fell and a remarkable improvement in behavior occurred. Although the special formula came too late to alter the child's mental retardation, the dramatic change in behavior in this child was the first demonstration of the profound effect of a low phenylalanine diet. This, and other similar experiences with affected children, led to the hope that such dietary manipulation might prevent the neurological as well as the behavioral problems so typical of the disease, if the diet were initiated early enough in life. The stage had been set for routine dietary treatment of PKU—if it could be detected soon after birth, before damage had occurred.

Once again, personal experience with PKU played a vital role, now in the development of the first successful screening test for PKU. This time, the personal experience was my own. My son John is mentally retarded, due to unknown causes. Through my activities with the local Association for Retarded Children, I made professional contacts that stimulated a career change. I left cancer research and became involved in human biochemical genetics research as it relates to causes and prevention of mental retardation. Two years later, a fantastic coincidence occurred. In another city, 1000 miles away, a niece of mine was found to have PKU at the age of 17 months. While I was already involved in basic research on PKU, it was certainly my niece who inspired me to develop a practical PKU screening test for newborns.

In 1961, my test method was first published. Unlike Dr. Følling's first urine-screening test, my test relies on the greater accuracy of testing for phenylalanine in blood. A national trial of the test was funded by the U.S. Children's Bureau in 1962–63, and with the success of that trial, it was parents from the many chapters of the National Association for Retarded Citizens who lobbied successfully for the state laws that mandated newborn screening of PKU. Newborn screening for PKU is now done throughout the United States and in many other parts of the world, commonly using the "Guthrie Test."

As a result of these screening efforts, coupled with early and continuing dietary treatment, we have learned that children with PKU can indeed develop normally and lead healthy and productive lives—something only dreamed of 30 years ago. Our children and young people with PKU today are the direct beneficiaries of the collaborative efforts of parents and professionals over the past several decades. These collaborative efforts are demonstrated not only in the history of PKU that I have outlined for you. This second edition of *Low Protein Cookery for Phenylketonuria* was written by a professional who has more than a decade of experience in helping families manage the diet, both in Wisconsin and through her contacts with families nationwide. The book was inspired by these families and their children, and has drawn on their day-to-day experiences with PKU.

The story of PKU has taken a new turn in recent years. Now the problem of preventing mental retardation in children is being augmented by the problem of preventing damage to unborn children of women who themselves have PKU. Additionally, there is a need to continue treatment for both young men and women with PKU in order to protect them from the adverse effects of elevated blood phenylalanine levels on mental performance and behavior. Regular use of this excellent resource book as part of a PKU treatment program should make continuing the diet possible on the long-term basis that is now recommended. It will help its users to take full advantage of the legacy of parent-professional collaboration and cooperation that has characterized the history of PKU.

Robert Guthrie, Ph.D., M.D.
Professor of Pediatrics
State University at Buffalo
Department of Pediatrics
Buffalo, New York

May 1986

Author's Note

Dr. Robert Guthrie died of congestive heart failure in Seattle, Washington, on June 18, 1995, four days short of his 80th birthday. He and his wife had moved to Seattle from his long-time home in Buffalo, New York, just two months earlier, to be closer to several of their children. I feel privileged to have been among those to see him in his final days, to say good-bye to this man who shaped the course of newborn screening for PKU and other inherited metabolic diseases.

From its beginning in 1989, Dr. Guthrie was a member of the Board of Directors of National PKU News. Beyond his single-minded dedication to preventing the mental retardation caused by PKU, throughout his life Dr. Guthrie was a devoted advocate for families living with it. I started National PKU News with his support and encouragement.

In his memory, National PKU News has started a higher education scholarship program—*The Robert Guthrie PKU Scholarship.* Early screening and diet treatment have allowed thousands of young people to grow up and lead normal lives. Now, thankfully, many are going to colleges and technical schools instead of living in institutions or group homes for the mentally retarded.

If you are interested in contributing to this program, or in applying for a scholarship, please contact National PKU News, 6869 Woodlawn Ave. NE #116, Seattle, WA 98115-5469. Scholarship applications will be available after September 1, 1997. The first scholarship will be awarded for the 1998 academic year.

Virginia Schuett
Seattle, Washington

November 1996

10

Preface

This third edition of *Low Protein Cookery for PKU* is being published exactly twenty years after the original 1977 version. In those two decades, the book has been used by thousands of families from all over the United States who are living with PKU. It also has found its way into the homes of families living in a number of other countries, even though our food supplies and habits are different. I am gratified that the book's appeal has been enduring and broad.

Through the Years with *Low Protein Cookery for PKU*

First Edition

I wrote the first edition while I was nutritionist for the inherited metabolic disease program at the Waisman Center in Madison, Wisconsin. The idea for the book arose from my involvement with a group of Wisconsin PKU mothers. Our little group met regularly for many years, sharing recipes and experiences living with PKU. The exchange was helpful for all of us. The recipes and ideas from that group formed the core of the original edition. Without the help of five mothers—Judy Brandt, Sonja Keesey-Berg, Nancy Reyzer, Sharon Swenson and Ann Van De Wiel—*Low Protein Cookery for PKU* might not exist. Their children, toddlers when we started the book, are all grown now—they are in college, are college graduates, or starting families.

Second Edition

Just over ten years later, the second edition was published, while I was still at the Waisman Center. The second edition evolved into what was essentially a new book. Only about 10% of the original recipes and materials were retained, and most of these were modified to some extent. While the first edition took advantage of all of the expertise in low protein cookery and diet management that we had at the time, in the following decade low protein cooking came a long way with the help of new products. The second edition took advantage of everything I learned in the ensuing ten years about low protein cookery and the PKU diet. It also drew on the collective experiences and expertise of people from all over the country. Approximately seventy of the recipes were selected from a collection submitted by families. I personally tested and standardized each of these recipes.

The remainder of the recipes, approximately four hundred, are ones that I developed specifically for the book, or adapted from the first edition or from my own extensive personal collection of cookbooks and recipes. The recipes were frequently evaluated by families and their children who came to the clinic for follow-up, and by the clinic staff. Also, on a very regular basis, my young neighbors at the time, Alice and Emily Pawley (then ages eight and six and now in college), were ever-ready kitchen helpers who never tired of "taste-testing," though neither has PKU. Approximately 20% of the recipes were further tested by a group of twenty-five mothers of children with PKU from all over the country.

The contributions of all of these people made the book the collaborative effort I had hoped it would be, and their support and enjoyment of the recipes made all of the many hours in my home "test kitchen" seem less overwhelming.

All of the foods in the photographs were made in my own kitchen, using low protein ingredients. I used no gimmicks and made no alterations of the food for the sake of photography—it was all prepared strictly according to the recipes in the book, to convince you that you can produce the same delicious-looking foods in your own kitchen.

Third Edition

In 1987 I left Wisconsin and moved to Seattle, Washington. Shortly thereafter I started National PKU News, a non-profit organization dedicated to providing news and information to PKU families and professionals. I suspect (and hope) that most people who use this cookbook are subscribers to the newsletter. Through the newsletter I keep everyone up-to-date on new food products, recipes, research and issues affecting everyone living with PKU.

Through National PKU News, I also have published several books, including *The Low Protein Food List for PKU* (1995). The new food list takes the place of the earlier version, *Low Protein Food List* (1981). The nutrient content of all recipes in the second edition of the cookbook was based on the old 1981 food list. For the cookbook's third edition, I have now updated all of the nutrient calculations based on the new food list. This is the major new feature of the third edition.

Like the original edition of *Low Protein Cookery for PKU*, the original food list was compiled using the best information we had at the time. But it had needed updating for a very long time. The available food supply changed greatly in the years since its publication. And the nutrient information that is available now is much better than it was in 1981. New food-labeling laws were the impetus for food manufacturers to do more extensive analyses, which I was able to obtain (with much effort) for the new food list. Also, the United States Department of Agriculture published updated data beginning in the late 1980s. Like the second version of *Low Protein Cookery for PKU*, the revision of the original 1981 food list became a whole new book.

12

There are many changes in the nutrient content of the recipes in this new edition, compared to the earlier version. We now know that some foods have more phenylalanine and protein than we thought, and others have less. For most of the recipes, the changes are fairly minor, but for a few, there are substantial changes. I felt that it was important for the new edition to reflect the most accurate information available.

For the third edition, I have also updated parts of the introductory material. And for some of the recipes, I have replaced ingredients that are no longer available with substitutes.

I have not altered the recipes themselves in any substantive way for this edition. Remarkably, they have stood the test of time. I continue to hear satisfying comments from people that the recipes work well. They tell me the recipes have made a big difference in the variety they are able to give to their children. I also know that parents and others have used many of the recipes as the basis for other creative variations. It seems the recipes in this book have become "classics" of low protein cookery. I could not be more pleased.

Changes in PKU Treatment Practices Bring Changes in How the Cookbook Is Used

In the years since the first cookbook was published, there has been a substantial change in our knowledge of PKU. That knowledge has had far-reaching effects on treatment and on who uses this book.

In 1977, most children with PKU stopped the diet during early school years. Most clinicians at the time believed this was a reasonable policy, since the majority of physical brain growth occurs by about age six. Therefore, the first edition of *Low Protein Cookery for PKU* was geared to the taste preferences and diet restrictions of a fairly young group of children.

In the 1980s, many clinics treating PKU in this country began recommending indefinite maintenance of diet. This change in attitude came about as clinical experience showed that children taken off the diet were at risk for developing a variety of significant problems. High phenylalanine levels were especially likely to affect intelligence and behavior. The problems were sometimes recognized only years after the diet was stopped. As a result of changes in clinic policy, we had to be dedicated to providing a varied, interesting, and high-quality diet for persons over a much greater age span. By the time of the second edition in 1988, many clinics nationwide had experience with older children, teens, and young adults on the diet. I kept this group in mind while preparing the second edition.

Now, in the 1990s, it has become standard practice for clinics throughout the United States and worldwide to maintain the diet "indefinitely." Indeed, "diet for life" is what parents are told to prepare for when their children are still infants.

In the 1990s we are also dealing with several burgeoning problems for young people with PKU. I hope these young people will benefit from using the book. One problem is the need to return teens and young adults with PKU to the diet. It is my strong belief that this is crucial to optimize their chances of becoming the most healthy and productive adults possible. I believe passionately, and many others agree, that all young persons with PKU who are off the diet should give serious consideration to returning to the diet—even those who do not currently believe they have suffered negative effects. A surprising number of young adults have told me that when they return to the diet, they recognize only then that they were indeed suffering a variety of ill effects from high phenylalanine levels. When they return to the diet, they commonly comment on how much better they feel, and on such changes as their increased energy, improved sleep, increased ability to focus, clearer thinking, and more even temperament.

Another problem that we are facing, as more young women with PKU become of child-bearing age, is the need to make sure all of them are on the diet before conception. Diet treatment before conception will optimize chances of a woman with PKU having a normal child. "Maternal PKU" is a concern for any young woman with elevated blood phenylalanine levels who is now pregnant or who may become pregnant. This includes any woman with a blood phenylalanine level above 6 mg/dl. Thus, even women who were not treated in infancy because their levels were thought not dangerous for development need to be concerned about modifying their diet during pregnancy. We still do not know everything we would like to about risks to young women and their babies from elevated blood phenylalanine levels. Research is ongoing.

Despite the continued "aging" of our PKU population, I believe that the recipes in this book are suitable for people of all ages. For young adults with more sophisticated taste-buds, the basic recipes can be modified with added herbs and spices. And they can provide inspiration for endless creative variations using low protein ingredients.

The ideas in the Helpful Hints section are unchanged and still geared to young children, with the thought that these are the "learning years" for both children and parents, and are of special importance. As time passes, most children and families learn to adapt to the needs of the diet in their own special ways, drawing on their years of previous experience to help them "improvise" in a variety of circumstances. I hope this ability to cope with the diet, learned over

14

time, will see our young adults through the trials and challenges the diet presents.

I hope this book will be a great source of continuing inspiration and support and bring you much pleasure in preparing truly delicious and satisfying low protein foods.

Virginia E. Schuett, M.S., R.D.
Director and Editor, National PKU News
Web site: www.pkunews.org

November 1996

Acknowledgments

Many people and organizations helped make this book possible. To all of them I express my deepest thanks and appreciation.

Publication of the original edition of *Low Protein Cookery for PKU* was funded by a grant from the National Headquarters of the March of Dimes Birth Defects Foundation. For the second edition, they again provided funds. Development costs of the book were also supported by funds from the Badger Bayland Chapter of the March of Dimes Birth Defects Foundation in Green Bay, Wisconsin. Special thanks goes to Dr. Mary Hughes, Vice President for Community Services at National Headquarters in 1988, for her strong interest in the book.

The following companies also made generous contributions toward publication of the first edition of the book:

  Anglo-Dietetics Limited (now Nutricia Dietary Products, Ltd.)
  Mead Johnson Nutritional Group
  Milupa Company
  Scientific Hospital Supplies, Ltd.

While the first edition was being prepared, the enthusiasm and support of Brenda Smith (Anglo-Dietetics), Karen Knauff (Mead Johnson), Dr. Ram Chaudhari and Robin Marks McCabe (Milupa), and David Whitelaw and Linda Edward (Scientific Hospital Supplies) were always encouraging. I am thankful for their genuine interest in the long-term welfare of persons with PKU.

Recipe creation and testing involved the use of many special low protein foods and recipe ingredients. Over 200 pounds of Wel-Plan Baking Mix, generously supplied by Anglo-Dietetics, was used; they also provided low protein pastas and crackers used in the recipes. Dietary Specialties, Inc., supplied wheat starch, low protein pastas, rusks, and Prono gelled desserts, for which I am grateful.

As recipes were developed and tested, I depended on a variety of local taste-testers to evaluate quality and acceptability, and to give suggestions for improvements. The recipes were frequently taste-tested by families and children with PKU as well as by staff in the metabolic clinic at the Waisman Center (Madison, WI). I am thankful for their excellent comments and their enthusiasm. Alice and Emily Pawley, my young Madison neighbors, were also very frequent visitors in my kitchen when I was testing recipes, and loved to help with preparations and sampling. They found great pleasure and interest in helping the "special children" (with PKU). I greatly enjoyed their assistance.

A selected group of mothers from all over the United States also prepared and sampled experimental recipes. Their comments were very important in shaping the final composition and form of many of the recipes. These dedicated and talented mothers (and their children who happily participated in taste-testing) are listed at the end of this section. The enthusiasm they showed for preparing and taste-testing so many of my recipes was a constant source of encouragement and inspiration. Their many creative suggestions for using the recipes and for dealing with the diet have been incorporated whenever possible. The book was enhanced by their extensive experience with low protein cookery and with managing the diets of their children in such a positive and successful way.

During the course of recipe testing, I received contributions of recipes from all over the United States and from Canada. Those that became the basis for recipes published in this book are from the persons listed at the end of this section. I also received "helpful hints" for managing the diet from people too numerous to name. I would like to gratefully acknowledge the contributions of these parents who had so many ideas to share by mail, by telephone, and at meetings.

In addition to the recipes provided by the persons listed, ideas for recipes in this book came from a variety of sources. I adapted many recipes from my extensive personal collection of cookbooks as well as from magazines, newspapers, and family recipes.

It is through my work as staff nutritionist of a large metabolic disease treatment center that I was able to establish contacts with families, contributors, and other professionals from across North America and beyond in the development of this book. I am grateful for the support of the Waisman Center on Mental Retardation and Human Development. I am especially indebted to the support of Dr. Stanley Berlow, now retired but then Director of the Metabolic Clinic, for providing the environment in which this long-term project could be carried out.

The food photography was done by Jim Wildeman, "on-location" in my Madison living room. I very much appreciate his skill and artistry in working with me to produce the inspirational images that appear in the book.

Finally, I would like to thank Mary Rasmussen, who is still on the staff at the Waisman Center Biochemical Genetics Clinic, for her patience and excellence in preparing many versions of the manuscript. My deepest thanks also to Elizabeth Steinberg, Chief Editor at the University of Wisconsin Press, for her enthusiasm over the book for all of these years and for her expertise in guiding preparation of the original manuscript and all later editions.

Recipe Testers

(Ages of children are their ages at the time of recipe testing—all are ten years older at the time of this third edition)

Edith McKeon Abbot and Matthew (age 12), Brookline, MA
Joyce Brubacher and Shayla (age 16), Goshen, IN
Jeanne Clark and Les (age 8), Stanton, NE
Evelyn Corwonski and Matthew (age 3), Franklinville, NJ
Ann Diffenderfer and Ben (age 5), Laytonsville, MD
Deborah Gorby and Joshua (age 6), Beaver Falls, PA
Gale Houston and Ross (age 12), Austin, TX
Donna Jahn and Elizabeth (age 10), Los Altos, CA
Janet W. Kean and Myra Jo (age 18), Louisville, KY
Cindy Koehlmoos, Jairren (age 9), and Jessica (age 7),
    Springfield, NE
Kathy Kuhry and Ashlee (age 6), Merrillan, WI
Earlene Lipowski and Steve (age 12), DeForest, WI
Kathy Malatesta and Mark (age 5), Dexter, ME
Linda A. Manzi and Eric (age 7), Methuen, MA
Dottie Miller and Jennifer (age 7), Havre de Grace, MD
Rose Gay Ostrowski and Melissa (age 10), Columbia, SC
Sandy Pedersen and Sarah (age 8), Neenah, WI
Shirley Roberts and John Jr. (age 4), Edgewood, MD
Judith Robinson and Margaret (age 10), Santa Maria, CA
Lorraine J. Russ and Kelly Lynn (age 4), Pittsfield, MA
Susanne Schumacher, Kristopher (age 7) and Lindsey (age 3),
    Appleton, WI
Tricia Simms and Eric (age 6), Carmichael, CA
Julie Simonson and Sarah (age 5), Port Deposit, MD
Nancy Stadter and Christopher (age 3), Gaithersburg, MD
Joyce Wright, Joshua (age 8) and Jamie (age 5), Townsend, MA

Recipe Contributors

Edith McKeon Abbot, Brookline, MA
Nariman Ajluni, San Jose, CA
Diana Boysen, Madison, WI
Jeanne Clark, Stanton, NE
Sandra Connor, Thunder Bay, Ontario, Canada
Linda Dallman, Greenwood, WI
Ann Diffenderfer, Laytonsville, MD
Bonnie Dooley, Tucson, AZ
Chris Emsley, Lilburn, GA
Jeanette Ertz, Grand Junction, CO
Beth Freeman, Derby, IA
Deborah Gorby, Beaver Falls, PA
Susan Hill, Savannah, GA
Gale Houston, Austin, TX
Mrs. R. S. Jensen, Kearney, MO

18

Barbara Johnson, Calgary, Alberta, Canada
Carolyn Johnson, Falls Church, VA
Carol Kaufman, Williamsville, NY
Mary Kemple, New Albany, IN
Sonja Keesey-Berg, Orfordville, WI
Alice Kennedy, Monroeville, NJ
Shawn Kingsford, San Leandro, CA
Earlene Lipowski, DeForest, WI
Kathy Malatesta, Dexter, ME
Teresa Mawhinney, Duluth, GA
Linda A. Manzi, Methuen, MA
Deb Martin, Mercersburg, PA
Bonnie McQuillin, Galeph, Ontario, Canada
Betty Meyer, Indianapolis, IN
Dottie Miller, Havre de Grace, MD
Darlene Mindrup, Glendale, AZ
Sandy Pedersen, Neenah, WI
Tammy Peters, Kingsport, TN
Lin Ries, Atkinson, NE
Lorraine Russ, Scottsville, NY
Susanne Schumacher, Appleton, WI
Nicky Schwartz, Donnellson, IA
Greg Schweitzer, Boise, ID
Tricia Simms, Carmichael, CA
Debbie Smith, Casselberry, FL
Mary Ann Stadel, Rapid City, SD
Rebekah Stout, Coeur d'Alene, ID
Lynn Stremer, Waunakee, WI
Dr. Rebecca Wappner, Indianapolis, IN
Tina Ward, San Marino, CA
Beverly Young, Cincinnati, OH

A Word to Users of this Book

This book is intended to be used primarily for persons with phenylketonuria (PKU), of any age, who are on a low phenylalanine diet. Your child with PKU may be an infant and you may just be learning about the tasks before you. Or you may have already dealt with your child's diet for a number of years. Or *you* may be the one on diet, a teenager or young adult with PKU.

If you are ready to use this book, by now you are probably aware of much of the information that will be discussed in this section. Use the basic information on PKU presented here as a review. (This book may also be used for diets other than the PKU diet—for any restricted protein diet used for treatment of an inherited metabolic disease affecting protein or amino acid metabolism. Because these diseases are rarer than PKU, information about them will not be presented here.)

The Disease

PKU is a rare, inherited disease of metabolism which affects approximately one in every 10,000 to 15,000 persons born in the United States (the incidence varies from country to country). Persons with this disease have a defect in their ability to utilize phenylalanine, an amino acid which is a component of all protein. Normally, when a person eats food containing protein, his or her body uses a small part of the amino acids from the protein for growth and for repair and maintenance of body tissues. The excess which is not needed is changed into other substances by means of body chemicals called enzymes. For persons with PKU, there is a genetically determined deficiency or absence of the enzyme necessary for changing excess phenylalanine into other substances. Without diet treatment, an abnormal amount of phenylalanine accumulates in the blood.

For infants and young children, the excess phenylalanine almost always causes severe damage to the developing brain and central nervous system. For older persons, the excess phenylalanine can also be harmful. Additionally, high blood phenylalanine levels in a woman who has PKU can severely damage any baby that she has, *before* the child is born (this has become known as the problem of "Maternal PKU").

Prior to the 1960s, most persons born with PKU became mentally retarded, suffered a variety of other serious neurological problems, and constituted approximately 1% of the population in institutions for the retarded. Today, approximately 200 infants with PKU are diagnosed in the United States each year, through newborn screening programs which have existed in nearly all states since the mid-1960s. Through early initiated, quality treatment with a special diet, these infants will have normal intelligence and will become fully productive members of society.

For women with PKU, it is also hoped that strict diet control throughout pregnancy will allow normal growth and development of their babies. Research is being carried out to assess the effectiveness of diet treatment during pregnancy.

The Treatment

The goal of the PKU diet, whether for a child, teenager, or adult, is to carefully limit the intake of phenylalanine—to provide only the amount necessary for normal growth and body processes, with no excess. The amount of phenylalanine allowed in the diet is different for each individual, and depends on each person's ability to utilize phenylalanine, as well as a variety of other factors. A diet prescription which provides a suitable amount of phenylalanine must be determined by an experienced physician or nutritionist through frequent checking of blood phenylalanine levels, height and weight, and diet intake records.

For children, especially during the period of most rapid growth and body change in infancy, the "right amount" of phenylalanine will change frequently. Phenylalanine needs will also continue to change slightly throughout the years, being altered by such things as growth and illness. It is very important that a local PKU treatment clinic be consulted for advice about necessary diet changes.

For women on diet during pregnancy, nutritional needs will change frequently as the pregnancy progresses. Maintaining very close contact with local PKU clinic professionals is crucial for monitoring the diet as well as for monitoring the pregnancy.

For the child with PKU, usually all high protein foods such as milk, cheese, meat, fish, and eggs, which contain a large amount of phenylalanine, are completely eliminated from the diet. For women during pregnancy, small amounts of high protein foods may be allowed in some cases. Foods low in protein such as fruits, vegetables, some grain products, special low protein foods, and protein-free foods can be eaten as recommended by a physician or nutritionist.

To provide the protein and other nutrients necessary, a special formula which is high in protein and essential nutrients, but contains little or no phenylalanine, is substituted for the naturally high protein foods which have been eliminated. This special formula—a powder that is mixed with water or fruit juice—will be one of a number currently available and described on pages 44–45.

For a young infant, establishing the proper balance of phenylalanine is accomplished by adding to the PKU formula small, measured amounts of either evaporated milk, homogenized milk, or regular infant formula. Solid foods low in protein are introduced at the same time as for any normal infant and these foods will gradually replace the milk added to the formula. It is at the time when the child has begun to eat solid foods that the "art" of dietary management really starts. It is beginning then, especially, that the recipes and ideas in this book are intended to provide assistance.

The amount of phenylalanine allowed on the PKU diet will be very small in comparison to amounts consumed on a normal diet (generally less than 10% of a normal intake). Since persons with PKU can utilize only a small amount of phenylalanine, foods eaten on the diet must be very carefully measured or weighed on a gram scale, following the advice of your local PKU treatment clinic. The food list recommended by your clinic should be utilized. (However, all nutrient calculations in this book are based on values from *The Low Protein Food List for PKU*, 1995*).

It is crucial that the diet prescription recommended by your clinic be followed, and that you maintain good control of blood phenylalanine levels. For infants and young children with PKU, and for women with PKU on the diet during pregnancy, maintaining good control is particularly imperative.

At this time, maintaining good control of blood phenylalanine levels through dietary restriction is the only method known for preventing mental retardation and ensuring optimal intellectual development of affected persons with PKU. In the future, however, the techniques of recombinant DNA and "genetic engineering" will perhaps revolutionize the treatment of PKU. We can all be hopeful that this will come about within our lifetimes. But in the meantime, it will be to your child's benefit (or to yours, if you have PKU) to do the best you possibly can with the diet, taking advantage of the helpful hints in this book and using the recipes regularly.

* May be purchased from Dietary Specialties, Inc. (a subsidiary of MenuDirect Corp.), 865 Piscataway, NJ 08854. Telephone: 1-888-MENU123 or 732-980-6700. Web site: www.menudirect.com.

General Instructions

For best results, read all of these *General Instructions* and the two following sections, *Using the Recipes* and *Special Ingredients*, before using any of the recipes in this book.

1. To Determine Nutrient Content When Serving Portion Size Is Different from Recipe

The serving size must be only as indicated in the recipe to maintain the stated amount of phenylalanine, protein, and calories per serving. If the number of servings you get varies from that listed on the recipe (that is, if you want a different portion size), divide the phenylalanine content stated for the whole recipe by the number of servings you get from the recipe. Do the same for protein and calories, if desired.

Example: If the recipe states there are 48 mg of phenylalanine per recipe and the recipe is intended to make 4 servings, but you want to make 6 servings, there would be 8 mg per serving instead of 12 mg (48 divided by 6 equals 8).

2. To Determine Nutrient Content When an Ingredient Substitution Is Made

For ingredient changes you wish to make, use *The Low Protein Food List for PKU*, 1995 (see page 22) to determine nutrient content of the item you wish to replace. *Subtract* these values from the nutrient content *per recipe.* Then, using *The Low Protein Food List for PKU* again, determine nutrient content of the item you wish to use instead. *Add* those values to the nutrient content per recipe. Recalculate *per serving* values, using the revised per recipe values (following the method described in #1). Many of the recipes will work equally well with minor alterations in ingredients, to suit taste preferences (for example substituting one vegetable for another, or omitting a minor ingredient).

Example: Hamburgerless Pie (page 243) calls for ⅓ cup green beans. If you want to replace the beans with frozen mixed peas and carrots and need the phenylalanine content of the altered recipe:

	Phenylalanine (mg)
Per recipe (current)	70
subtract ⅓ cup green beans	– 23
	47
add ⅓ cup peas and carrots	+ 53
	100

So there is now 100 mg phenylalanine per recipe instead of 70 mg. If you still want to make 2 servings, each serving of the revised recipe will contain 50 mg phenylalanine (100 divided by 2 equals 50), which is approximately 3½ exchanges.

3. To Determine Exchange Content of a Serving Portion

Since the phenylalanine content of the recipes is stated in mg, if a phenylalanine "exchange" (or "equivalent") system is used for diet management in your clinic, do the following:

a. Find out from your clinic (if you don't already know) how many mg of phenylalanine are in each exchange. This is *15 mg* in most parts of the United States.

b. If one exchange is 15 mg of phenylalanine, you may use the conversion table below for figuring exchanges, which uses ½ of an exchange as the smallest fraction.

milligrams (mg) of phenylalanine	number of exchanges
0–3	"free"*
4–7	½
8–15	1
16–22	1½
23–30	2
31–37	2½
38–45	3
46–52	3½
53–60	4
61–67	4½
68–75	5
76–82	5½
83–90	6
91–97	6½
98–105	7
106–112	7½
113–120	8

*If several servings worth 2 or 3 mg are consumed during the day, the amount of phenylalanine should be counted.

c. If one exchange in your clinic is different from 15 mg of phenylalanine, or if you want to be more precise than "rounding" up or down to ½ exchange, do the following:

● When the total phenylalanine content per serving for a recipe is *greater than* the total mg of phenylalanine equal to one exchange, divide the total phenylalanine content per serving by the number of mg of phenylalanine equal to one exchange. *Your answer will give you the number of exchanges contained in one serving.*

Example: If the recipe states that there are 49 mg of phenylalanine in one serving, and one exchange is equal to 15 mg of phenylalanine, then one serving contains 3¼ exchanges (49 divided by 15 equals 3.27 or about 3¼).

● When the total phenylalanine content per serving for a recipe is *less than* the total mg of phenylalanine equal to one exchange, divide the mg of phenylalanine equal to one exchange by the total phenylalanine content per serving. *Your answer will give the number of servings containing one exchange.*

Example: If the recipe states that there are 10 mg of phenylalanine in one serving, and one exchange is equal to 15 mg of phenylalanine, then 1½ servings contain one exchange (15 divided by 10 equals 1.5 or 1½).

4. Measuring Instructions

All measurements should be made with standard household measuring cups and spoons. Do not use coffee cups, glasses, or serving spoons for measuring. All measurements should be level unless stated otherwise in the recipe.

There are two types of measuring cups: one type for dry ingredients and one for liquid ingredients. A measuring cup for dry ingredients is made with the upper edge straight across so that the ingredients can be leveled with the edge of a spatula or knife. These cups are available in sets of graduated measurement sizes, including ¼ cup, ⅓ cup, ½ cup, and 1 cup measures, and they are usually made of metal or plastic.

Liquid measuring cups have a rim that extends above the top measurement mark to prevent liquids from spilling as they are measured. They also have a "lip," which makes pouring easier. These cups are usually found in 1 cup, 2 cup, and 4 cup sizes, and they are usually made of glass or plastic.

Measuring Recipe Ingredients

Wel-Plan Baking Mix and wheat starch should be lightly spooned into a dry measuring cup and leveled off with the straight edge of a spatula or knife. Do not tap cup or pack down. Do not sift before measuring.

Cake Flour. Sift cake flour only if the recipe calls for sifting. Nutrient content of recipes containing cake flour are calculated based on the weight of flour that you would scoop directly from the box (9 gm/tablespoon), or in recipes calling for sifted cake flour, nutrient content is based on the weight after sifting (6 gm/tablespoon). For convenience, sifting is called for only when the amount to be used is greater than several tablespoons.

White granulated sugar needs sifting only if it has lumps. Spoon the sugar into a dry measuring cup and level off with the straight edge of a spatula or knife.

Confectioner's sugar (powdered sugar) should be sifted before measuring for best results. Lumps that won't sift out may be removed by pressing with a spoon through a sieve. Spoon the sugar lightly into a dry measuring cup and level off with the straight edge of a spatula or knife.

Brown sugar should be firmly packed into a dry measuring cup and leveled off. When it is packed firmly, the sugar will hold its shape when turned out of the measuring cup.

Spices, salt, baking powder, and baking soda should be leveled off with the straight edge of a spatula or knife after the measuring spoon is dipped into the container.

Vegetable shortening, margarine, and butter should be firmly packed into a dry measuring cup and leveled off with the straight edge of a spatula or knife. If less than ¼ cup is required, pack into a measuring spoon in the same manner. Remove with the tip of a rubber spatula.

Water and other liquid ingredients should be measured in a liquid measuring cup; or a measuring spoon for amounts less than ¼ cup. Place the cup on a level surface. Pour liquid into the cup until it is level with the required measurement.

5. Use of a Gram Scale

A gram scale was used throughout recipe testing, wherever a gram weight appears.

What are grams? Grams are simply a metric unit of weight. There are about twenty-eight grams in one ounce. You don't have to understand the metric system to weigh a food in grams as long as you have a scale that weighs in grams. Grams are used because gram weights are more accurate and can measure weights much smaller than one ounce.

Over the years, more and more families have become "gram scale converts," finding that it is actually much easier to weigh on a gram scale than using a standard measuring utensil. I highly recommend using a gram scale to replace or to augment measuring when possible.

There are several important reasons for using a gram scale:

• *Accuracy* of portion sizes and phenylalanine/protein content is greater. This is especially important for items relatively "high," where small deviations from the intended portion could make a large difference in phenylalanine/protein content. It is also much more accurate to weigh hard-to-measure foods (foods which are lumpy, chunky, etc.).

• *Reproducibility* of recipes, especially those using Wel-Plan Baking Mix or wheat starch, is more assured when these items are weighed.

• *Convenience*—using a scale minimizes the number of measuring cups and spoons used, and speeds measuring for many items.

Recommended Gram Scales. At the time of printing the third edition, the gram scale I recommend is either the Ohaus (model LS2000) or the Polder (model 936-90). These compact, precise, and easy-to-use digital counter-top scales weigh in increments of 1 gram for foods weighing up to 2000 grams (just over four pounds).

The Ohaus scale has somewhat greater accuracy and is more expensive than the Polder scale, but the Polder weighs precisely enough for most diets. Both are available from the New England Connection for PKU & Allied Disorders (a non-profit organization) at a discounted price. Or you can write or call the U.S. distributors for information about where to buy the scales locally. Over the years, model numbers and features are sometimes changed, and new scales will become available. The New England Connection for PKU & Allied

Disorders will have any updated models or other scales that I recommend in future years.

New England Connection for PKU
   & Allied Disorders
c/o John Sullivan
5 Jones Lane
East Sandwich, MA 02537
Telephone: 508-888-2295
E-mail: lophechef@capecod.net

U.S. Scale Distributors:
Ohaus Corporation
29 Hanover Rd./PO Box 900
Florham Park, NJ 07932-0900
Telephone: Call toll-free 1-800-526-0659 or 973-377-9000
Web site: www.ohaus.com

Polder, Inc.
200 Central Park Ave.
Hartsdale, NY 10530
Telephone: Call toll-free 1-800-431-2133 or 914-937-8200
Web site: www.polder.com

Other brands of grams scales are available in the United States. However, most are not accurate enough for our purposes, even if they claim to be very accurate and precise.

Consult your nutritionist or other clinic staff if you have questions about how to use the scales. Both scales are simple to operate, even for a child. Do remember that they are not play things, though. They should be handled with care to maintain their accuracy.

From a young age, children can be taught to use the scale for weighing their formula powder and other foods, to become familiar with the concept that "all foods on my diet need to be weighed or measured."

Using Your Gram Scale

After turning on the scale, place your plate or other container on the scale. Press the bar on the scale so it reads "0," then add your food until you have the desired weight. If you have more foods to weigh that will go on the same plate or in the same recipe, you can then continue to re-zero the scale, adding foods to the plate, re-zeroing and adding.

The Polder scale has a nice feature that allows you to preset a food weight that you want, and a beep then alerts you when you are close to the desired weight.

Using the Recipes

Check the labels of all ingredients that might contain a substance called "aspartame," which is used as a sweetener. Aspartame is composed of two amino acids, aspartic acid and *phenylalanine.* Any item that contains aspartame should be avoided by anyone on a PKU diet. Foods that potentially contain it include carbonated beverages, drink mixes, Jell-O and gelatin-type products, pudding and pie fillings, whipped toppings, and cold cereals. Aspartame can also be found in chewing gum, instant tea and coffee, chewable vitamin supplements, and some medicines. On food items, look for the warning on the package label: "Phenylketonurics: contains phenylalanine." NutraSweet is one trade name for aspartame. Many items containing aspartame have the NutraSweet logo stamped on the label. However, there are now other trade names for aspartame, since the Nutra-Sweet Company's patent on aspartame production ran out several years ago.

The Low Protein Food List for PKU (1995) was used for all nutrient calculations (see page 22 for ordering). Whenever the phenylalanine content of the recipe or of a given serving size was less than 1 mg or the protein content was less than 0.05 gm, the amount is indicated as a "trace." When the phenylalanine or protein content was zero, based on available data, "0" is indicated. Phenylalanine and calorie content have been rounded off to the nearest whole number and protein content to the nearest tenth.

Gram weights of some recipe ingredients are given in addition to common household measurements. This was done in cases where accurate measurements are especially important because of relatively high phenylalanine/protein content of the ingredient, where success of the recipe depends on reasonably accurate measurement (especially for Wel-Plan Baking Mix and wheat starch), or when it might be more convenient and accurate to weigh an item than to measure it (especially chunky vegetables and fruits). See page 27 for purchasing a gram scale.

When a recipe specifies a brand name for a particular ingredient, use only the brand indicated (except for cake flour, as noted below) to ensure that the phenylalanine content of the recipe will be as indicated in the nutrient analysis for the recipe. In some cases, other brand names also may be acceptable to use but should not be used unless the exact nutrient content is known and can be compared with the nutrient analysis of the brand ingredient specified in the recipe.

Use only Wel-Plan Baking Mix when it is indicated in the recipes. Do not try to substitute another brand of baking mix, unless you are prepared for some failures. Success of the recipes depends on the particular ingredients in the Wel-Plan Baking Mix. However, in the years since the second edition was published, the price of Wel-Plan Baking Mix has skyrocketed. I know parents are looking for ways to decrease the costs of preparing low protein baked items. Parents frequently have told me that they have successfully substituted dp Baking Mix (Dietary Specialties, Inc.) for some recipes calling for Wel-Plan Baking Mix or wheat starch and Wel-Plan Baking Mix combinations. These include cake, quick bread and muffin recipes. Some people have told me these recipes turn out better using dp Baking Mix. This substitution does not work well for most other recipes in the book, however, including yeast breads (my experiences with yeast breads and dp Baking Mix were disastrous). For each 1 cup measurement of Wel-Plan Baking Mix, substitute 1 *packed* cup of dp Baking Mix (dp Baking Mix contains fat, which means you need to use more to get the same amount of wheat starch).

In recipes calling for wheat starch, use wheat starch from Dietary Specialties, Inc., if you can. All of the recipes containing wheat starch were developed using the Dietary Specialties product. Other brands will behave similarly, but the texture or flavor of the product may be slightly different.

Cake flour is used in several of the recipes, to optimize texture of the finished product. Cake flour is considerably lower in protein and phenylalanine than regular flour. Regular flour should not be substituted. Cake flour comes in a box rather than a bag, and can usually be found in the flour section or next to the cake mix section in a grocery store. The recipes specify "Softasilk," since many people can readily identify "Softasilk" but not cake flour. Other brands, such as "Swansdown," also can be used.

In recipes calling for an egg, be sure to use a medium-sized egg, as specified in the recipe. The average weight of a medium-sized egg is

50 gm, including shell. Using a large or extra large egg would significantly increase the amount of phenylalanine and protein in the recipe.

Regular margarine and butter are used interchangeably in the recipes. To lower the phenylalanine content of a given recipe, there are several "free" margarines available:

Gregg's Gold'n Soft Spread (tub, not the margarine sticks)
Janet Lee Spread (tub)
Mother's Margarine
Nucoa Margarine
Parkay Spread (tub, not the margarine sticks)
Saffola Unsalted Margarine
Weight Watcher's Margarine

For each tablespoon of regular margarine or butter that is replaced with one of these brands, subtract 6 mg of phenylalanine and 0.1 gm protein from the phenylalanine/protein content of the total recipe. Remember that reduced-calorie diet margarines are not suitable for use in baked products such as cakes or cookies.

Rich's Richwhip Topping and Rich's Coffee Rich are frequently used in the recipes as cream and milk substitutes. Richwhip Topping, in the liquid form that can be whipped at home, is "free." In some parts of the United States, prewhipped Richwhip Topping is sold in plastic tubs, but the phenylalanine/protein content is similar to that of Coolwhip. If Rich's Coffee Rich is unavailable where you live, Mocha Mix Non-Dairy Creamer is available on the West Coast and several other western states and may be substituted for Coffee Rich. Other non-dairy creamers can also be substituted (use *The Low Protein Food List for PKU*, 1995, to identify other non-dairy creamers).

All of the non-dairy products can be frozen for a number of months. For convenience in using small portions, freeze in an ice cube tray, then place frozen cubes in a plastic freezer bag.

Instructions for using a microwave oven are given for some recipes. A 675-watt oven was used in testing these recipes. Depending on the power of your oven, the timing in the recipes may need to be adjusted slightly. When you have some experience using a microwave oven, you will learn that many other recipes can be prepared in part or in whole in your oven even when no specific instructions are given. For all recipes indicating that a microwave oven can be used, use only microwave oven-safe utensils (non-metal).

Special Ingredients

Following is a list of special ingredients used in the recipes or mentioned elsewhere In the book. This includes special low protein products and other ingredients that are low in protein and commonly available, but perhaps unfamiliar. See *The Low Protein Food List for PKU* (page 22 for ordering) for nutrient content of these items.

Special Low Protein Products

1. Dietary Specialties, Inc.
    865 Piscataway, NJ 08854
    Telephone: Call toll-free 1-888-MENU123 or 732-980-6700
    Web site: www.menudirect.com

    Purchase products directly from the company (call for a current order form). This company sells several brands of low protein products. Their Wel-Plan brand products are made in England by Nutricia Dietary Products, Ltd. (these products in Canada and Europe may have the name Rite-Diet). Dietary Specialties' product line includes, but is not limited to, the following items:

    Wel-Plan Baking Mix (recipes in this book use only Wel-Plan brand baking mix)

    Wel-Plan pastas (Spaghetti Ring Style, Macaroni and Short-Cut Spaghetti)

    Wel-Plan cookies (Cream-Filled Wafers, Sweet Cookies, Cream-Filled Chocolate Flavored Cookies)

    Wel-Plan crackers

    dp wheat starch and dp Baking Mix

    dp cookies (several varieties)

    Aproten pastas and Dietary Specialties pastas (a variety of shapes of each)

    Aproten rusks and crackertoast

    Prono Gelled Dessert Mix (strawberry, cherry, orange, lime)

    Dietary Specialties Graham Cracker Cookies (these can be used as a substitute for homemade low protein *Cinnamon Graham Crackers* in recipes calling for low protein graham cracker crumbs)

    Dietary Specialties Porridge

    Dietary Specialties Cheese Flavored Sauce, Almost Chocolate Sauce, Tomato Flavored Sauce, Lemon Herb Sauce and Garlic Herb Sauce

    Dietary Specialties Wheat Starch Bread and Bread Machine Mix

2. Ener-G Foods, Inc.
    P.O. Box 84487
    Seattle, WA 98124-5787
    Telephone: Call toll-free 1-800-767-6660 or 206-767-6660
    Web site: www.ener-g.com

Purchase directly from the company (call for a current order form). This company also sells several brands of low protein products, including some also carried by Dietary Specialties. In addition, they have their own line of baked products and pasta products. They also sell egg replacer, almond bark (used in numerous candy recipes in this book), as well as low protein cheese.

3. Med-Diet
   3050 Ranchview Lane
   Plymouth, MN 55447
   Telephone: Call toll-free 1-800-633-3438 or 612-550-2020
   Web site: www.med-diet.com
   Purchase directly from the company (call for a current order form). Med-Diet distributes many of the same products that Dietary Specialties handles, usually at a somewhat higher price. They also now carry their own cheese-flavored sauce mix, Lo Pro brand cookies, Hunt's Lemon Snack Pack Pudding (a phe-free product difficult to locate in grocery stores) and a vegetarian tomato cup-a-soup style product by Manichewitz. They also sell some Kingsmill products.

4. SHS North America
   P.O. Box 117
   Gaithersburg, MD 20884-0117
   Telephone: Call toll-free 1-888-LOPROGO or 301-315-5500
   Web site: www.shsna.com
   Purchase directly from the company (call for a current order form, or see their Web site). SHS distributes the Loprofin range of low protein products, including pastas, cookies, bread, crackers, cereal, and other items. According to many families who have used it, the Loprofin Baking Mix, introduced long after this book was originally published, can replace Wel-Plan Baking Mix in some but not all recipes. The author has no personal experience with this product. Typically, it can be used for cakes, muffins, pancakes, and cookies, based on family reports.

5. Kingsmill Food Col, Ltd.
   1399 Kenndey Road, Unit 17
   Scarborough, Ontario
   Canada M1P 2L6
   Telephone: 416-755-1124
   Web site: www.kingsmill.com
   Purchase products directly from the company (call for a current order form). This company distributes a number of brands of low protein products, including some products from the U.S.-based low protein food companies.

Other Low Protein Ingredients

1. Rich Products Corp.
    P.O. Box 245
    1145 Niagara Street
    Buffalo, NY 14240
    Telephone: Call toll-free 1-800-822-7555
       Rich's Richwhip Topping (8 oz carton)
       Rich's Coffee Rich (8 oz and 16 oz cartons)
       (See page 31 for description of a Coffee Rich substitute.)
    Products made by Rich are now sold exclusively by Morningstar, 2515 McKinney Avenue, Suite 1200, Dallas, TX 75201 (telephone: 1-800-236-1014 or 214-303-3528). You may also purchase these products from a grocery store, usually in the frozen foods section or sometimes in the dairy case. These products are not readily available in some parts of the country. If unavailable in local grocery stores, these products are widely used in hospitals, restaurants, and bakeries. Try calling a local hospital dietary department, restaurant, or bakery and ask if it is possible to purchase Rich products through them. If so, you will probably need to purchase them by the case and you may wish to contact another family to share a case. Any willing retailer in the US also can order these products for you by calling Customer Service at Morningstar. The UPC code for Richwhip is #49800 01214. The UPC code for Rich's Coffee Rich is #49800 01839. The products also may be purchased through a local restaurant supplier, Gordon Foods. In many cities they have outlet-type stores where the public can purchase bulk items, such as Rich's products. Check out their Web site at www.gfs.com, then go to http://www.gfs.com/marketplace/location.html. You also may call Morningstar to find out where the products are distributed in your area.

2. International Home Foods, Inc.
    1633 Littleton Road
    Parsippany, NJ 07054
    Telephone: Call toll-free 1-800-544-5680 or 973-359-9920 for information about where to find it in your state
       G. Washington's Seasoning and Broth (Golden or Rich Brown flavors are "free"). Purchase these products from a grocery store, in or near the soups section. The broth comes in a small box.

Using Low Protein Products

Although low protein products are expensive, using them regularly should be viewed as a necessity rather than a luxury for most persons on the diet. It is highly recommended that you begin introducing low protein products very early in your child's life—preferably within the first year, when table foods are first introduced. While it may be tempting to use relatively higher protein foods when appetites are small, it is difficult later to withhold these things and introduce low protein substitutes when appetites have grown. Starting to use low protein foods when your child is young also gives you an opportunity to become familiar with them before it is an absolute necessity, removing some of the pressures.

Suggested low protein products and recipes from this book to introduce during the first year of life include:
- low protein bread (very small pieces to start with, fresh or toasted)
- Prono low protein gelled dessert
- low protein pasta (especially Aproten Anellini or Wel-Plan Spaghetti Ring Style, plain or with a little margarine and a dash of salt)
- Aproten rusks for teething; Wel-Plan crackers and cookies
- *Cinnamon Graham Crackers*
- *Crispy Chips*
- instant pudding made with non-dairy creamer (page 399)

If you are not "at home" in the kitchen or are short of time, perhaps a nearby grandparent or even a friend might be able to help with low protein cooking and baking.

A positive attitude towards these special foods by parents (and siblings) is very important. This cannot be overemphasized. Although there may be slight differences in taste or texture compared with the equivalent "regular" product, for many of the low protein products and recipes in this book there are no noticeable differences. In fact, other family members or neighbor children may be interested in eating low protein baked goods regularly—you may need to decide whe er the additional cost is a constraining factor in "allowing" others to partake.

Wel-Plan Baking Mix, wheat starch, and all of the low protein pasta products will keep indefinitely when stored in an area that is not subject to extremes in heat. Commercially made low protein cookies, crackers, and canned bread also keep well for many months. Order your low protein products directly from the company which distributes them (see page 33–34). You may order as much or as little as you like, though it is sometimes convenient to order a full case for products which are used frequently. Consider the family budget. Order steadily so that huge orders are unnecessary.

Recipe Adaptation

There is a large selection of recipes in this book from which to choose, all of which were painstakingly developed and tested to yield optimal results. Still, you may have the creative urge and wish to create or adapt your own recipes occasionally. Following are some suggestions for doing this.

- Wel-Plan Baking Mix and/or wheat starch, or a combination of Baking Mix and wheat starch can be substituted for flour in approximately equal amounts. But remember, since it is the protein component of regular flour that gives it most of the properties important for baked goods, a very special combination of ingredients is typically necessary to make the baked item similar in texture, appearance, and taste to regular baked goods. For baked goods, you will have more predictable results if you take one of the recipes already in the book and modify minor ingredients to produce a new flavor, rather than starting "from scratch."
- Substitute Rich's Richwhip Topping or Rich's Coffee Rich for milk or other similar liquids. Dilute Rich's Richwhip Topping 2 : 1 with water for the consistency of milk, or dilute Rich's Coffee Rich 1 : 1 with water for the consistency of milk or to reduce sweetness.
- Reduce the quantity of high phenylalanine ingredients (for example, chocolate chips). Omit other ingredients entirely (for example, nuts).
- Substitute a lower phenylalanine ingredient for a higher one (for example, substitute raisins or maraschino cherries for chocolate chips).
- Substitute G. Washington's Seasoning and Broth for bouillon (Rich Brown and Golden varieties are "free").
- Substitute low protein pasta for regular pasta.
- Use low protein croutons or bread crumbs in casseroles or on top of casseroles.

To calculate the phenylalanine content of the recipe you have adapted:

Step 1: Using *The Low Protein Food List for PKU* (1995), determine the phenylalanine content in milligrams (mg) of each ingredient and add to find the total.

Step 2: When appropriate, measure the total amount of food the recipe yields in a measuring cup or other standard measuring device, or weigh on a gram scale.

Step 3: Decide how many servings this total can be divided into and record the number of servings and size and/or weight of serving on the recipe. If the recipe is for cookies, record the number of cookies the recipe made.

Step 4: Divide the total phenylalanine content (from step 1) by the number of servings to get phenylalanine content in mg per serving.

Step 5 (optional): Convert phenylalanine content in mg per serving to exchanges according to directions on page 24–25.

Once you've developed a recipe, repeat it once or twice to check for consistently good results, and then pass it on to other families or to your PKU clinic for a newsletter!

Apple Coconut Cupcakes

½ c. butter	1¼ c wheat starch
1 c. sugar	2 t. baking powder
½ t. vanilla	½ t. salt
½ c. Coffee Rich	½ c. coconut
¼ c. water	1½ c. chopped
1¼ c. Baking Mix	apple

Preheat oven to 350°. Cream the butter and sugar in a bowl. over →

Standard Household Measurement Equivalents

Liquid and Solid Measures

3 teaspoons equal 1 tablespoon
2 tablespoons equal ⅛ cup
4 tablespoons equal ¼ cup
5 tablespoons plus 1 teaspoon
   equal ⅓ cup
8 tablespoons equal ½ cup

10 tablespoons plus 2
   teaspoons equal ⅔ cup
16 tablespoons equal 1 cup
1 cup equals ½ pint
2 cups equal 1 pint
4 cups equal 1 quart

Liquid Measures

2 tablespoons equal 1 fluid
   ounce

1 cup equals 8 fluid ounces
4 cups equal 32 fluid ounces

Metric Measures

28 grams equal 1 ounce
454 grams equal 1 pound

1 gram equals 1000 milligrams

Cooking Terms and Definitions

Baste: To brush juices or liquids over food while it cooks.

Beat: To make a mixture smooth or to introduce air by using a regular motion that turns the mixture over and over.

Blend: To thoroughly combine two or more ingredients.

Boil: To heat to the boiling point (until bubbles form).

Chill: To refrigerate until cold.

Chop: To cut into small pieces with a knife.

Cream: To blend one or more foods until mixture is soft.

Cube: To cut into small, square pieces.

Cut: To divide into pieces with a knife or scissors.

Dice: To cut into cubes approximately ¼ inch in size.

Dissolve: To melt or liquefy.

Fold: To incorporate a food ingredient into a mixture by blending with a spoon or wire whisk, using an up-and-over motion.

Garnish: To add a decorative touch to food, usually with other foods.

Grate: To pulverize by rubbing on a grater.

Grease: To rub the inside of a baking pan with vegetable fat or oil.

Knead: To work dough with the hands by folding, turning, and pressing down until it becomes smooth and elastic.

Mince: To cut or chop into tiny particles.

Mix: To combine or blend ingredients in any way that evenly distributes them.

Pare: To trim off the outside skin or covering of a food.

Peel: To strip off the outer skin or covering of a food.

Purée: To render foods into a mash, using a grinder, food mill, electric blender, or sieve.

Sauté: To fry quickly in a small amount of hot fat.

Shred: To cut finely in strips with a grater or knife.

Sift: To put through a sifter or sieve.

Simmer: To cook in liquid below or just at the boiling point.

Stir: To mix with a circular motion for the purpose of blending.

Toss: To mix gently until well coated with a dressing.

Whip: To beat rapidly by hand or in a mixer.

RECIPES

Beverages

Most of the recipes in this section either call for adding PKU formula, or give the option for adding it (either powder or already mixed), since this is by far the most important beverage for anyone on the diet and since there are such a variety of "free" or very low protein drinks already commercially available.

The formula-included beverages are nice for variety—or for those who have difficulty drinking formula. Most of the drinks are prepared using ice, which minimizes the formula taste, and flavorings which also mask the taste. The recipes provided can be used as inspiration for creating your own interesting formula-included beverages.

Special Tips

Any of the available PKU formulas can be used in the recipes and the amounts indicated are only a general guideline—use as much or as little as you wish.

The formula-included beverages are designed to be consumed right after preparation, though they could also be frozen, thawed partially, and reblended until slushy.

An easy way to crush ice cubes for the formula-included beverages, is to put them in a double or triple layer of heavy plastic freezer bags, or a cloth bag (preferable) and pound with a rolling pin. Crushing ice cubes in a blender can be done, but with difficulty, and it is not advised for a food processor.

PKU Formulas

There is now an array of formulas available for management of PKU. The flavor, composition, and potential use of the formulas are variable. Because of these differences, there is considerable flexibility in meeting individual nutritional needs and accommodating taste and volume preferences. A formula can be used individually, or several formulas can be successfully mixed together to best suit specific needs. Sometimes by combining formulas, the advantages of several formulas can be incorporated and any disadvantages minimized.

Selection of a single formula, or a combination of formulas, will depend on a number of factors and should always be discussed and planned with professionals at a PKU clinic. *The correct amount of phenylalanine to meet individual needs must be added to any of the formulas, or to the diet in other ways, as prescribed by your PKU clinic.* Other nutrients may also need to be added, as indicated on the chart on pages 43–45.

When the time becomes appropriate for a formula change, mixing small amounts of the new formula together with the old formula and gradually increasing the amounts of the new and decreasing amounts

Nutrient Content*

	Most Suitable Ages	Phe	Protein (gm/100gm)	Fat (gm/100gm)	Carbohydrate (gm/100gm)	Vitamins/ Minerals	Total Calories (cal/100gm)	Comments
Applied Nutrition Corp. 273 Franklin Road Randolph, NJ 07869								
Phenylade	all ages over one year	none	moderate (25)	moderate (14)	moderately high (45)	adequate	moderately high (410)	A "complete" formula.
Phenylade Amino Acid Bar	older children to adults	none	moderate (10 gm/bar)	moderate (18)	low (17/bar)	none added	high (260/ bar)	Use together with a complete formula.
Mead Johnson Nutritionals 2400 W. Lloyd Expressway Evansville, IN 47721-0001								
Lofenalac (to be discontinued sometime after 2000)	infants and young children	low	moderate (15)	moderate (18)	high (60)	adequate	high (460)	A "complete" formula.
Phenyl-Free	children to adults	none	moderate (20)	low (7)	high (66)	adequate	moderately high (410)	A "complete" formula.
PKU 1	infants to 1 year	none	high (50)	none	low (19)	adequate	low (270)	Fat source and extra carbohydrate must be added.
PKU 2	1 year to teenagers	none	high (67)	none	low (7)	adequate	low (290)	Fat source must be added. Extra carbohydrate may be desirable.
PKU 3	teenagers to adults (also pregnancy)	none	high (68)	none	low (3)	adequate	low (280)	Fat source must be added. Extra carbohydrate may be desirable.

Ross Products Division
625 Cleveland Ave.
Columbus, OH 43215

Phenex-1	infants and toddlers	none	moderate (15)	moderately high (24)	moderately high (46)	adequate	high (480)	A "complete" formula.
Phenex-2	children and adults	none	moderately high (30)	moderate (16)	moderate (30)	adequate	moderately high (410)	A "complete" formula.

SHS North America
P.O. Box 117
Gaithersburg, MD 20884

XP Analog	infants up to 1 year	none	moderate (13)	moderate (21)	high (59)	adequate	high (475)	A "complete" formula.
XP Maxamaid	2 to 8 years	none	moderately high (25)	none	high (62)	adequate	moderate (350)	Fat source must be added. Extra carbohydrate may be desirable.
XP Maxamum	8 years to adult (including pregnancy)	none	moderately high (39)	none	moderately high (45)	adequate	moderate (340)	Fat source must be added. Extra carbohydrate may be desirable.
Periflex	over 1 year of age	none	moderate (20)	moderate (17)	moderate (41)		moderately high (395)	

* Descriptive terms (for example, "moderate") are based on relative comparisons between the formulas.

** For pregnancy, there are many special considerations not indicated on the chart, including the need for vitamin/mineral supplements in some cases. Women with PKU who are on the diet during pregnancy must keep in very close contact with PKU clinic professionals, since nutritional needs change as the pregnancy progresses.

For infants, children, teens, and non-pregnant adults, the various formulas can supply adequate vitamins and minerals when consumed in sufficient volume, but in some cases a supplement may be desirable. This should be determined by professionals at a PKU clinic.

of the old over a period of weeks, or even months, is generally the optimal approach to a formula transition for children over the age of 1 year.

The information provided in the chart is designed to provide a basic description of what is available in the United States. The terms "high," "moderately high," "moderate," and "low" have been used to describe certain characteristics of the formulas. These terms are used to compare the amount of something in one formula to the same characteristic in the other formulas.

Frosted Orange Creme

5 to 6 crushed ice cubes
2 tablespoons orange Tang
    powder
1 tablespoon granulated sugar
½ cup water
2 tablespoons Rich's Coffee
    Rich

drop of vanilla
2 to 6 scoops (20 to 60 gm)
    PKU formula powder
    (optional)

Blend all ingredients in a blender for 1 minute. Serve immediately.

Yield: one 14 oz serving.

	Phenylalanine (mg)	Protein (gm)	Calories
Per serving (not including formula)	6	0.1	293

Birthday Party Punch

four 12 oz cans strawberry or
    orange soda

3 cups unsweetened pineapple
    juice

Mix soda and juice together in a beverage container. Chill.

Yield: 9 cups (72 oz).

	Phenylalanine (mg)	Protein (gm)	Calories
Per recipe	60	2.4	996
Per ½ cup (4 oz) serving	3	0.1	55

Orange Freeze

4 crushed ice cubes
3 tablespoons orange Tang
    powder
2 drops peppermint flavoring

1 cup (8 oz) PKU formula,
    prepared according to diet
    prescription

Blend all ingredients in a blender for 1 minute. Serve immediately.

Yield: one 10 oz serving.

	Phenylalanine (mg)	Protein (gm)	Calories
Per serving (not including formula)	0	0	166

Strawberry Orange Freeze

½ cup orange juice
½ cup water or ½ cup (4 oz)
    PKU formula, prepared
    according to diet
    prescription
1 teaspoon honey

½ medium banana (40 gm)
½ cup (50 gm) frozen
    unsweetened loose-pack
    strawberries
crushed ice

Put all ingredients except ice in a blender container. Cover and whirl at high speed until smooth. With blender motor running, gradually add as much crushed ice as necessary for desired thickness.

Yield: one serving.

	Phenylalanine (mg)	Protein (gm)	Calories
Per serving (not including formula)	34	1.5	130

Strawberry Shake

2 to 3 crushed ice cubes
½ cup liquid Rich's Richwhip
   Topping
1½ tablespoons Nestlé
   Strawberry Quik

2 drops vanilla or almond
   flavoring
2 to 6 scoops (20 to 60 gm)
   PKU formula powder
   (optional)

Blend all ingredients in a blender for 1 minute. Serve immediately.

Yield: one 10 oz serving.

	Phenylalanine (mg)	Protein (gm)	Calories
Per serving (not including formula)	4	trace	403

Variation

Chocolate Shake

Replace Strawberry Quik with 1½ tablespoons Chocolate Quik.

	Phenylalanine (mg)	Protein (gm)	Calories
Per serving (not including formula)	43	1.0	410

Apple Snow Spooner

½ cup water
6 tablespoons frozen apple
   juice concentrate (¼ of 12 oz
   can)
5 to 6 crushed ice cubes

2 to 4 scoops (20 to 40 gm)
   PKU formula powder
   (optional)
1 drop red food coloring
   (optional)

    Pour water into electric blender container. Add frozen apple juice concentrate, crushed ice, and formula powder (if desired). Blend on high for several minutes. As the mixture gets thick, you may need to start and stop the blender several times. Serve immediately with a spoon, as a slushy drink.

Yield: one 12 oz serving.

	Phenylalanine (mg)	Protein (gm)	Calories
Per serving (not including formula)	trace	trace	180

Mock Pink Champagne

A nice party beverage for adults and children alike.

¼ cup granulated sugar
¾ cup water
1 cup cranberry juice cocktail

½ cup pineapple juice
¼ cup orange juice
1 cup (8 oz) 7-Up

    In a saucepan, boil sugar and water until sugar dissolves; transfer to a beverage container. Stir in cranberry, pineapple, and orange juices. Chill. Add 7-Up just before serving.

Yield: 3½ cups (28 oz).

	Phenylalanine (mg)	Protein (gm)	Calories
Per recipe	18	0.8	507
Per ½ cup (4 oz) serving	3	0.1	72

Hot Chocolate

4 teaspoons Hershey's
   chocolate syrup
½ cup Rich's Coffee Rich and
   ¼ cup water, or ¼ cup
   liquid Rich's Richwhip
   Topping and ½ cup water

drop of peppermint flavoring
   (optional)
6 mini marshmallows

Mix chocolate syrup, Coffee Rich or Richwhip, and water in a small saucepan and heat (or microwave in a mug on High for 1½ to 2 minutes, or until as hot as desired). Add a drop of peppermint flavoring if desired. Put marshmallows on top and serve.

Yield: one 6 oz serving.

Note
If you wish, mix in several scoops of PKU formula powder after hot chocolate has cooled to drinking temperature.

	Phenylalanine (mg)	Protein (gm)	Calories
Using Richwhip			
Per serving	23	0.6	231
Using Coffee Rich			
Per serving	45	0.9	243

Banana Smoothie

2 to 3 crushed ice cubes
3-inch section (40 gm) banana,
   frozen
1 cup (8 oz) PKU formula,
   prepared according to diet
   prescription

1 teaspoon honey or sugar
½ teaspoon vanilla

Blend all ingredients in a blender for 1 minute. Serve immediately.

Yield: one 12 oz serving.

Note
Non-frozen fruits can also be used, but the drink will not become as thick. For versions using banana, the drink should be made just prior to serving, as the banana will darken over time.

	Phenylalanine (mg)	Protein (gm)	Calories
Per serving (not including formula)	15	0.4	59

Variations

Banana Strawberry Smoothie

Add ½ cup (90 gm) loose-pack frozen strawberries.

Yield: one 12 oz serving.

	Phenylalanine (mg)	Protein (gm)	Calories
Per serving (not including formula)	23	1.0	86

Peach Smoothie

Replace banana with ½ cup (50 gm) loose-pack frozen peaches.

Yield: one 12 oz serving.

	Phenylalanine (mg)	Protein (gm)	Calories
Per serving (not including formula)	11	0.4	43

Pineapple Smoothie

Replace banana with ½ cup (140 gm) frozen, crushed pineapple.

Yield: one 12 oz serving.

	Phenylalanine (mg)	Protein (gm)	Calories
Per serving (not including formula)	13	0.5	97

Strawberry Smoothie

Replace banana with ½ cup (90 gm) loose-pack frozen strawberries.

Yield: one 12 oz serving.

	Phenylalanine (mg)	Protein (gm)	Calories
Per serving (not including formula)	8	0.6	49

Sauces, Dips, and Dressings

Special Tips

All of the recipes in this section are suitable for the whole family.

Relatively few salad dressing recipes are included because there are many commercially available "free" dressings that can conveniently be used (see the *Low Protein Food List*).

Most dip recipes and commercially prepared dips are notoriously high in protein and phenylalanine, being made from sour cream and/or cream cheese. "Low" alternatives are difficult to devise, but the recipes in this section using Miracle Whip Dressing are good and quite "low." *Guacamole* is also a great dip for *Taco Chips,* low protein crackers, or raw vegetables.

To prepare low protein gravy use the *Gravy Anytime* recipe. Strained meat drippings *may* be comparable in protein/phenylalanine to commercial bouillon in some cases, but may also be much "higher" (any meat juices that become partially solidified after cooling may be especially high).

A satisfactory low protein white sauce recipe that could be used as a "lower" alternative to canned soups in some of the main dish recipes would be highly desirable, but so far attempts to prepare such a recipe using non-dairy creamers have not been successful.

French Dressing

½ cup catsup   2 tablespoons vinegar
½ cup vegetable oil   1 tablespoon lemon juice
¼ cup granulated sugar

Shake all ingredients in a tightly covered jar or bottle, or blend for one minute in a blender. Chill. Shake before using.

Yield: 1¼ cups.

	Phenylalanine (mg)	Protein (gm)	Calories
Per recipe	56	1.8	1243
Per tablespoon	2	trace	62

Simple Vinaigrette Dressing

¼ cup white wine vinegar or salt and pepper to taste
 herb vinegar   ½ cup olive oil or vegetable oil
1 tablespoon lemon juice
¼ teaspoon dry mustard or 1
 teaspoon prepared Dijon
 mustard

In a small bowl, mix together the vinegar, lemon juice, mustard, salt, and pepper. Add oil, a little at a time, beating with a whisk until the mixture emulsifies. This dressing may also be made in a blender. Simply put all ingredients into a blender container and blend at high speed for a short time.

Yield: ¾ cup.

	Phenylalanine (mg)	Protein (gm)	Calories
Per recipe	15	0.4	983
Per tablespoon	1	trace	82

Lori's Red Tornado Salad Dressing

¼ cup Miracle Whip Salad
    Dressing
1 tablespoon granulated sugar

1 tablespoon sweet or dill
    pickle juice
dash of paprika for red coloring

Mix all ingredients together with a wire whip in a small bowl. Chill.

Yield: ⅓ cup.

	Phenylalanine (mg)	Protein (gm)	Calories
Per recipe	12	0.2	330
Per tablespoon	2	trace	62

Creamy Dressing

Excellent over low protein noodles, vegetables, or potatoes as well as for salad.

½ of 1 oz pkg Hidden Valley
    Ranch Dressing Mix (the
    variety that normally calls
    for adding buttermilk)

1 cup Miracle Whip Salad
    Dressing
1 cup Rich's Coffee Rich

Mix all ingredients in a small bowl or in a blender. Chill.

Yield: 2 cups.

	Phenylalanine (mg)	Protein (gm)	Calories
Per recipe	197	3.6	1492
Per tablespoon	6	0.1	47

Summer Salad Dressing and Dip

Good as a fresh vegetable dip, or over a fresh vegetable salad made of raw cauliflower, broccoli, celery, cucumbers, carrots, tomato, and green pepper (or vegetables of your choice).

½ cup Miracle Whip Salad
    Dressing
2 tablespoons bottled French
    dressing
¼ cup sour cream

2 tablespoons granulated sugar
2 teaspoons vinegar
chopped fresh herbs of your
    choice

Mix all ingredients together in a small bowl or jar and chill.

Yield: 1 cup.

	Phenylalanine (mg)	Protein (gm)	Calories
Per recipe	96	1.9	8⸱⸱
Per tablespoon	6	0.1	55

Creamy Dip

¼ cup Miracle Whip Salad
    Dressing
3 tablespoons Coolwhip or
    whipped Rich's Richwhip
    Topping

½ to 1 teaspoon Hidden Valley
    Salad Dressing Mix (from a
    1 oz pkg)
1 teaspoon lemon juice

Mix all ingredients in a small bowl or refrigerator container. Chill.

Yield: ½ cup.

	Phenylalanine (mg)	Protein (gm)	Calories
Using Richwhip			
Per recipe	35	0.7	348
Per tablespoon	4	0.1	44
Using Coolwhip			
Per recipe	44	0.8	315
Per tablespoon	5	0.1	39

Gravy Anytime

½ cup cold water
2 teaspoons cornstarch

½ bouillon cube, 1 teaspoon
granulated bouillon, or
½ package G. Washington's
Golden or Rich Brown
Seasoning and Broth

In a small dish, mix 2 tablespoons of the water with cornstarch; set aside. In a small saucepan, dissolve broth in remaining water (6 tablespoons). Bring to a boil; add cornstarch mixture and stir vigorously until thickened and smooth.

Yield: ½ cup.

	Phenylalanine (mg)	Protein (gm)	Calories
Using G. Washington's Broth			
Per recipe	0	0.0	14
Per tablespoon	0	0.0	2
Using bouillon			
Per recipe	16	0.3	14
Per tablespoon	2	trace	2

Fresh Cranberry Relish

1 small apple (about
130 gm), cored, unpeeled
1 medium orange (about
160 gm), unpeeled

12 oz bag (3 cups) fresh or
frozen cranberries
1¼ cups granulated sugar

Quarter apple and orange, removing seeds. Put apple, orange, and cranberries through a food grinder (or chop in a food processor using the steel blade, processing orange and apple first, then adding cranberries). Add sugar and mix well. Chill several hours or overnight.

Yield: 2¾ cups (900 gm).

Storage Tip
Keeps well in refrigerator for several weeks. Also freezes well.

	Phenylalanine (mg)	Protein (gm)	Calories
Per recipe	50	2.0	1238
Per 2 tablespoons (20 gm)	2	0.1	56

Guacamole

Delicious as a tortilla filling or as a dip for low protein *Taco Chips.*

⅔ cup (150 gm) mashed
avocado (about 1 medium)
2 teaspoons lemon juice
1 tablespoon Old El Paso
taco sauce

2 teaspoons grated onion
¼ teaspoon salt

In a small bowl, mix mashed avocado with lemon juice, taco sauce or salsa, onion, and salt. Place 1½ tablespoons in a baked low protein *Tortilla* and roll up, or use as a dip with low protein *Taco Chips,* or with other chips or crackers. Use within several hours of preparing as the avocado will darken.

Yield: ⅔ cup (150 gm).

	Phenylalanine (mg)	Protein (gm)	Calories
Per recipe	102	3.0	271
Per tablespoon (14 gm)	15	0.4	40

59

Salsa Fresca

Serve with *Taco Chips* or *Burritos.*

1 cup (180 gm) peeled, seeded, and chopped fresh tomatoes
½ cup (70 gm) finely chopped onions
1 jalapeño chili, seeded and finely chopped, or 1 canned chili, chopped

2 teaspoons olive oil
1 teaspoon vinegar
1 teaspoon lemon or lime juice
½ teaspoon dried leaf oregano, crushed or 2 tablespoons chopped fresh oregano
½ teaspoon salt

In a medium bowl, combine tomatoes, onion, and chili. Add oil, vinegar, lemon or lime juice, oregano, and salt. Mix well. Let sauce stand for at least 2 hours to blend flavors. Serve at room temperature.

Yield: 1 cup plus 2 tablespoons.

	Phenylalanine (mg)	Protein (gm)	Calories
Per recipe	65	2.5	151
Per tablespoon	4	0.1	8

Sweet and Sour Sauce

Serve with *Mock Egg Rolls* or *French Fried Veggies.*

⅓ cup cold water
2 teaspoons cornstarch
2 teaspoons brown sugar
⅓ cup catsup

2 teaspoons vinegar
1 teaspoon La Choy soy sauce
dash of salt

In a small saucepan, stir together water, cornstarch, and sugar. Stir in catsup, vinegar, soy sauce, and salt. Cook and stir until thickened and bubbly; cook and stir for an additional 1 to 2 minutes. Serve warm.

Yield: ⅔ cup.

	Phenylalanine (mg)	Protein (gm)	Calories
Per recipe	45	1.4	112
Per tablespoon	7	0.2	17

Microwave Hot Fudge Sauce

A rich and chocolatey favorite.

½ cup granulated sugar
2 tablespoons Hershey's
  unsweetened cocoa (not
  instant)
2 tablespoons cornstarch

dash of salt
½ cup plus 2 tablespoons water
2 tablespoons margarine or
  butter
1 teaspoon vanilla

In a one-quart casserole, mix sugar, cocoa, cornstarch, and salt. Add several tablespoons of the water and mix until well blended; gradually add remaining water while stirring. Microwave on High for about 2 minutes, stirring twice during cooking time (any lumps which form during the later stages of cooking can be easily stirred out). Blend in margarine. Microwave on High for 45 seconds, or until margarine is melted and sauce is thickened and glossy, stirring half-way through cooking time. Blend in vanilla. Serve immediately over ice cream or cake, or chill and rewarm in microwave oven. Keeps well, refrigerated, for up to 1 week.

Yield: 1 cup.

	Phenylalanine (mg)	Protein (gm)	Calories
Per serving	142	2.8	700
Per tablespoon	9	0.2	44

Caramel Marshmallow Sauce

Great over low protein ice cream or unfrosted cake.

1½ cups packed brown sugar
⅔ cup light Karo corn syrup
⅓ cup water
⅓ cup margarine or butter

6 large marshmallows, diced
¼ cup Rich's Coffee Rich
¼ cup water

Combine sugar, syrup, and water in a medium saucepan. Cook over medium heat, using a candy thermometer, until soft ball stage (230°) is reached, stirring occasionally during cooking. Mix in margarine and marshmallows, stirring until melted. Add Coffee Rich and water; mix well. Chill. Sauce will separate during storage; stir before serving. Keeps well in refrigerator or freezer for several months.

Yield: 2 cups.

For Microwave Oven
Combine sugar, corn syrup, and water in a 1½-quart casserole. Microwave on High for 9 to 10 minutes, stirring occasionally during cooking. Mix in remaining ingredients as for original recipe.

	Phenylalanine (mg)	Protein (gm)	Calories
Per recipe	50	1.2	2452
Per tablespoon	2	0.1	77

62

Ruby Strawberry Sauce

A favorite sauce and a great way to use your rhubarb harvest.

¾ cup granulated sugar
2 tablespoons cornstarch
10 oz pkg frozen strawberries

4 cups (480 gm) sliced, fresh or
frozen rhubarb

Combine sugar and cornstarch. Put rhubarb and thawed strawberries in a 1½ quart casserole; sprinkle sugar mixture over and mix. Microwave on High for 10 to 12 minutes or until mixture boils, stirring several times during cooking. Sauce will become thickened when done. If your rhubarb is not the red type, add a few drops of red food coloring if desired. Serve warm or chilled, as a dessert or for a breakfast fruit.

Yield: 3 cups (780 gm).

Note
Fresh strawberries may be substituted for frozen. Add ¼ cup additional sugar if desired and decrease cooking time slightly.

	Phenylalanine (mg)	Protein (gm)	Calories
Per recipe	189	5.8	1020
Per ¼ cup (65 gm) serving	16	0.5	85

Breads

Notes about Low Protein Yeast Breads

It has been said that good bread is the most fundamentally satisfying of all foods. For children and others on the diet, this thought takes on special importance. Good low protein breads added to the diet on a regular basis can provide variety and bulk that would otherwise be lacking. And what person of any age can resist a warm roll or slice of freshly baked bread? The result of baking low protein bread can be especially rewarding, since you cannot simply buy a fresh loaf at the grocery store.

There are two basic methods for preparing low protein breads: either the traditional method of mixing, kneading, and rising; or a far quicker and simpler method using one of the marvels of technology, the automatic bread baker. This machine has caused a "revolution" in low protein bread making and allowed families to bake bread on a regular basis with almost no bother. General tips for preparing low protein breads and tips for using either of these methods are given on the next pages.

The low protein breads you can bake from the recipes in this book are excellent—in fact, some people would not be able to distinguish them from regular bread. But several special ingredients used in low protein breadmaking are unique, and their characteristics in baking need some explanation:

Wheat starch, and **Wel-Plan Baking Mix** (which is composed mainly of wheat starch). These are used in place of flour. Wheat starch is the part of regular flour that remains after the protein has been removed. It contains no gluten, the special wheat protein which normally gives bread its structure and enhances browning.

Metamucil.® This is a natural fiber compound that is added to the low protein bread doughs to compensate for the lack of gluten. It imparts the elasticity and structure that would otherwise be missing; it is the "miracle ingredient" that allows you to make low protein bread with properties very similar to regular bread. In the quantity used, the natural fiber addition is a healthy one for the PKU diet, which provides lesser amounts of natural fiber than normal diets. Use only plain flavor Metamucil, found in grocery and drug stores, with no added Nutrasweet. Other generic brands of Metamucil-type products may be used but may impart a slightly different flavor to the bread.

Another thing to keep in mind is that because "browning" of regular baked products depends largely on the presence of protein, low protein breads and baked goods have a tendency to brown less well than those made with wheat flour. Brushing on a little melted margarine or butter may be called for in the recipes, either prior to baking (rolls only) or midway through. Never brush melted margarine or butter on raw bread dough as a proper crust will not form. Also avoid too much on the partially-baked loaf of bread or the cooled crust will become "wrinkled" (though this affects only the appearance).

Finally, remember that the recipes for low protein breads were developed very carefully to take best advantage of the special ingredients and enable you to produce the best possible breads and rolls. So be sure that you follow the instructions exactly. The results will be well worth your effort!

General Tips for Preparation of Low Protein Yeast Breads

Ingredients

- Use only fresh, dry yeast. Be sure to check that the expiration date has not passed. Do not use Quick-Rise yeast, as it rises too quickly for this bread and leaves large air holes. Fleischmann's active dry yeast was used in developing the bread recipes, but other brands can also be used. A good way to keep yeast fresh is in the refrigerator or freezer.
- Do not try to substitute other baking mixes for the breads indicated in the recipes. The success of the recipes is very much dependent on using the specific breads listed.
- Weighing Wel-Plan Baking Mix and wheat starch on a gram scale is the best way to ensure consistently good results with your bread.

Cooling

- The bread should be left to cool on its side on a cooling rack. Leaving the bread upright to cool may cause it to become deformed.

Cutting

- Use an electric knife if you want very thin slices or very even slices. Or take your bread to a bakery in a local grocery store where they can slice it using a commercial machine. If you explain the nature of the bread, they will generally be very accommodating. Alternatively, you can purchase a "deli-slicer" for about $30-50 from a department or discount store. This will be well worth the investment.

Storage

- The bread or rolls keep well in the refrigerator or at room temperature for 3-5 days. Bread made in the automatic bakers tends to stay fresher longer than that made by the traditional method. Freshness can be preserved by freezing. Use foil or plastic wrap inside of a heavy freezer-type plastic bag (such as Ziploc) or plastic container.

- For convenience when appetites are small, slice bread when cool and wrap individual slices or several slices per package with slices separated by waxed paper, then freeze.
- Frozen bread slices thaw well in a microwave oven after unwrapping (30 to 45 seconds on 50% power); or remove from wrapping and thaw at room temperature (if bread thaws in a closed plastic bar or plastic wrap, moisture may accumulate on the crust and cause it to become soggy). A solidly frozen whole loaf can be quick-thawed by placing it in a 300° oven for 25 to 40 minutes (cover it with foil first to prevent drying out).

Making Low Protein Bread the "Traditional" Way

Ingredients

- For *Best White Bread,* a convenient way to measure the Wel-Plan Baking Mix is to begin with an unopened box (400 gm). Remove $^1/_3$ cup (42 gm) and use the rest (358 gm) for the bread; the extra $^1/_3$ cup will be partially used for kneading the bread.

Utensils

- Keep mixing utensils warm for best yeast activity: Warm bowl/mug in which yeast is dissolved by first running hot water over it, then drying it and adding the $^1/_4$ cup warm water. In the same manner, warm bowl in which bread will be mixed (if it is cold) to keep dough warm initially.
- Buy an oven thermometer if you are unsure of the temperature control on your oven. The 120 to 130° temperature that begins the rising process is important. The optimal rising temperature is very warm to start with, but not hot. The oven will cool down naturally as rising progresses, but it should not be rewarmed.
- Use an $8^1/_2 \times 4^1/_2$ inch pan rather than the more standard 9×5 inch pan for bread slices that are most like commercial bread.
- Your bread pan may be any kind of metal (black, shiny, or dull metal).

Preparation

- Plan on approximately $2^1/_4$ hours to produce a loaf of bread (only about 30 minutes of actual preparation time and clean-up—the rest of the time the bread is rising or baking).
- Water for the bread should be quite warm, but not hot to the touch. A dough thermometer may be helpful if you are a novice bread-baker, or use the temperature probe on your microwave oven to bring the water up to temperature.
- When "proofing the yeast" (that is, dissolving it in warm water and causing it to become activated), if after 10 minutes the dis-

solved yeast looks only bubbly and does not have a dense layer of creamy foam on top, the bread may not rise properly. If this occurs, it would be advisable to buy some fresh yeast and start again. Adequate kneading (the full 3 minutes) gives a beautiful, smooth crust and helps the bread to rise optimally. For high altitudes, rising time will probably need to be reduced somewhat.

Making Low Protein Bread in an Automatic Bread Machine

Preparing low protein breads in an automatic bread machine will not only save you preparation and clean-up time, but will produce consistently good bread with a light, soft texture. Purchasing an automatic baker may be one of the best investments you will make to help in management of PKU. Imagine only 5 minutes of your time to make a great loaf of fresh bread, whenever you want. You can measure out the ingredients in the morning, go to work, and program your bread baker to have the loaf finished by dinner-time! It is so simple that even a child of age 7 or 8 can learn to make bread.

Recommended Bread Machine for Low Protein Bread

"Breadman" by Salton-Maxim (model TR500)

• This is my favorite bread machine as this edition is printed (1997). It is similar to a bread machine I once preferred that is no longer sold, the Mister Loaf (also sold as Chefmate when it was sold at Target discount stores). It makes a nice-sized loaf of bread for sandwiches. The bread has good texture and the cycle is only approximately 2$\frac{3}{4}$ hours from start to finished loaf. The price is also very reasonable. At the time of the printing of this book, the Breadman machine is available at a discount through The New England Connection for PKU & Allied Disorders, c/o John Sullivan, 5 Jones Lane, East Sandwich, MA 02537 (telephone: 508-888-2295, e-mail: lophechef@capecod.net). Beware that bread machine models are constantly changing. If the TR500 model is discontinued, The New England Connection will have a replacement to recommend, based on my personal testing experience. At present, the Breadman machine seems to produce the most consistently good results compared to other machines I have tested.

Other Bread Machines

I do not specifically recommend any other brands of bread machines, although I have tried many. Low protein bread is very "sensitive" and simply does not work well in many machines I have tried. In some cases the results have been "acceptable," but in other cases, the results were disastrous. I cannot account for the differences in the machines that would cause such variability in results, and therefore cannot give you any hints about which of any of the new machines that come on the market will make successful low protein bread. Unless you are prepared for failure, I advise that you purchase the Breadman machine (or a replacement that I will recommend to The New England Connection for PKU and Allied Disorders).

General Tips

• For low protein breads, when you are not using the delay timer, you need to add all of the dry ingredients to the pan with the dough hook in place, mixing them briefly with a spoon. (This is not what the machine instructions will tell you to do.) Then insert the pan in the machine, add the liquid ingredients *all at once,* and immediately start the machine. Be sure that the pan is properly in place in the machine before you add the liquid ingredients to the dry ingredients, so that you begin the kneading process without delay (important so that the Metamucil mixes in properly). You can even start the machine first, then add the liquid.

• If you are using the delay timer, the crucial thing is that you do not let the water come in contact with either the yeast or the Metamucil while the ingredients are waiting for the bread-making process to begin. The best way to do this is to *first* add the water, then carefully add the baking mix, followed by the apple fiber (for County Style Bread), salt, sugar, yeast, and Metamucil.

• When set to be finished in 10-12 hours, the bread may rise about an inch or so higher than when the process is started immediately, making bread that is lighter in texture (this may or may not be an advantage, depending on your texture preference).

• If you find that your bread doesn't rise well, or has a very lumpy top, add a little more water (1 to 2 tablespoons) the next time. The bread is very sensitive to changes in water content, so measure accurately, using the measuring utensil provided with the machine (which is much more accurate than most household measuring cups). Note exactly how much water you added and add that amount each time you make the bread, using the same measuring utensil.

• Another trick to try if you are not pleased with how the bread rises is to "proof" the yeast before adding it to the bread maker: dissolve the yeast in about ⅓-½ cup of the water specified in the recipe (using water quite warm to the touch) along with ½ teaspoon of sugar and let stand for 10 minutes. The yeast should produce a dense foam. Pour into the bread baker along with the remaining water.

• If you find that your bread rises well but turns out with a bumpy or uneven top, you may find that opening the lid of the baker to smooth the bread while it is rising will help. (It is all right briefly to open the lid of the machine at any time).

• Buy yeast in bulk (for example, the brown jars of Fleischmann's or Red Star)—more convenient than little packages, since the recipes use less than a small packet. Keep the yeast in your freezer for freshness, but allow it to come to room temperature before using. One of the most important keys to properly risen bread (in addition to the water content) is to use fresh, active yeast.

• The machine has different settings for crust darkness. For the Breadman, I use the light setting (the dark setting produces a tougher crust). The crust will not brown much.

• If you want a more golden crust, you can open the lid about 20 minutes before the bread is done and brush on a little melted butter or margarine.

• To remove the bread from the pan after baking, you will need to rap the pan firmly several times on a hard surface to shake it loose from the kneading blade which will be imbedded in the baked bread. The kneading blade may become completely imbedded in the bread and will come out with the bread as you remove it from the pan; remove hook when bread is cool. (Unavoidably, with any bread machine, one slice of bread will be adversely affected by the dough hook impression.) To facilitate removal of the kneading blade, you may rub it with a little vegetable oil or shortening in advance of using the machine.

• Using the "rapid bread" cycle on the machines produces unacceptably holey low protein bread.

• To make any of the rolls, pizza, unusually shaped loaves, or other recipes in this book that require shaping of dough, you may still use a bread machine. Use the recipes for making bread the *traditional way*, however. *Do not use the recipes for automatic bread machines, since the latter will produce dough that is too sticky to shape*. Use the "Dough" setting on your machine. When the dough cycle is complete, remove dough to a surface lightly dusted with wheat starch or baking mix, knead a few times with your hands if it has risen during the dough cycle, and shape as desired. Let rise and bake as per recipe instructions, in your own preheated oven.

• You may also want to remove dough from the machine and freeze individual balls of dough to use later for fresh fry bread, rolls, or other recipes (although the rising may be somewhat less than when using unfrozen dough). If you are keeping up with very small appetites, you also can purchase small bread pans (5 ¾ × 2 ½ inches), place the dough from any of the full-size recipes into 4 pans, and freeze for later.

• For a complete discussion of low protein bread making in bread machines, and for an extensive collection of recipes, please consult *Low Protein Bread Machine Baking for PKU* by Virginia E. Schuett, 1993. (Available from Dietary Specialties, Inc. [a subsidiary of MenuDirect Corp.], 865 Piscataway, NJ 08854. Telephone: 1-888-MENU123 or 732-980-6700.)

Best White Bread

¼ cup very warm water (105° to 115°)
½ teaspoon granulated sugar

1 pkg or 2¼ teaspoons active dry yeast (not "quick-rise")

Pour water into a small bowl or large coffee mug; add sugar, then yeast. Stir briefly, then let sit for 10 minutes (mixture should develop a good "head" of creamy foam on top). Meanwhile, mix together dry ingredients in a medium bowl:

3¼ cups (358 gm) Wel-Plan Baking Mix
2½ tablespoons (25 gm) Metamucil

1 teaspoon salt
1 tablespoon granulated sugar

When yeast mixture is ready, pour it into a large mixing bowl. Then add: 1 cup plus 3 tablespoons very warm water (105° to 115°).

Mix together the yeast and water just until well combined. Now stir in the premeasured or preweighed dry ingredients all at once, mixing vigorously for a few seconds until smooth (dough will remain very sticky at this point).

Tightly cover bowl of dough with plastic wrap (Saran Wrap works best) to prevent drying out. Warm oven to about 120° to 130° (very warm but not hot) by turning oven on to 350° for 1 to 2 minutes, then turning off. Place covered dough in oven and let rise for 30 minutes.

Remove dough from bowl to a kneading surface dusted with Baking Mix (bread board or pastry cloth works well). Knead dough for a full 3 minutes using regular bread kneading technique. Add 2 to 4 tablespoons (16 to 32 gm) additional Baking Mix during kneading, just enough to keep dough from sticking to hands and kneading surface.

Form dough into a rectangular loaf shape and place in a lightly greased 8½ × 4½-inch bread plan; cover with a cloth and set in oven, again warmed to 120° to 130°. Let rise for 30 to 45 minutes, or until dough is about 1 inch above top of pan at its highest point, then remove from oven. Preheat oven to 375°. Remove cloth and bake bread 15 minutes. Brush lightly with melted margarine or butter, then continue baking for 15 to 25 minutes. Place pan on a cooling rack for several minutes, then remove bread from pan and turn on its side to cool on the rack. Let bread cool completely before cutting or storing.

Yield: 15 slices.

	Phenylalanine (mg)	Protein (gm)	Calories
Per recipe	164	3.6	1333
Per slice	11	0.2	89

Best White Bread for Automatic Bread Bakers

3¼ cups (354 gm) Wel-Plan
  Baking Mix
1 tablespoon plus 2 teaspoons
  Metamucil

1¾ teaspoons active dry yeast
1 tablespoon sugar
¾ teaspoon salt
1¼ cups plus 3 tablespoons
  warm water

Pour dry ingredients into bread baker pan, making sure that the dough hook is in place. Mix dry ingredients with a spoon. Insert pan into the machine. Pour liquid ingredients into pan and immediately turn machine on. Close cover and let machine continue until bread is baked. When cool, cut into 15 slices.

	Phenylalanine (mg)	Protein (gm)	Calories
per recipe	130	3.0	1356
per slice	9	0.2	90

Variation

Best White Bread for Automatic Bread Bakers II

This variation has a fine, soft texture and is a favorite of many families.

Follow instructions for *Best White Bread for Automatic Bread Bakers,* except increase sugar to 2½ tablespoons, add 3 tablespoons Cremora or Coffee Mate non-dairy creamer powder and increase water to 1½ cups plus 3 tablespoons. Cut into 15 slices.

	Phenylalanine (mg)	Protein (gm)	Calories
per recipe	148	3.3	1536
per slice	10	0.2	102

Country Style Bread for Automatic Bread Bakers

This bread is my favorite, for its earthy color, lovely texture, and especially good flavor.

1 box (400 gm) Wel-Plan Baking Mix
3 tablespoons Tastee Apple Fiber
3 tablespoons Metamucil
1¾ teaspoons active dry yeast

1 tablespoon sugar
1 teaspoon salt
1 tablespoon vegetable oil
1 tablespoon molasses or honey
1¾ cups warm water

Follow instructions for *Best White Bread for Automatic Bread Bakers.* Cut into 15 slices.

Note

Apple fiber is a wonderful addition to low protein breads, but is not readily available in most cities. You can order it directly by mail in 1 lb. boxes (enough for 20 loaves of bread) for a reasonable price: Tastee Apple Inc., 60810 CR 9, Newcomerstown, OH 43832. Tele: 1-800-262-7753 or 740-498-8316. Web site: http://web.tusco.net/tastee. Some health food stores also carry it.

	Phenylalanine (mg)	Protein (gm)	Calories
per recipe	170	3.2	1708
per slice	11	0.3	114

Best Homestyle Bread

A light golden brown bread.

¼ cup very warm water (105° to 115°)
½ teaspoon granulated sugar

1 pkg or 2¼ teaspoons active dry yeast (not "quick-rise")

Pour water into a small bowl or large coffee mug; add sugar, then yeast. Stir briefly, then let sit for 10 minutes (mixture should develop a good "head" of creamy foam on top). Meanwhile, mix together dry ingredients in a medium bowl:

1⅓ cups (147 gm) Wel-Plan Baking Mix
1⅔ cups (183 gm) wheat starch
¼ cup (40 gm) Metamucil

2 teaspoons baking powder
1 teaspoon baking soda
1 teaspoon salt
1 tablespoon granulated sugar

When yeast mixture is ready, pour it into a large mixing bowl. Then add:

1 cup very warm water (105° to 115°)

¼ cup (60 gm) applesauce

Mix together the yeast, water, and applesauce just until well combined. Now stir in premeasured or preweighed dry ingredients all at once, mixing vigorously for a few seconds until smooth (dough will remain very sticky at this point).

Cover bowl of dough with plastic wrap (Saran Wrap works best) to prevent drying out. Warm oven to about 120° to 130° (very warm but not hot) by turning oven on to 350° for 1 to 2 minutes, then turning off. Place covered dough in oven and let rise for 30 minutes.

Remove dough from bowl to a kneading surface dusted with Baking Mix (bread board or pastry cloth works well). Knead dough for a full 3 minutes using regular bread kneading technique. Add 2 to 4 tablespoons (16 to 32 gm) additional wheat starch or Baking Mix during kneading, just enough to keep dough from sticking to hands and kneading surface.

Form dough into a rectangular loaf shape and place in a lightly greased 8½ × 4½-inch bread pan; cover with a cloth and set in oven, again warmed to 120° to 130°. Let rise for 30 to 45 minutes, or until dough is about 1 inch above top of pan at its highest point, then remove from oven. Preheat oven to 375°. Remove cloth and bake bread 15 minutes. Brush lightly with melted margarine or butter, then continue baking for 15 to 25 minutes. Place pan on a cooling rack for several minutes, then remove bread from pan and turn on its side to cool on the rack. Let bread cool completely before cutting or storing.

Yield: 15 slices.

	Phenylalanine (mg)	Protein (gm)	Calories
Per recipe	174	3.4	1642
Per slice	12	0.2	109

Variation

Molasses and Honey Bread

A slightly sweet, dark golden brown bread.

For either automatic or regular recipes, replace the 1 cup warm water with only ³/₄ cup warm water. Add 2 tablespoons dark molasses and 3 tablespoons honey along with the water.

Yield: 15 slices.

	Phenylalanine (mg)	Protein (gm)	Calories
Per recipe	174	3.4	1967
Per slice	12	0.2	131

Best Homestyle Bread for Automatic Bread Bakers

1 cup (110 gm) Wel-Plan
   Baking Mix
1¾ cups (190 gm) wheat starch
3 tablespoons Metamucil
1½ teaspoons active dry yeast

1 tablespoon sugar
¾ teaspoon salt
3 tablespoons applesauce
1¼ cups minus 1 tablespoon
   warm water

Follow instructions for *Best White Bread for Automatic Bread Bakers*. Cut into 15 slices.

	Phenylalanine (mg)	Protein (gm)	Calories
per recipe	126	2.6	1312
per slice	8	0.2	87

Bread in a Can

Perfect for a quick pizza.

1 recipe *Best White Bread* or *Best Homestyle Bread*	two 1 lb coffee cans

Prepare *Best White Bread* or *Best Homestyle Bread* as directed, forming dough into two balls after it has been kneaded. Place dough balls into greased coffee cans and let rise as directed, except check rising after 20 to 30 minutes; dough should not rise more than about 1 inch above the top of the can. Bake as directed for *Best White Bread* or *Best Homestyle Bread*. Remove bread from cans to a cooling rack immediately after baking. Slice when completely cool, into 11 slices per loaf; or for a very smooth pizza base, slice when frozen, as needed.

Yield: 22 slices.

Note

For a quick and delicious little pizza, toast a slice of *Bread in a Can*, then add 1 tablespoon tomato sauce and topping of your choice and broil 3 to 4 minutes until sauce is hot.

	Phenylalanine (mg)	Protein (gm)	Calories
Using Best White Bread			
Per recipe	164	3.6	1333
Per slice	7	0.2	61
Using Best Homestyle Bread			
Per recipe	174	3.4	1642
Per slice	8	0.2	75

Cinnamon Rolls

1 recipe *Best White Bread* or
   Best Homestyle Bread
3 tablespoons melted
   margarine or butter

½ cup granulated sugar
3 to 4 teaspoons cinnamon

Icing

1 cup sifted confectioner's
   sugar
1 tablespoon melted margarine
   or butter

1½ to 2 tablespoons water
½ teaspoon vanilla

Prepare dough, let rise for 30 minutes, and knead as directed for *Best White Bread* or *Best Homestyle Bread.* Instead of forming into a loaf shape, divide dough into 2 parts. On a surface lightly dusted with Wel-Plan Baking Mix or wheat starch, roll one piece of dough into a rectangle approximately 12 × 7 inches. Brush surface with 1½ tablespoons of the melted margarine. Mix together sugar and cinnamon. Sprinkle dough with one half of the cinnamon-sugar mixture.

Roll dough by lifting the long edge of the rectangle with your hands and curling it over the filling. Pressing the dough tightly with both hands, roll the rectangle into a compact cylinder. Seal by pinching the long edge of the dough to the roll. With a sharp bread knife, cut the cylinder into 12 equal slices. Repeat this process with remaining dough.

Place rolls, cut side down, in two lightly greased 8- or 9-inch cake pans, 12 rolls per pan, or on a cookie sheet, nearly edge to edge. Cover rolls with a kitchen towel or cloth and let rise in an oven warmed to 120° to 130° (turn oven on for several minutes, then turn off) for about 30 to 45 minutes. Remove rolls, then preheat oven to 375°. Uncover rolls and brush lightly with a little melted margarine. Bake 18 to 20 minutes, until lightly browned. Remove to a cooling rack. While still warm, spread with *Icing:* In a small mixing bowl, combine confectioner's sugar, melted margarine, water, and vanilla and mix until smooth.

Yield: 24 rolls.

Storage Tip
   The rolls freeze well, especially unfrosted, in an airtight container.

	Phenylalanine (mg)	Protein (gm)	Calories
Using Best White Bread			
Per recipe	188	3.6	2127
Per roll	8	0.2	89
Using Best Homestyle Bread			
Per recipe	198	3.8	2436
Per roll	8	0.2	102

Caramel Rolls

1 recipe *Best White Bread* or
   Best Homestyle Bread
¼ cup melted margarine or
   butter

⅔ cup packed brown sugar
1 tablespoon cinnamon

Glaze

¾ cup packed brown sugar
3 tablespoons melted
   margarine or butter

½ cup light Karo corn syrup

Prepare dough, let rise for 30 minutes, and knead as directed for *Best White Bread* or *Best Homestyle Bread.* Instead of forming into a loaf shape, divide dough into 2 parts. On a surface lightly dusted with wheat starch or Wel-Plan Baking Mix, roll one piece of dough into a rectangle approximately 12 × 7 inches. Brush with 2 tablespoons of the melted margarine. Sprinkle with one-half of a mixture of the brown sugar and cinnamon. Lightly press filling mixture into the dough, using a rolling pin. Roll dough into a cylinder and cut, as for *Cinnamon Rolls.* Repeat this process with remaining dough.

Prepare *Glaze* by mixing together the brown sugar, melted margarine, and syrup in a small bowl. Coat two 8-inch cake pans with this mixture, spreading with a knife to evenly distribute (heat pans slightly if necessary to get an even coating). Put the dough slices nearly edge to edge in the pans, 12 rolls per pan; cover with a kitchen cloth or towel and let rise in an oven warmed to 120° to 130° (turn oven on for several minutes, then turn off) for about 30 to 45 minutes. Remove rolls, then preheat oven to 375°. Uncover rolls, then bake 18 to 20 minutes.

To cool the rolls, first place an inverted wire rack over the pan. Holding the rack and pan together at both sides with pot holders, flip the assembly over onto a plate (the plate will catch any dripping caramel). Lift off the pan. Let the rolls cool for at least 10 minutes before serving.

Yield: 24 rolls.

	Phenylalanine (mg)	Protein (gm)	Calories
Using Best White Bread			
Per recipe	211	4.7	3786
Per roll	9	0.2	158
Using Best Homestyle Bread			
Per recipe	215	4.3	3525
Per roll	9	0.2	147

Hot Cross Buns

1 recipe *Best White Bread* or *Best Homestyle Bread* to which you have added, along with the dry ingredients:

1 to 2 teaspoons cinnamon
¼ teaspoon cloves
¼ teaspoon nutmeg

grated rind of 1 orange or lemon
½ cup (80 gm) raisins or
currants

Icing

1½ cups sifted confectioner's
sugar
5 to 6 teaspoons water
¾ teaspoon vanilla
½ teaspoon almond flavoring
(optional)

Prepare dough, adding the spices, citrus rind, and raisins or currants along with dry ingredients; let rise for 30 minutes and knead as directed for *Best White Bread* or *Best Homestyle Bread*. Instead of forming into a loaf, divide dough into 2 parts, then cut each part into 12 equal pieces. Form each piece into a round bun shape. Place buns in 2 lightly greased 8- or 9-inch cake pans, 12 buns per pan, or on a cookie sheet, nearly edge to edge. Cover with a kitchen cloth or towel and let rise in an oven warmed to 120° to 130° (turn oven on for a few minutes, then turn off) for about 30 to 45 minutes. Remove rolls, then preheat oven to 375°. Uncover rolls and brush lightly with a little melted margarine. Bake 18 to 20 minutes. Remove to a cooling rack.

Prepare *Icing* by mixing confectioner's sugar, water, and flavoring in a small bowl. Icing should be quite stiff. When buns are completely cool, pipe icing through a pastry tube to form a cross on each bun; or make cross with icing using a spoon or knife.

Yield: 24 buns.

Storage Tip
The buns freeze well, without icing, in an airtight container.

	Phenylalanine (mg)	Protein (gm)	Calories
Using Best White Bread			
Per recipe	217	6.3	2275
Per bun	9	0.3	95
Using Best Homestyle Bread			
Per recipe	228	6.2	2583
Per bun	9	0.3	108

Filled Coffee Braid

Nice for a holiday or special occasion.

1 recipe *Best White Bread* or *Best Homestyle Bread*
1 cup canned Wilderness or Comstock pie filling (any fruit variety)

Prepare dough, let rise for 30 minutes, and knead as directed for *Best White Bread* or *Best Homestyle Bread*. Instead of forming into a loaf shape, divide dough into 2 parts. On a surface lightly dusted with Wel-Plan Baking Mix or wheat starch, roll one piece of dough into a rectangle approximately 10 × 8 inches. Spread ½ cup pie filling down the middle one-third of the rectangle, leaving 2-inch margins at either end.

Cut out the corners and make slanting cuts to within ½ inch of the filling, at 1-inch intervals down the long sides (see diagram). Completely remove the corners that were cut away. Using both hands, fold the rectangular end flaps up and over the filling. Then, starting at one end, fold one diagonal strip of dough over the filling. Cross the opposite strip over the first, continue to bring strips from alternate sides over the filling forming a braid down the length of the dough. Tuck loose ends of the last pair of strips under the coffee cake. Repeat this process with the remaining dough, making a second braid.

Place the braids on a greased baking sheet, cover with a kitchen cloth or towel and let rise in an oven warmed to 120° to 130° (turn oven on for a few minutes, then turn off) for about 30 to 45 minutes. Remove braids from oven, then preheat to 375°. Uncover braids, brush with a little melted margarine, then bake for 20 to 25 minutes. Remove to a cooling rack. Brush again with a little margarine. Cut into slices. These freeze well (for convenience wrap slices individually).

Yield: 2 braids (18 slices each).

	Phenylalanine (mg)	Protein (gm)	Calories
Using Best White Bread			
Per recipe	188	4.5	1645
Per slice	5	0.1	46
Using Best Homestyle Bread			
Per recipe	198	4.3	1954
Per slice	5	0.1	54

Rosettes or Bowknot Rolls

1 recipe *Best White Bread* or *Best Homestyle Bread*

Prepare dough, let rise for 30 minutes, and knead as directed for *Best White Bread* or *Best Homestyle Bread*. Instead of forming into a loaf shape, divide dough into 18 equal pieces. With your hands, roll each piece into a strip about 8 inches long; tie each in a loose knot. For *Bowknot rolls*, lay long ends out as you place on greased baking sheet; for *Rosettes*, tuck one long end inside the knot and one underneath. Space rolls 1 to 2 inches apart on a lightly greased baking sheet.

Cover rolls with a kitchen towel or cloth and place in an oven warmed to 120° to 130° (turn oven on for a few minutes, then turn off) for about 30 to 45 minutes. Remove rolls, then preheat oven to 400°. Uncover rolls and brush lightly with a little melted margarine. Bake for 13 to 15 minutes. Remove to a cooling rack. Brush again with a little margarine.

Yield: 18 rolls.

	Phenylalanine (mg)	Protein (gm)	Calories
Using Best White Bread			
Per recipe	164	3.6	1333
Per roll	9	0.2	74
Using Best Homestyle Bread			
Per recipe	174	3.4	1642
Per roll	10	0.2	91

Bowknot　　　　Rosette

Cloverleaf Rolls

1 recipe *Best White Bread* or *Best Homestyle Bread*

Prepare dough, let rise for 30 minutes, and knead as directed for *Best White Bread* or *Best Homestyle Bread*. Instead of forming into a loaf shape, divide dough into 3 parts. Divide each part into 6 pieces, then each of the 6 pieces into 3 pieces (total of 54 small pieces). Form dough pieces into small walnut-size balls. Place 3 balls together for each roll in a greased 2½-inch muffin cup.

Cover rolls with a kitchen towel or cloth and let rise in an oven warmed to 120° to 130° (turn oven on for a few minutes, then turn off) for about 30 to 45 minutes. Remove rolls, then preheat oven to 400°. Uncover rolls and brush lightly with a little melted margarine. Bake for 13 to 15 minutes. Remove to cooling rack. Brush again with a little margarine.

Yield: 18 rolls.

	Phenylalanine (mg)	Protein (gm)	Calories
Using Best White Bread			
Per recipe	164	3.6	1333
Per roll	9	0.2	74
Using Best Homestyle Bread			
Per recipe	174	3.4	1642
Per roll	10	0.2	91

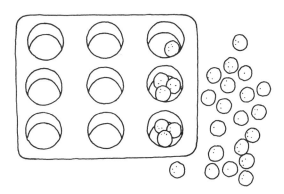

Butterflake Rolls

1 recipe *Best White Bread* or
    Best Homestyle Bread

3 tablespoons melted
    margarine or butter

Prepare dough, let rise for 30 minutes, and knead as directed for *Best White Bread* or *Best Homestyle Bread*. Instead of forming into a loaf shape, divide dough into 2 parts. Roll one part into approximately a 12-inch square. Brush with melted margarine, then:

1. Cut square into six 2-inch strips.
2. Stack strips into two piles of three dough strips.
3. Cut each pile of strips into nine 1½-inch lengths.
4. Put two stacks of 1½-inch strips together (total of 6 layers) vertically in greased 2½-inch muffin cups.
5. Repeat this process with remaining dough.

Cover rolls with a kitchen towel or cloth and place in an oven warmed to 120° to 130° (turn oven on for a few minutes, then turn off) for about 30 to 45 minutes. Remove rolls, then preheat oven to 400°. Uncover rolls and brush lightly with a little melted margarine. Bake for 13 to 15 minutes. Remove to cooling rack. Brush again with a little margarine.

Yield: 18 rolls.

	Phenylalanine (mg)	Protein (gm)	Calories
Using Best White Bread			
Per recipe	182	3.9	1638
Per roll	10	0.2	91
Using Best Homestyle Bread			
Per recipe	192	3.8	1947
Per roll	11	0.2	108

Variation

Will have approximately the same nutrient content as the original recipe.

Cinnamon Butterflake Rolls

Prepare *Butterflake Rolls*, sprinkling as desired with a mixture of cinnamon and sugar after brushing tops of unbaked rolls with melted margarine.

Yield: 18 rolls.

Crescent Rolls

1 recipe *Best White Bread* or
   Best Homestyle Bread

3 tablespoons melted
   margarine or butter

Prepare dough, let rise for 30 minutes, and knead as directed for *Best White Bread* or *Best Homestyle Bread*. Instead of forming into a loaf shape, divide dough into 3 parts. On a surface lightly dusted with Wel-Plan Baking Mix or wheat starch, roll one piece of dough into a circle, approximately 9 inches in diameter. Brush surface with 2 teaspoons melted margarine.

Cut circle into 8 pie-shaped pieces. Roll each wedge, starting with wide end and rolling to the point. Place on greased baking pan or cookie sheet 1 to 2 inches apart, point side down on the pan. Curve ends in a little to form a wide U-shape if desired. Repeat this process with remaining 2 pieces of dough. Cover rolls with a kitchen towel or cloth and let rise in an oven warmed to 120° to 130° (turn oven on for a few minutes, then turn off) for about 30 to 45 minutes. Remove rolls, then preheat oven to 400°. Uncover rolls and brush lightly with a little melted margarine. Bake for 13 to 15 minutes. Remove to cooling rack. Brush again with a little margarine.

Yield: 24 rolls.

	Phenylalanine (mg)	Protein (gm)	Calories
Using Best White Bread			
Per recipe	182	3.9	1638
Per roll	8	0.2	68
Using Best Homestyle Bread			
Per recipe	192	3.8	1947
Per roll	8	0.2	81

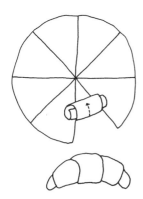

Burger Buns

Serve with *Broccoli Burgers* (page 236), *Mushroom Burgers* (page 234), or as part of a "Sloppy Joe" using seasoned tomato sauce for a topping.

1 recipe *Best White Bread* or *Best Homestyle Bread*

Prepare dough, let rise for 30 minutes, and knead as directed for *Best White Bread* or *Best Homestyle Bread*. Instead of forming into a loaf shape, divide dough into 12 pieces. Form each piece into a smooth ball. Place on a lightly greased cookie sheet 2 inches apart. Flatten each bun slightly with your hand.

Cover buns with a kitchen towel or cloth and place in an oven warmed to 120° to 130° (turn oven on for a few minutes, then turn off) for about 30 to 45 minutes. Remove buns, then preheat oven to 400°. Uncover buns and brush all over lightly with a little melted margarine. Bake for 18 to 20 minutes. Remove to a cooling rack. Slice as for hamburger buns when completely cool.

Yield: 12 rolls.

Note

By making 12 buns from the recipe, they will be rather small, but just right for the vegetable burgers. Make 9 buns per recipe if you want a larger, traditional-size bun. For a young child, you may want to make 14 or 15 buns from the recipe.

	Phenylalanine (mg)	Protein (gm)	Calories
Using Best White Bread			
Per recipe	164	3.6	1333
Per bun	14	0.3	111
Using Best Homestyle Bread			
Per recipe	174	3.4	1642
Per bun	14	0.3	137

Fry Bread

Puffy and golden brown, *Fry Bread* is delicious and sure to become a favorite.

1 recipe *Best White Bread*   vegetable oil for frying

Prepare dough for *Best White Bread*. After the 30-minute rising, knead for 3 minutes as directed. Heat vegetable oil to 375° in a skillet or deep-fat fryer. Pull off small pieces of dough (about 25 gm each) and form into a circular shape; then pull and press dough with hands to an approximately ⅛-inch thickness. Drop circular pieces of dough in hot oil and fry, one or more at a time, for approximately 45 seconds on each side. Remove to paper toweling to drain and cool slightly, then serve warm with butter.

The *Fry Bread* is best when eaten soon after frying but can also be reheated in a toaster oven (heating in a microwave oven will leave it limp).

For convenience, after kneading, prepared bread dough can be frozen in a plastic freezer bag. When ready to make *Fry Bread*, thaw size portion of dough desired (either on lowest setting of microwave oven or at room temperature) and shape and fry dough as directed above.

Yield: 25 fry breads.

	Phenylalanine (mg)	Protein (gm)	Calories
Per recipe	164	3.6	1813
Per fry bread	7	0.1	73

Bagels

These look very much like regular bagels and also have a similar chewy texture. Excellent toasted, with butter and jam or with pre-whipped sweet unsalted butter (which is uncolored) as a cream cheese substitute.

1 recipe *Best White Bread*

Prepare dough, let rise for 30 minutes, and knead as directed for *Best White Bread*. Instead of forming into a loaf shape, divide dough into 10 pieces. Form each piece into a round ball and place on a Baking Mix dusted surface. Flatten each ball slightly with your hand. Dip your index finger into Baking Mix, then bore a hole in the center of each ball to form a ring shape. Twirl the dough on your finger to widen the hole, until the hole is about ⅓ of the bagel's diameter (somewhat larger than a 50-cent piece).

Place bagels on a lightly greased cookie sheet, 5 per sheet. Cover with a kitchen cloth or towel and let rise in a warm oven or warm stove top for 10 to 15 minutes. Meanwhile, preheat oven to 375° and also heat a large kettle of water to boiling. After bagels have risen, drop three to four at a time into boiling water. Boil for a total of 3 minutes, turning over once after about 1½ minutes. Bagels will become puffed and somewhat elastic. Remove from water with a slotted spoon onto a kitchen towel to drain, then place back on your lightly greased cookie sheets. Bake for approximately 25 minutes, until golden brown. Remove to a cooling rack.

Yield: 10 bagels.

	Phenylalanine (mg)	Protein (gm)	Calories
Per recipe	164	3.6	1333
Per bagel	16	0.4	133

Variation

Cinnamon and Raisin Bagels

Add 2 teaspoons cinnamon and ½ cup (80 gm) raisins to the bread dough during the initial mixing stage.

Yield: 10 bagels.

	Phenylalanine (mg)	Protein (gm)	Calories
Per recipe	217	6.2	1573
Per bagel	22	0.6	157

Breadsticks or Soft Pretzels

1 recipe *Best White Bread*   coarse salt
melted margarine or butter

Prepare dough for *Best White Bread*. After the 30-minute rising, knead for 3 minutes as directed. Preheat oven to 450°.

Breadsticks

Cut dough into 30 small pieces (about 25 gm each). With hands, roll each piece into a rope about 6 inches long and twist with your hands to get a "corkscrew" effect. Brush each strip with a little melted margarine, then sprinkle with coarse salt. Place strips on an ungreased cookie sheet. Do not let rise a second time, but immediately bake for 15 to 18 minutes, until light golden brown. The breadsticks will be chewy-soft; if you want crispy breadsticks, dry them in a 200° oven for 30 to 45 minutes more.

Soft Pretzels

Cut dough into 30 small pieces. With hands, roll each piece into a rope about 10 inches long. Twist into a pretzel shape, pinching ends down. Brush each pretzel lightly with melted margarine using a pastry brush and sprinkle with a little coarse salt. Place on an ungreased cookie sheet. Bake for 15 to 18 minutes, until light golden brown.

Yield: 30 breadsticks or pretzels.

Note

Coarse salt can be found at gourmet food stores or many grocery stores. Morton is one brand commonly available.

	Phenylalanine (mg)	Protein (gm)	Calories
Per recipe	176	3.8	1537
Per breadstick or pretzel	6	0.1	51

French Toast

2½ tablespoons Rich's Coffee
   Rich
1 teaspoon Wel-Plan Baking
   Mix
drop of vanilla
dash of salt

1 drop yellow food coloring
cinnamon to taste
2 slices low protein bread of
   your choice
margarine or butter for frying

Mix all ingredients except bread and margarine in a small bowl or gravy shaker until smooth; pour into a shallow dish. Dip each slice of bread in mixture for a few seconds on each side, turning with a fork. Add a little margarine to a medium-hot frying pan or pancake griddle. Fry bread for several minutes on each side, until light golden brown. Serve hot with syrup or powdered sugar.

Yield: dip for 2 slices.

Note

Breads especially good for *French Toast* are *Best White Bread* or *Bread in a Can* (using *Best White Bread*). You may substitute an equal amount of prepared PKU formula for the Coffee Rich if desired, for a "free" batter.

	Phenylalanine (mg)	Protein (gm)	Calories
Per recipe	11	0.2	131
Per slice (not including bread)	5	0.1	65

Coconut Caramel Toast

2 slices *Best White Bread* or
    Best Homestyle Bread,
    toasted
1 tablespoon margarine or
    butter

1 tablespoon packed brown
    sugar
2 teaspoons shredded coconut

Preheat oven to broil (550°). Melt margarine and brown sugar in a small saucepan; bring to a boil over medium heat, stirring constantly. Continue boiling over medium-low heat for 1½ minutes. Pour 1 tablespoon of brown sugar–margarine mixture over each piece of toast. Sprinkle each with 1 teaspoon coconut. Place on a cookie sheet and broil for 1 minute, or until coconut is lightly browned (watch carefully so coconut does not burn).

Yield: 2 slices.

Note
Nutrient analysis is based on *Best White Bread.* Add 2 mg phenylalanine per slice if using *Best Homestyle Bread.*

	Phenylalanine (mg)	Protein (gm)	Calories
Per recipe	33	0.7	350
Per slice	17	0.4	175

Broiled Pineapple Toast

1 slice *Best White Bread* or
  Best Homestyle Bread,
  toasted
1½ tablespoons (26 gm)
  drained crushed pineapple

2 teaspoons packed brown
  sugar

Preheat oven to broil (550°). Top toast with pineapple, spreading evenly; sprinkle with brown sugar. Place on a cookie sheet and broil for 2 minutes, or until sugar is melted.

Yield: 1 slice.

Note
Nutrient analysis is based on *Best White Bread.* Add 2 mg phenylalanine per slice if using *Best Homestyle Bread.*

	Phenylalanine (mg)	Protein (gm)	Calories
Per slice	14	0.3	139

Banana Breakfast Toast

1 slice *Best White Bread* or
  Best Homestyle Bread,
  toasted

¼ of a medium banana (20 gm)
2 teaspoons jam (any flavor)
cinnamon to taste

Preheat oven to broil (550°). Spread jam over toast; place on a cookie sheet. Slice banana and arrange slices evenly over top of jam. Sprinkle with a little cinnamon. Broil for 1½ to 2 minutes.

Yield: 1 slice.

Note
Nutrient analysis is based on *Best White Bread.* Add 2 mg phenylalanine per slice if using *Best Homestyle Bread.*

	Phenylalanine (mg)	Protein (gm)	Calories
Per slice	21	0.5	139

Peachy Toast

1 slice *Best White Bread* or
Best Homestyle Bread,
toasted
1 canned peach half (50 gm)

1 teaspoon packed brown
sugar
cinnamon to taste

Preheat oven to broil (550°). Pat peach half dry with a paper towel. Slice thinly and arrange slices over top of toast. Sprinkle with brown sugar and a little cinnamon. Place on a cookie sheet and broil for about 2 minutes.

Yield: 1 slice.

Note
Nutrient analysis is based on *Best White Bread*. Add 2 mg phenylalanine per slice if using *Best Homestyle Bread*.

	Phenylalanine (mg)	Protein (gm)	Calories
Per slice	18	0.5	118

Crunchy Herb Toast

1 slice *Best White Bread* or
Best Homestyle Bread
2 teaspoons margarine or
butter
garlic powder or garlic salt to
taste

onion powder or onion salt to
taste
1 teaspoon dried parsley or any
desired herb

Preheat oven to broil (550°). Toast one side of bread in broiler. Turn bread over; spread with margarine. Sprinkle on herbs. Place on a cookie sheet and broil about 2 minutes or until lightly browned.

Yield: 1 slice.

Note
Nutrient analysis is based on *Best White Bread*. Add 2 mg phenylalanine per slice if using *Best Homestyle Bread*.

	Phenylalanine (mg)	Protein (gm)	Calories
Per slice	15	0.3	157

Low Pro Croutons

8 cups (330 gm) low protein bread cubes, from *Best White Bread* or
Best Homestyle Bread

Cut off crusts of bread. Cut into ⅜-inch cubes. Put in an ungreased
13 × 9-inch baking pan in an evenly distributed layer. Dry in a 250°
oven for 1½ to 2 hours, until crispy. Use for soups, casserole toppings, salads, *Zucchini Stuffing Casserole* or *Low Pro Snack Mix*.

Yield: 5 cups (180 gm).

Note
Approximately 8 cups of low protein bread cubes can be made from
1 loaf of bread after crusts are removed.

	Phenylalanine (mg)	Protein (gm)	Calories
Per recipe	98	2.2	801
Per ¼ cup (9 gm) serving	5	0.1	40

Garlic Snack Croutons

1⅓ cups (85 gm) ⅜-inch bread
  cubes from *Best White
  Bread* or *Best Homestyle
  Bread*

2 tablespoons melted
  margarine or butter
½ teaspoon garlic salt

Take approximately two ½-inch thick slices of low protein bread and cut off crusts. Cut into cubes to measure 1⅓ cups. Dry in a single layer in a 300° oven for 30 to 40 minutes, or until very dry. Mix melted margarine with garlic salt, then dribble over the dry bread cubes. Place on a paper towel to absorb any excess margarine. Serve either warm or at room temperature.

Yield: 1 cup (115 gm).

Storage Tip
Keeps well in an airtight container for up to 2 weeks or longer, or can be frozen in an airtight container. Make a triple batch or more and freeze in individual labeled portions.

	Phenylalanine (mg)	Protein (gm)	Calories
Per recipe	43	0.9	456
Per ½ cup (58 gm) serving	21	0.5	228

Toasted Cinnamon Sticks

2 slices *Best White Bread* or
   Best Homestyle Bread
1 tablespoon vegetable oil

2 teaspoons Rich's Coffee Rich
2 tablespoons granulated sugar
½ teaspoon cinnamon

Preheat oven to 400°. Cut crusts from bread. Brush both sides of bread with oil, then Coffee Rich, using a pastry brush. Cut each slice into 6 strips; roll in a mixture of the sugar and cinnamon. Lay strips on a cookie sheet and toast for 10 to 15 minutes or until crisp, turning over once during baking.

Yield: 12 sticks.

Note
Nutrient analysis is based on *Best White Bread.* Add 2 mg phenylalanine per slice if using *Best Homestyle Bread.*

	Phenylalanine (mg)	Protein (gm)	Calories
Per recipe	24	0.5	408
Per 3 sticks	6	0.1	102

Toasted Honey Sticks

2 slices *Best White Bread* or
   Best Homestyle Bread
1½ tablespoons melted
   margarine or butter

2 tablespoons honey

Preheat oven to 400°. Brush both sides of bread with melted margarine, then with honey, using a pastry brush. Cut each slice into 6 strips; lay on a cookie sheet and toast in oven for 10 to 15 minutes, or until crisp and golden brown, turning over once during baking.

Yield: 12 sticks.

Note
Nutrient analysis is based on *Best White Bread.* Add 2 mg phenylalanine per slice if using *Best Homestyle Bread.*

	Phenylalanine (mg)	Protein (gm)	Calories
Per recipe	30	0.7	457
Per 3 sticks	9	0.3	114

Low Pro Snack Mix

A crunchy munchy "low" snack, very similar to the standard "party mix" in flavor.

½ cup (14 gm) Rice Chex cereal
½ cup (14 gm) Corn Chex cereal
3 cups (108 gm) ⅜-inch *Low Pro Croutons*

⅓ cup margarine or butter
1 tablespoon Worcestershire sauce
¼ teaspoon salt
½ teaspoon chili powder

In a 13 × 9-inch baking pan, mix together cereal and croutons. Melt margarine and mix with Worcestershire sauce, salt, and chili powder; pour over cereal and croutons and toss to coat. Spread in pan fairly evenly. Bake at 250° for 45 minutes, stirring several times during baking.

Yield: 4 cups (260 gm).

Storage Tip
Keeps well in an airtight container for up to 2 weeks or longer, or can be frozen in an airtight container. Make a double or triple batch and freeze in individual labeled portions.

	Phenylalanine (mg)	Protein (gm)	Calories
Per recipe	181	3.9	1112
Per ½ cup (33 gm) serving	23	0.5	139

Savory Dressing

1⅓ cups (85 gm) ⅜-inch bread cubes from *Best White Bread* or *Best Homestyle Bread*

⅓ cup (35 gm) finely chopped fresh mushrooms

1 teaspoon margarine or butter

1 tablespoon (9 gm) chopped onion or green onions

2 tablespoons (13 gm) diced or thinly sliced celery

⅛ to ¼ teaspoon sage or poultry seasoning

1 tablespoon melted margarine or butter

¼ cup hot water

salt and pepper to taste

Take approximately 2 slices of low protein bread and cut off crusts. Cut into cubes to measure 1⅓ cups. Dry in a single layer in a 300° oven for 30 to 40 minutes, or until very dry.

Meanwhile, prepare vegetables. Sauté mushrooms in margarine in a small skillet or saucepan for 2 minutes. Combine mushrooms, celery, and onions with dry bread cubes and seasoning in a small greased baking pan. Dribble melted margarine over all, then dribble hot water over to moisten (use slightly more or less depending on whether you like drier or more moist dressing, realizing that it will become somewhat more moist in baking). Add salt and pepper to taste. Bake at 350° for 40 to 45 minutes.

Yield: 1⅓ cups (140 gm).

	Phenylalanine (mg)	Protein (gm)	Calories
Per recipe	73	1.8	403
Per ⅓ cup (35 gm) serving	18	0.5	101

Apple and Raisin Dressing

1⅓ cups (85 gm) ⅜-inch bread cubes from *Best White Bread* or *Best Homestyle Bread*

1 tablespoon (9 gm) chopped onion or green onions

2 tablespoons (13 gm) diced or thinly sliced celery

⅓ cup (42 gm) finely diced apples

1 tablespoon (10 gm) raisins

1 tablespoon melted margarine or butter

¼ cup hot water

salt and pepper to taste

Prepare bread as for *Savory Dressing*. Combine onion, celery, apple, and raisins with dry bread cubes in a small greased baking dish. Dribble melted margarine over all, then dribble hot water over to moisten (use slightly more or less depending on whether you like drier or more moist dressing, realizing that it will become somewhat more moist on baking). Add salt and pepper to taste. Bake at 350° for 40 to 45 minutes.

Yield: 1⅓ cups (150 gm).

	Phenylalanine (mg)	Protein (gm)	Calories
Per recipe	51	1.4	415
Per ⅓ cup (37 gm) serving	13	0.4	104

Snack Crackers

Delicious, crispy little crackers that can be seasoned according to taste preference.

1½ cups (165 gm) Wel-Plan
  Baking Mix
1½ teaspoons baking powder
½ teaspoon paprika
¼ to ½ teaspoon garlic or
  onion powder, taco
  seasoning mix, or seasoning
  of your choice

½ to ¾ teaspoon salt
⅓ cup margarine or butter
¼ cup plus 1 tablespoon water

Preheat oven to 500°. In a medium bowl, stir together Baking Mix, baking powder, paprika, garlic or onion powder (or taco seasoning or seasoning of your choice) and salt. Mix in margarine with tips of fingers, a fork, two knives, or a pastry blender until like coarse crumbs; sprinkle water over, mixing with a fork until well blended. Knead with Baking Mix—dusted hands to make a smooth ball.

Divide dough in half. Roll out each half until very thin (about ¹⁄₁₆ inch thick) using a wooden surface, a pastry cloth—covered surface dusted with Baking Mix, or rolling onto waxed paper. Sprinkle Baking Mix on top of dough before you roll out if it is at all sticky. Cut out with tiny cookie or sandwich cutters (about 1 to 1¼ inch in size), re-rolling and cutting scraps, or cut in 1-inch squares or size desired with a knife or pizza cutter. Prick each cracker with a fork several times. Place on an ungreased baking sheet (crackers can be put very close together as they do not spread).

Bake for 4 to 5 minutes, depending on thickness of crackers (check after 4 minutes as they can become too dark very quickly, but if underbaked they will not be optimally crispy). Immediately remove to a wire rack to cool. Crackers should be light golden and very crisp after cooling.

Yield: about 110 small crackers.

Store in airtight container for up to several weeks. They also freeze well. Cracker dough can also be made in bulk and frozen, portions to be thawed and baked at your convenience; or dough can be made up to several days in advance, refrigerated, then baked when you have time.

	Phenylalanine (mg)	Protein (gm)	Calories
Per recipe	38	1.1	1113
Per cracker	trace	trace	10

Cinnamon Graham Crackers

Very similar in taste and texture to regular graham crackers, with a fraction of the protein.

½ cup margarine or butter
½ cup packed brown sugar
1 tablespoon molasses or dark
   Karo corn syrup
3 tablespoons light Karo
   corn syrup or honey (or 2
   tablespoons corn syrup plus
   1 tablespoon honey is good)

¼ cup vegetable oil
1 box (400 gm) Wel-Plan
   Baking Mix
1 teaspoon baking soda
1 teaspoon cinnamon
½ teaspoon salt

Preheat oven to 425°. In a large bowl, mix margarine and brown sugar until thoroughly creamed (no lumps of sugar should remain). Mix in molasses, corn syrup and/or honey, and vegetable oil until well blended. You may add 2 drops of yellow food coloring here to make crackers that more closely approximate the color of commercial graham crackers. Stir together Baking Mix, baking soda, cinnamon, and salt; gradually blend into creamed mixture (dough will look very dry at first, but will become clay-like with additional mixture; work dough with your hands to this stage if you like).

Divide dough into 2 parts; for each part, pat dough into a small 4- to 5-inch square on an ungreased standard size cookie sheet (13 × 11 inches) without sides. Dust with a little Baking Mix or wheat starch, then roll out evenly, to approximately a 13 × 11-inch rectangle (dough should just fill the cookie sheet). If you have any trouble with sticking, roll out dough using plastic wrap or waxed paper on top of the dough.

Cut with a pizza cutter or sharp knife into 30 squares, leaving on baking sheet. You will probably have some ragged edges but cut so that you have nice squares. Bake the ragged edges as they are; later they can be made into crumbs for a variety of uses. Prick each cracker 3 times with a fork (or so that they will look very much like commercial crackers, score each cracker very lightly down the center with a pizza cutter, being careful not to cut all the way through, then prick each half 3 times).

Bake at 425° for 7 to 8 minutes (do not overbake; they are most like regular graham crackers when slightly underbaked; they will crisp up nicely as they cool even though soft when right from the oven). Crackers may "bubble" slightly in baking; press flat with a spatula right after removing from oven if this happens. Recut with pizza cutter while hot, if necessary. Let crackers sit on pan for a minute or two, then remove to a cooling rack.

Yield: 60 crackers.

Note

Recipes using *Cinnamon Graham Cracker* crumbs are *Low Pro Graham Cracker Crust, Low Orange Balls, Quick and Low Apple Dessert,* and *Peppermint Crunch Dessert.*

Storage Tip

Store in an airtight container for up to several weeks. Crackers also freeze well. Cracker dough can also be made in bulk and frozen, portions to be thawed and baked at your convenience; or dough can be made up to several days in advance, refrigerated, then baked when you have time.

	Phenylalanine (mg)	Protein (gm)	Calories
Per recipe	63	2.2	3345
Per cracker	1	trace	56

Tortillas

These take less work than you might imagine and the results are rewarding—they are very much like authentic flour tortillas.

1⅔ cups (180 gm) Wel-Plan Baking Mix
¾ teaspoon dry taco seasoning mix
½ teaspoon salt

2 tablespoons vegetable oil
6 to 7 tablespoons water with a scant drop yellow food coloring

Stir together Baking Mix, taco seasoning, and salt in a mixing bowl; dribble oil over and mix in with a fork. Add colored water, 1 tablespoon at a time, continuing to mix with a fork. Dough will look a little dry, but pick up with hands and work in the drier portion, kneading to form a smooth ball. Dough should feel a little moist, but not at all sticky. Cut dough into 9 pieces (about 30 gm each); shape into small balls, then press with hands into small flat discs.

Pressing firmly, roll each disc on a Baking Mix–dusted surface or wax paper, into a 5- to 6-inch circle (dough will be thin, but flexible and not fragile). Cut off any ragged edges with a sharp knife. Stack tortillas after you roll them, with a piece of wax paper between each one.

Heat a skillet to high (do not grease). Cook each tortilla 30 seconds on first side, 30 seconds on the second. After cooking each tortilla, keep tortilla stack covered with a towel or plastic wrap so they do not dry out; they should remain nice and flexible. Rewarm either on a hot ungreased skillet, wrapped in foil in the oven, or on a paper plate in a microwave oven.

Yield: 9 tortillas.

For a Crispy Taco Shell

Heat ½ inch vegetable oil to 375°-400° in a skillet. Fry a *pre-baked* soft tortilla for 5 to 8 seconds per side. Drain on paper toweling. Fold in half immediately, before the tortilla cools, if you want a nice taco shape for filling, or put in metal taco holder.

Note

For a filling, try shredded lettuce, chopped olives or mushrooms, onions, and taco sauce or salad dressing (see *Tacos*).

For a snack or desert a soft tortilla can be spread with softened margarine, sprinkled with cinnamon and sugar, rolled up, and baked at 400° for 10 minutes. A fried tortilla could also be sprinkled with cinnamon and sugar right after frying.

For an edible salad "bowl" (as served in Mexican restaurants), fry tortilla lightly, then immediately place between two cereal bowls until cool. Fill with a mixed green salad or filling of your choice.

Storage Tip

You can freeze the unbaked tortillas (making a double or triple batch if desired), with waxed paper between them; place in a plastic freezer bag on a heavy paper plate to preserve shape. Remove number desired, thaw, then fry and/or bake as directed. You can also freeze the soft, cooked tortillas; rewarm on a hot skillet for a few seconds on each side after thawing, or wrap and heat in oven. The fried tortillas do not reheat well once they have been frozen.

	Phenylalanine *(mg)*	*Protein* *(gm)*	*Calories*
Per recipe	11	0.6	874
Per tortilla	1	0.1	97

Taco Chips

Light and crispy, almost like potato chips. A treat that could easily replace other "high" snack foods.

1 recipe *Tortillas* dough to
    which you have added an
    extra:
¼ teaspoon paprika, ¼
    teaspoon seasoned salt, or
    ¼ teaspoon chili powder

vegetable oil for deep-frying

Roll tortillas as directed in recipe, rolling into 6- to 6½-inch circles. Cut each tortilla into 8 or more pie-shaped pieces using a knife or pizza cutter. In a large skillet, heat about ½ inch of vegetable oil to 375°. Fry 6 to 8 taco chips at a time, for less than a minute, turning once with a fork after about 15 to 20 seconds. Chips will "bubble" as they fry. Be careful not to get them too dark as lighter chips will have the best flavor (they will darken slightly on cooling). Remove to paper toweling to drain. Immediately sprinkle with extra salt if desired. Chips should be light and very crispy.

Yield: 72 chips.

Note

For variety, omit seasonings from dough. Immediately after frying, sprinkle chips with a mixture of cinnamon and sugar; cinnamon could also be added to the dough.

Storage Tip

Store in an airtight container at room temperature for up to a month. They also freeze well.

	Phenylalanine (mg)	Protein (gm)	Calories
Per recipe	11	0.6	1354
Per chip	trace	trace	19

Crispy Chips

1 cup (120 gm) cornstarch
1½ tablespoons (8 gm)
  Metamucil*
1 teaspoon salt or garlic salt, or
  other seasoning of your
  choice

½ to 1 teaspoon paprika
6 tablespoons softened
  margarine or butter
¼ cup water with 1 drop yellow
  food coloring

Preheat oven to 450°. Mix together cornstarch, Metamucil, seasoning, and paprika. Blend in margarine with a fork, 2 knives, or a pastry blender until mixture is like coarse crumbs; sprinkle colored water over all, mixing first with a fork, then with your hands to finish the mixing. Press and work dough with your hands until it is clay-like and smooth.

Form dough into a ball, then shape into a small rectangle on an ungreased standard size cookie sheet without sides (13 × 11 inches). Sprinkle a little extra cornstarch or wheat starch on top to prevent sticking, then roll out with a rolling pin to fill the entire cookie sheet, pressing together any cracked edges as you roll. Try to roll dough out to fairly even thickness.

Cut rolled dough with a sharp knife, pizza cutter, or fluted pastry wheel, into as many small cracker or chip shapes as you like. Bake for about 8 minutes. Remove pan from oven and let cool for a few minutes, then remove chips to a cooling rack. Chips should become very crisp on cooling.

Yield: about 80 chips.

	Phenylalanine (mg)	Protein (gm)	Calories
Per recipe	35	0.7	1149
Per chip	trace	trace	14

*See discussion on pages 65–66.

Applesauce Pancakes

A good and very "low" pancake.

½ cup (55 gm) wheat starch
½ teaspoon baking powder
⅛ teaspoon salt
⅛ teaspoon cinnamon

⅓ cup (80 gm) applesauce
1 teaspoon vegetable oil
¼ cup water

In a small mixing bowl, mix together wheat starch, baking powder, salt, and cinnamon. Blend applesauce, oil, and water together in a liquid measuring cup and add all at once to dry ingredients. Mix until smooth. Spoon or pour batter from a measuring cup onto a hot griddle which has been greased with margarine. Fry until bubbles form and top side looks set around edges (underside will brown only lightly); turn and fry briefly on second side.

Yield: eight 3-inch pancakes.

	Phenylalanine (mg)	Protein (gm)	Calories
Per recipe	10	0.3	326
Per pancake	1	trace	41

Variation

Banana Pancakes

Replace the applesauce with ¼ cup (58 gm) mashed banana. Add an extra 1 tablespoon water.

Yield: eight 3-inch pancakes.

	Phenylalanine (mg)	Protein (gm)	Calories
Per recipe	27	0.8	318
Per pancake	3	0.1	40

Old-Fashioned Pancakes

What could make a more appealing and satisfying breakfast than these tasty, light, and golden brown pancakes?

3 tablespoons (22 gm) wheat starch

2 tablespoons (14 gm) Wel-Plan Baking Mix

1 tablespoon (9 gm) Softasilk cake flour (do not use regular flour)

½ teaspoon baking powder

dash of salt

¼ teaspoon cinnamon or ¼ teaspoon vanilla

1 teaspoon granulated or brown sugar

2 teaspoons vegetable oil

3 tablespoons Rich's Coffee Rich

2 tablespoons water

In a small bowl, stir together wheat starch, Baking Mix, cake flour, baking powder, salt, and cinnamon. Mix together vegetable oil, Coffee Rich, and water in a liquid measuring cup; add to dry ingredients, mixing well. Batter should be quite thin. If you like thicker pancakes, add 1 teaspoon Baking Mix; if you like thinner pancakes, add 1 teaspoon water.

Heat griddle or frying pan. Brush bottom with a little margarine or shortening. For convenience, scrape batter into a glass measuring cup with pouring spout and pour batter into 3-inch circles. Turn after about 1½ minutes, or when bubbles have formed, top side looks set around edges, and bottom side is browned; turn over and brown other side for ½ to 1 minute.

Yield: six 3-inch pancakes.

Storage Tip

For convenience, measure out dry ingredients for more than one batch; store in a plastic bag or other container; for each 6 tablespoons mix (1 recipe) simply add 2 teaspoons oil, 3 tablespoons Coffee Rich, and 2 tablespoons water when you're ready to make pancakes.

Prepared batter will also keep for 24 hours, and prepared pancakes can be reheated in a toaster oven or microwave oven for a quick meal the next day. Pancakes can also be frozen and reheated in a micro-wave oven.

	Phenylalanine (mg)	Protein (gm)	Calories
Per recipe	46	1.0	328
Per pancake	8	0.2	55

Variations

Apple Pancakes

Add 3 tablespoons (30 gm) finely chopped, pared apple to pancake batter. Fry as for *Old-Fashioned Pancakes,* making sure you cook them long enough, as the apple imparts extra moisture.

Yield: six 3-inch pancakes.

	Phenylalanine (mg)	Protein (gm)	Calories
Per recipe	47	1.0	346
Per pancake	8	0.2	58

Bear Cakes

Make 4 pancakes, pouring small drops of batter to top of cakes for ears. Add raisin eyes, nose, and mouth.

Yield: 4 bear cakes.

	Phenylalanine (mg)	Protein (gm)	Calories
Per recipe	46	1.0	328
Per pancake	11	0.2	82

Blueberry Pancakes

Add ¼ cup (40 gm) small sized fresh or frozen, slightly thawed blue-berries to pancake batter. Fry as for *Old-Fashioned Pancakes,* making sure you cook them long enough, as the blueberries impart extra moisture.

Yield: seven 3-inch pancakes.

	Phenylalanine (mg)	Protein (gm)	Calories
Per recipe	56	1.2	351
Per pancake	8	0.2	50

115

Waffles

Golden brown and delicious, these waffles look and taste like regular home-made or commercial frozen waffles. Try one of the tasty variations, too.

3 cups (330 gm) Wel-Plan
   Baking Mix
1 cup (110 gm) wheat starch
4 teaspoons baking powder
½ teaspoon salt
1 teaspoon granulated sugar
1 teaspoon cinnamon
   (optional)

⅔ cup vegetable oil
1⅓ cups Rich's Coffee Rich
1¼ cups water
¼ teaspoon vanilla
1 medium egg white
   (1 tablespoon plus
   2 teaspoons, 29 gm)

In a large mixing bowl, mix together Baking Mix, wheat starch, baking powder, salt, sugar, and cinnamon. Combine oil, Coffee Rich, water, and vanilla in a large liquid measuring cup or small bowl; add to dry ingredients, mixing until smooth.

Separate egg to get white. Put white in a small bowl and beat with an electric mixer until stiff but not dry. The total volume will be about ¾ cup. Gently mix beaten white into waffle batter. Thin batter with a little water if it seems too thick to spread on waffle iron.

Brush vegetable oil lightly on both top and bottom of a hot waffle iron to prevent any sticking (even if iron is Teflon coated). Use a 1-cup measure to dip out batter, scraping out quickly onto hot iron (1 cup of batter will make a nice, full 4-square waffle).

Bake 3 to 5 minutes. Lid should open easily when done. Open iron and remove waffle with a fork. Serve immediately, or cool completely on a wire rack and freeze.

Yield: 5 waffles (4 squares per waffle).

Note

To lower phenylalanine content, this recipe turns out very satisfac-torily by deleting the egg white, though the waffles will not be quite as light in texture. To lighten the texture, mix batter with an electric mixer on medium speed for 1 to 1½ minutes. If you delete the egg white, subtract 180 mg phenylalanine, 3.2 gm protein, and 15 calo-ries from the basic recipe or any of the variations.

Storage Tip

This recipe makes a large batch, since waffles freeze very well. For an exceptionally convenient breakfast or supper, freeze one or more waffles in individual-size plastic freezer bags; pop into a toaster or toaster oven when ready to use (a microwave oven could also be used, but waffles will be soft rather than a little crisp).

	Phenylalanine (mg)	Protein (gm)	Calories
Per recipe	263	5.4	3369
Per ¼ waffle (1 square)	13	0.3	168

Variations

Applesauce Waffles

Add 1 cup (240 gm) applesauce to the waffle batter and add only ½ cup water.

Yield: 5 waffles (4 squares per waffle).

	Phenylalanine (mg)	Protein (gm)	Calories
Per recipe	275	5.8	3551
Per ¼ waffle (1 square)	14	0.3	178

Banana Waffles

Add ⅔ cup (152 gm) mashed ripe banana to the waffle batter.

Yield: 5 waffles (4 squares per waffle).

	Phenylalanine (mg)	Protein (gm)	Calories
Per recipe	320	7.0	3509
Per ¼ waffle (1 square)	16	0.3	175

Blueberry Waffles

Add ¾ cup (120 gm) fresh or frozen and partially thawed small blueberries to the waffle batter.

Yield: 5 waffles (4 squares per waffle).

	Phenylalanine (mg)	Protein (gm)	Calories
Per recipe	291	6.2	3437
Per ¼ waffle (1 square)	15	0.3	172

Chocolate Waffles

Add ¼ cup Hershey's unsweetened cocoa (not instant), ½ cup granulated sugar, and 1 teaspoon vanilla to the waffle batter before folding in egg white. These are really dessert waffles. For a special chocolate-lovers' treat, serve warm with powdered sugar sprinkled on top and chocolate sauce over all, with a dollop of whipped non-dairy topping or low protein vanilla ice cream.

Yield: 5 waffles (4 squares per waffle).

	Phenylalanine (mg)	Protein (gm)	Calories
Per recipe	523	10.6	3839
Per ¼ waffle (1 square)	26	0.5	192

Chocolate Chip Waffles

Add ⅓ cup (67 gm) Nestlé mini semisweet chocolate chips to the waffle batter.

Yield: 5 waffles (4 squares per waffle).

	Phenylalanine (mg)	Protein (gm)	Calories
Per recipe	398	8.2	3727
Per ¼ waffle (1 square)	20	0.4	186

Applesauce Bread

1⅓ cups (147 gm) Wel-Plan
  Baking Mix
½ cup granulated sugar
2½ teaspoons baking powder
¼ teaspoon salt

1 teaspoon cinnamon
¼ cup vegetable oil
⅓ cup plus 1 tablespoon water
½ cup (120 gm) applesauce
¼ cup (40 gm) raisins

Preheat oven to 350°. In a mixing bowl, stir together Baking Mix, sugar, baking powder, salt, and cinnamon. Add oil and water to dry ingredients and mix until smooth. Add applesauce and raisins and blend well. Pour batter into a greased 7½ × 3¾-inch bread pan. Bake for 50 to 55 minutes.

Yield: 16 slices.

	Phenylalanine (mg)	Protein (gm)	Calories
Per recipe	39	2.0	1589
Per slice	2	0.1	99

Carrot Bread

1⅓ cups (147 gm) Wel-Plan
  Baking Mix
½ cup granulated sugar
1½ teaspoons baking powder
½ teaspoon baking soda
¼ teaspoon salt

1 teaspoon cinnamon
¼ cup vegetable oil
½ cup plus 1 tablespoon water
1 cup (114 gm) shredded or
  grated carrots

Preheat oven to 350°. In a mixing bowl, stir together Baking Mix, sugar, baking powder, baking soda, salt, and cinnamon. Add oil and water to dry ingredients and mix until smooth. Add grated carrot and blend well. Pour batter into a greased 7½ × 3¾-inch bread pan. Bake for 50 to 55 minutes.

Yield: 16 slices.

	Phenylalanine (mg)	Protein (gm)	Calories
Per recipe	43	1.6	1427
Per slice	3	0.1	89

Pumpkin Bread

1⅓ cups (147 gm) Wel-Plan
  Baking Mix
½ cup granulated sugar
2 teaspoons baking powder
1 teaspoon baking soda
¼ teaspoon salt
1 teaspoon cinnamon

¼ teaspoon nutmeg
¼ teaspoon cloves
¼ cup vegetable oil
½ cup water
¼ cup (50 gm) canned
  pumpkin

Preheat oven to 350°. In a mixing bowl, stir together Baking Mix, sugar, baking powder, baking soda, salt, cinnamon, nutmeg, and cloves. Add oil and water to dry ingredients and mix until smooth. Add pumpkin and blend well. Pour batter into a greased 7½ × 3¾-inch bread pan. Bake for 45 to 50 minutes.

Yield: 16 slices.

	Phenylalanine (mg)	Protein (gm)	Calories
Per recipe	23	1.0	1394
Per slice	1	0.1	87

Variations

Pumpkin Chocolate Chip Bread

Add ¼ cup (45 gm) Nestlé mini semisweet chocolate chips to batter.

Yield: 16 slices.

	Phenylalanine (mg)	Protein (gm)	Calories
Per recipe	114	2.9	1635
Per slice	7	0.2	102

Pumpkin Raisin Bread

Add ⅓ cup (53 gm) raisins to batter.

Yield: 16 slices.

	Phenylalanine (mg)	Protein (gm)	Calories
Per recipe	59	2.7	1553
Per slice	4	0.2	97

Date Bread

½ cup (100 gm) chopped dates
½ cup vegetable shortening
1½ teaspoons baking soda
¼ teaspoon salt
⅔ cup boiling water

½ cup granulated sugar
1½ cups (165 gm) Wel-Plan
   Baking Mix
1 teaspoon vanilla

Preheat oven to 350°. In a small bowl, mix together dates, shortening, baking soda, salt, and boiling water; let sit for 15 minutes. Meanwhile, in a medium bowl, stir together sugar and Baking Mix. Add date mixture to dry ingredients and mix well. Add vanilla. Pour batter into a greased 7½ × 3¾-inch bread pan. Bake for 50 to 55 minutes.

Yield: 16 slices.

	Phenylalanine (mg)	Protein (gm)	Calories
Per recipe	56	2.5	2195
Per slice	4	0.2	137

Zucchini Bread

1⅓ cups (147 gm) Wel-Plan
   Baking Mix
½ cup granulated sugar
1½ teaspoons baking powder
½ teaspoon baking soda
¼ teaspoon salt
1 teaspoon cinnamon

¼ cup vegetable oil
½ cup water
¾ cup (135 gm) shredded or
   grated zucchini squash
   (skin left on)

Preheat oven to 350°. In a mixing bowl, stir together Baking Mix, sugar, baking powder, baking soda, salt, and cinnamon. Add oil and water to dry ingredients and mix until smooth. Add zucchini and blend well. Pour batter into a greased 7½ × 3¾-inch bread pan. Bake for 50 to 55 minutes.

Yield: 16 slices.

	Phenylalanine (mg)	Protein (gm)	Calories
Per recipe	59	2.1	1406
Per slice	4	0.1	88

Strawberry Bread

1½ cups (165 gm) Wel-Plan
    Baking Mix
½ cup granulated sugar
½ teaspoon baking powder
1½ teaspoons baking soda

¼ teaspoon salt
1 teaspoon cinnamon
¼ cup vegetable oil
10 oz pkg frozen strawberries,
    thawed and mashed

Preheat oven to 350°. In a mixing bowl, stir together Baking Mix, sugar, baking powder, baking soda, salt, and cinnamon; add oil and mashed, undrained strawberries and mix until smooth. Pour batter into a greased 7½ × 3¾-inch bread pan. Bake for 50 to 55 minutes.

Yield: 16 slices.

	Phenylalanine (mg)	Protein (gm)	Calories
Per recipe	28	2.0	1709
Per slice	2	0.1	107

Banana Bread

1⅓ cups (147 gm) Wel-Plan
    Baking Mix
½ cup granulated sugar
2½ teaspoons baking powder
1 teaspoon baking soda
¼ teaspoon salt

1 teaspoon cinnamon
¼ cup vegetable oil
⅓ cup water
½ cup (115 gm) mashed ripe
    banana (about 1 banana)
1 teaspoon vanilla

Preheat oven to 350°. In a mixing bowl, stir together Baking Mix, sugar, baking powder, baking soda, salt, and cinnamon. Add oil and water to dry ingredients and mix until smooth. Add mashed banana and vanilla and blend well. Pour batter into a greased 7½ × 3¾-inch bread pan. Bake for 50 to 55 minutes.

Yield: 16 slices.

	Phenylalanine (mg)	Protein (gm)	Calories
Per recipe	49	1.6	1484
Per slice	3	0.1	93

Cranberry Bread

1½ cups (165 gm) Wel-Plan
   Baking Mix
½ cup granulated sugar
2 teaspoons baking powder
½ teaspoon baking soda
¼ teaspoon salt
¼ cup vegetable oil

¼ cup orange juice
⅓ cup water
¾ cup (75 gm) quartered fresh
   or frozen cranberries
1 teaspoon grated orange rind
   (optional)

Preheat oven to 350°. In a mixing bowl, stir together Baking Mix, sugar, baking powder, baking soda, and salt. Add oil, orange juice, and water to dry ingredients and mix until smooth. Add cranberries and grated orange rind. Pour batter into a greased 7½ × 3¾-inch bread pan. Bake for 55 to 60 minutes.

Yield: 16 slices.

	Phenylalanine (mg)	Protein (gm)	Calories
Per recipe	19	1.0	1505
Per slice	1	0.1	94

Variation

Blueberry Bread

Replace cranberries with ¾ cup (120 gm) fresh or frozen blueberries.

Yield: 16 slices.

	Phenylalanine (mg)	Protein (gm)	Calories
Per recipe	43	1.7	1536
Per slice	3	0.1	96

Applesauce Muffins

Light-textured, beautifully browned muffins.

1 cup (110 gm) Wel-Plan
   Baking Mix
3 tablespoons granulated sugar
2 teaspoons baking powder
½ teaspoon baking soda

½ teaspoon cinnamon
¼ teaspoon salt
3 tablespoons vegetable oil
⅓ cup water
⅓ cup (80 gm) applesauce

Preheat oven to 400°. In a medium mixing bowl, stir together Baking Mix, sugar, baking powder, baking soda, cinnamon, and salt. Mix together oil, water, and applesauce in a liquid measuring cup; add all at once to dry ingredients and mix by hand, 20 to 30 seconds until smooth (do not use an electric mixer). Spoon batter into six greased 2½-inch muffin cups (they will tend to stick to cupcake liners). Bake for 15 to 18 minutes.

Yield: 6 muffins.

	Phenylalanine (mg)	Protein (gm)	Calories
Per recipe	8	0.5	948
Per muffin	1	0.1	158

124

Variation

Pineapple Muffins

These are excellent!

Replace applesauce with ½ cup (140 gm) crushed, undrained pine-apple and add only 1 tablespoon water.

Yield: 6 muffins.

	Phenylalanine (mg)	Protein (gm)	Calories
Per recipe	17	0.9	979
Per muffin	3	0.1	163

Blueberry Muffins

1 cup (110 gm) Wel-Plan
   Baking Mix
3 tablespoons granulated sugar
2 teaspoons baking powder
¼ teaspoon baking soda
¼ teaspoon salt
½ teaspoon cinnamon

2½ tablespoons vegetable oil
¼ cup Rich's Coffee Rich
⅓ cup plus 2 tablespoons water
½ cup (80 gm) fresh, or frozen
   and partially thawed
   blueberries

Preheat oven to 400°. In a medium mixing bowl, stir together Baking Mix, sugar, baking powder, baking soda, salt, and cinnamon. Mix together oil, Coffee Rich, and water in a liquid measuring cup; add all at once to dry ingredients and mix on medium speed of electric mixer for 1½ minutes. Gently mix in blueberries by hand. Spoon batter into six greased 2½-inch muffin cups (they will tend to stick to cupcake liners). Bake for 15 to 18 minutes.

Yield: 6 muffins.

Note
Mixing with an electric mixer, as directed, is important for producing muffins with a light texture.

	Phenylalanine (mg)	Protein (gm)	Calories
Per recipe	35	1.0	955
Per muffin	6	0.2	159

Variations

Apple Muffins

Replace the blueberries with ½ cup (60 gm) pared and finely diced apple.

Yield: 6 muffins.

	Phenylalanine (mg)	Protein (gm)	Calories
Per recipe	18	0.6	945
Per muffin	3	0.1	157

Cinnamon Raisin Muffins

Replace the blueberries with ⅓ cup (53 gm) raisins. If desired, "plump" raisins by pouring ½ cup boiling water over them and let sit about 5 minutes; drain well before adding to muffin batter.

Yield: 6 muffins.

	Phenylalanine (mg)	Protein (gm)	Calories
Per recipe	51	2.2	1068
Per muffin	8	0.4	178

Orange Date Muffins

Delete cinnamon. Replace the blueberries with ½ cup (100 gm) chopped dates. Add 1 teaspoon grated orange rind to liquid ingredients. To soften dates, pour ½ cup boiling water over them and let sit about 5 minutes; drain well before adding to muffin batter.

Yield: 6 muffins.

	Phenylalanine (mg)	Protein (gm)	Calories
Per recipe	71	2.5	1184
Per muffin	12	0.4	197

Coffee Cake Muffins

½ cup (55 gm) Wel-Plan
Baking Mix
3 tablespoons (21 gm) wheat
starch
2 tablespoons (18 gm) Softasilk
cake flour (do not use
regular flour)
⅓ cup granulated sugar

1 teaspoon baking powder
⅛ teaspoon salt
2 tablespoons vegetable oil
or melted shortening
⅓ cup water
½ teaspoon vanilla
1 drop yellow food coloring

Streusel Topping

2 tablespoons plus 1 teaspoon
packed brown sugar
1 teaspoon Wel-Plan Baking
Mix

1 teaspoon cinnamon
2½ teaspoons melted
margarine or butter

Preheat oven to 350°. In a mixing bowl, stir together Baking Mix, wheat starch, cake flour, sugar, baking powder, and salt. Mix together oil or melted shortening, water, vanilla, and drop of yellow coloring in a liquid measuring cup; add all at once to dry ingredients and mix on medium speed of electric mixer for 1½ minutes. Spoon batter into six greased 2½-inch muffin cups (they will tend to stick to cupcake liners). Mix together all ingredients for *Streusel Topping* in a small bowl. Sprinkle topping over each muffin. Bake for 20 to 25 minutes.

Yield: 6 muffins.

Note
Mixing with an electric mixer, as directed, is important for producing muffins with a light texture.

	Phenylalanine (mg)	Protein (gm)	Calories
Per recipe	79	1.8	1048
Per muffin	13	0.3	175

Honey Bran Muffins

1 cup (110 gm) Wel-Plan
   Baking Mix
1 teaspoons baking powder
¼ teaspoon baking soda
¼ teaspoon salt
½ cup (24 gm) Raisin Bran
   cereal, crushed

2½ tablespoons vegetable oil
3 tablespoons Rich's Coffee
   Rich
⅓ cup plus 2 tablespoons water
3 tablespoons honey

Preheat oven to 400°. In a medium mixing bowl, stir together Baking Mix, baking powder, salt, and crushed cereal (you can crush the cereal right in your measuring cup, with your hands). Mix together oil, Coffee Rich, and water in a liquid measuring cup; add all at once to dry ingredients. Mix on medium speed of electric mixer for 1½ minutes. Add honey and mix until smooth. Spoon batter into six greased 2½-inch muffin cups (they will tend to stick to cupcake liners). Bake for 15 to 18 minutes.

Yield: 6 muffins.

Note
   Mixing with an electric mixer, as directed, is important for producing muffins with a light texture.

	Phenylalanine (mg)	Protein (gm)	Calories
Per recipe	78	2.0	1014
Per muffin	13	0.3	169

Jiffy Drop Biscuits

⅔ cup (73 gm) Wel-Plan Baking Mix
1½ teaspoons baking powder
¼ teaspoon cream of tartar
¼ teaspoon salt

3 tablespoons vegetable shortening
3½ tablespoons Rich's Coffee Rich

Preheat oven to 400°. In a medium bowl, mix together Baking Mix, baking powder, cream of tartar, and salt. Cut in shortening with a fork, two knives, or a pastry blender until like coarse meal. Add Coffee Rich all at once and stir until smooth. Drop batter by tablespoon onto a lightly greased cookie sheet or other baking pan. Bake for 15 minutes. Let cool for 5 to 10 minutes before removing from pan. These are best served at room temperature or just slightly warm as they are fragile when very hot.

Yield: 6 biscuits.

Note

Use a yellow shortening such as Fluffo or Butter-Flavored Crisco for a nice color, or add a drop of yellow food coloring to Coffee Rich.

	Phenylalanine (mg)	Protein (gm)	Calories
Per recipe	12	0.4	689
Per biscuit	2	0.1	115

Variations

All of the variations have approximately the same nutrient content as the original recipe.

Christmas Biscuits

Add ½ cup (50 gm) candied mixed fruit or finely chopped red and/or green candied cherries to the biscuit dough.

Yield: 7 biscuits.

	Phenylalanine (mg)	Protein (gm)	Calories
Per recipe	19	0.6	859
Per biscuit	3	0.1	123

Jam Biscuits

Add 2 tablespoons orange marmalade or any flavor jam and only 1½ tablespoons Rich's Coffee Rich to the biscuit dough.

Yield: 6 biscuits.

	Phenylalanine (mg)	Protein (gm)	Calories
Per recipe	13	0.5	742
Per biscuit	2	0.1	124

Thumbprint Biscuits

After dropping biscuit dough onto baking sheet, indent the top of each biscuit with a finger or ½ teaspoon measuring spoon dipped in Baking Mix, to a depth of about ½ inch. Fill indentation with a scant ¼ teaspoon jam or jelly.

Yield: 6 biscuits.

	Phenylalanine (mg)	Protein (gm)	Calories
Per recipe	13	0.4	693
Per biscuit	2	0.1	116

Biscuit Topper

These tasty "biscuits" become golden brown in baking. Excellent for topping stews or pot pies, or served warm with butter.

⅔ (73 gm) cup Wel-Plan
  Baking Mix
1½ teaspoon baking powder
¼ teaspoon cream of tartar
¼ teaspoon salt
3 tablespoons vegetable
  shortening

2 tablespoons Rich's Coffee
  Rich or water
melted margarine or butter
  (optional)

In a small mixing bowl, combine Baking Mix with baking powder, cream of tartar, and salt. Cut in shortening with a fork, 2 knives, or a pastry blender until like coarse meal. Add Coffee Rich or water and stir with a fork until dough is evenly moistened.

Press dough out with your hand or roll out with rolling pin to ⅜-inch thickness on a surface dusted with Baking Mix, dusting top of dough with a little Baking Mix to keep from sticking. Cut out with a 2½-inch diameter biscuit cutter, rerolling scraps until you have 6 biscuits. Brush lightly with melted margarine or butter before baking, if desired.

Place dough rounds on top of stew or pot pie filling in an individual casserole. Bake at 425° for 10 to 12 minutes, or bake alone on a cookie sheet for 8 to 10 minutes and serve on top of any stew. These biscuits are more like pastry than traditional biscuits and will rise only slightly on baking. They are excellent served warm with butter and jelly, for a snack or meal accompaniment.

Yield: 6 biscuits.

Note

Use a yellow shortening such as Fluffo or Butter-Flavored Crisco for a nice color, or add a drop of yellow food coloring to Coffee Rich or water.

	Phenylalanine (mg)	Protein (gm)	Calories
Per recipe	8	0.3	657
Per biscuit	1	0.1	110

Soups

All of the recipes in this section can be enjoyed by the whole family. They either contain no special low protein ingredients, or have instructions for preparing a family version alongside the diet version.

Any of the soups can provide a satisfying meal, especially when combined with bread and a salad. The "chowders" are especially hearty and warming in colder months.

The homemade soups in this section are not only lower in phenylalanine and protein than canned soups, but are also superior in taste, more nutritious, and less salty than canned soups. While canned soups are convenient, they don't compare to soups made in your own kitchen with fresh ingredients.

Special Tips

Most of the soups freeze well, so a larger portion could be prepared for the diet and frozen in individual portions. See *Freezing and Storage Tips* for advice about freezing foods.

G. Washington's Seasoning and Broth mix is a frequent ingredient in the recipes. The Rich Brown and Golden flavors of this broth powder are phenylalanine/protein free and are a nice alternative to the relatively "high" bouillon cubes or granules. The mix can be found in many grocery stores, near the canned soups or various bouillons. Because the broth mix is not readily available everywhere, it is listed as an optional ingredient. It provides flavor and seasoning that could be replaced by extra salt and/or dried or fresh herbs of your choice. Regular bouillon could also be used, but do remember to add the extra phenylalanine/protein to the nutrient content of the recipe (see *The Low Protein Food List for PKU*).

To "extend" canned soups, add G. Washington's Broth and extra water, and/or cooked low protein pasta to broth-based soups.

To dilute canned cream-style soups, add a little Rich's Coffee Rich to the water for extra richness.

It is easy to create your own simple, broth-based soups using G. Washington's Seasoning and Broth mix or bouillon, low protein pasta of any desired shape, and cut-up vegetables of your choice. (See the directions on page 134.)

For a thickened soup that is hearty, tasty, and exceptionally easy to make, cook the pasta and vegetables right in the broth. Both pasta and vegetables will be tender after simmering for about 8 to 12 minutes, for an "instant soup" that can be very low in phenylalanine/ protein. If you prefer a thinner soup, cook the pasta first, then add to vegetables which have been simmered until tender in broth.

A guideline for your own "created" soups:

1 pkg G. Washington's Seasoning and Broth, *or* 1 teaspoon granules *or* 1 cube regular bouillon
1½ to 2 cups water
¼ to ½ cup diced vegetables of your choice (one vegetable or a mixture of several)

¼ to ½ cup uncooked pasta of your choice (Wel-Plan Short-Cut Spaghetti or Spaghetti Ring Style are especially nice; the Short-Cut Spaghetti–based soups will look like canned noodle soups).

Use *The Low Protein Food List for PKU* to calculate nutrient content of your "created" soups.

Cream of Mushroom Soup

Far superior in taste to canned soup and lower in protein too. The whole family will enjoy it.

1⅓ cups (100 gm) sliced fresh mushrooms
¼ cup (35 gm) chopped onion
2 tablespoons margarine or butter
1½ tablespoons cornstarch dissolved in 1 cup cold water

1 pkg G. Washington's Rich Brown Seasoning and Broth, or extra salt to taste
1 cup Rich's Coffee Rich
½ teaspoon salt

In a medium skillet, sauté mushrooms and onions in margarine for 2 to 3 minutes. Add cornstarch-water mixture to skillet, along with remaining ingredients. Cook over medium heat several minutes until soup bubbles and thickens, stirring constantly.

Yield: 2⅓ cups (608 gm).

	Phenylalanine (mg)	Protein (gm)	Calories
Per recipe	146	3.4	643
Per ½ cup (130 gm) serving	24	0.6	107

Creamy Tomato and Carrot Soup

An unusual and delicious soup that is well worth the effort. Something nice to do with all of those garden tomatoes.

¼ cup margarine or butter
1 tablespoon vegetable oil
1 cup (140 gm) coarsely
    chopped onion
2½ cups (360 gm) coarsely
    chopped carrots
1¼ cups (150 gm) peeled,
    coarsely chopped, tart
    apples
1 clove garlic, minced
1 tablespoon packed brown
    sugar
3½ cups (672 gm) peeled,
    seeded, and coarsely
    chopped fresh tomatoes

3 pkg G. Washington's Golden
    Seasoning and Broth, or
    salt to taste
4 cups water
1 tablespoon lemon juice
1 teaspoon curry powder
4 whole cloves
2 bay leaves
¼ teaspoon thyme
½ cup Rich's Coffee Rich (*Diet
    Portion* only)
1 cup cream or evaporated milk
    (*Family Portion* only)

Melt margarine with oil in a large saucepan or stockpot. Add onion and cook over medium heat until just translucent, stirring occasionally, about 5 minutes. Add carrots, apples, and garlic and cook, stirring occasionally until softened, about 10 minutes. Blend in brown sugar and cook 2 minutes. Add tomatoes, broth powder or salt, water, lemon juice, spices, and herbs. Reduce heat; cover partially, and simmer until thickened, about 45 minutes, stirring occasionally.

Discard cloves and bay leaves. Purée soup in blender or food processor until almost smooth (a little texture should remain).

Diet Portion

Remove 1½ cups (333 gm) purée and put in a small saucepan. Add Coffee Rich and rewarm over low heat. Add salt to taste.

Family Portion

Transfer remaining purée back to original saucepan or stockpot. Blend in 1 cup cream or evaporated milk and rewarm over low heat. Add salt to taste.

Yield: 2 cups (445 gm) *Diet Portion*, 7 cups *Family Portion*.

	Phenylalanine (mg)	Protein (gm)	Calories
Per diet recipe	88	2.8	344
Per ½ cup (111 gm) serving	22	0.7	86

Golden Carrot Soup

A tasty, Vitamin-A–rich soup.

⅓ cup margarine or butter
1 tablespoon vegetable oil
2 cups (220 gm) shredded
   or grated carrots
½ cup (70 gm) chopped onion
¼ cup cornstarch mixed in
   1¾ cups cold water
2 pkg G. Washington's Golden
   Seasoning and Broth, or
   salt to taste

2 tablespoons Rich's Coffee
   Rich plus 2 tablespoons
   water (*Diet Portion* only)
¾ cup milk (*Family Portion*
   only)

Heat margarine and oil in a large saucepan or stockpot; cook carrots and onion until tender, about 10 minutes. Mix cornstarch and broth powder into water; add to saucepan. Cook over medium heat until soup is thickened, stirring frequently.

Diet Portion
Remove 1 cup (232 gm) of soup mixture to a smaller saucepan. Add the 2 tablespoons Coffee Rich and 2 tablespoons water and rewarm over low heat.

Family Portion
Add the ¾ cup milk to remaining soup mixture and rewarm over low heat. If desired, add 2 tablespoons crumbled, cooked bacon bits prior to serving.

Yield: 1¼ cups (290 gm) *Diet Portion*, 3¾ cups *Family Portion*.

	Phenylalanine (mg)	Protein (gm)	Calories
Per diet recipe	42	1.0	320
Per ½ cup (111 gm) serving	16	0.4	123

Garden Vegetable Chowder

A main dish soup with a wonderful flavor. Sure to be a family favorite.

¼ cup margarine or butter
1 tablespoon vegetable oil
1 cup (140 gm) chopped onion
1½ cups (210 gm) zucchini
 squash, sliced and cut
 into smaller pieces
1 cup (135 gm) carrots, sliced
 and cut into smaller pieces
2 pkg G. Washington's Golden
 Seasoning and Broth
 (optional)
4 cups water
¼ cup (8 gm) chopped fresh
 parsley or 1 tablespoon
 dry parsley
1 tablespoon chopped fresh
 basil or 1 teaspoon dry basil

1½ teaspoons salt
⅓ cup (60 gm) fresh or
 frozen corn
1¼ cups (240 gm) peeled,
 seeded, and coarsely
 chopped fresh tomatoes
¼ cup cornstarch dissolved
 in ½ cup cold water
½ cup Rich's Coffee Rich
 (*Diet Portion* only)
13 oz can evaporated milk or
 1½ cups cream (*Family
 Portion* only)

Melt margarine with oil in a large saucepan or stockpot. Add onion and cook until just translucent, stirring occasionally, about 5 minutes. Add zucchini, carrots, broth powder, water, parsley, basil, and salt. Simmer until vegetables are tender, about 10 minutes. Add corn and tomatoes and continue simmering for another 5 minutes. Add cornstarch-water mixture and cook several minutes until soup is thickened, stirring constantly.

Diet Portion

Remove 1½ cups (396 gm) soup and put in a small saucepan. Add ½ cup Coffee Rich and rewarm over low heat.

Family Portion

Blend in evaporated milk or cream with remaining soup; if desired, add 4 to 8 oz shredded cheddar cheese or ½ cup grated Parmesan or Romano cheese for a satisfying main dish soup. Rewarm over low heat.

Yield: 2 cups (508 gm) *Diet Portion,* 7 cups *Family Portion.*

	Phenylalanine (mg)	Protein (gm)	Calories
Per diet recipe	92	2.4	360
Per ½ cup (127 gm) serving	23	0.6	90

Hearty Vegetable Soup

Easy and satisfying.

½ cup (70 gm) chopped onion
2 tablespoons margarine or
butter
¼ cup (28 gm) uncooked
Ditalini or Wel-Plan
Macaroni (*Diet Portion* only)
½ cup (55 gm) uncooked
regular elbow macaroni
(*Family Portion* only)
¼ cup (8 gm) chopped fresh
parsley or 1 tablespoon
dried parsley
1 tablespoon chopped fresh
basil or 1 teaspoon dried
basil (optional)

¼ teaspoon salt
⅛ teaspoon pepper
1 can condensed Campbell's
Old Fashioned Vegetable
Soup
1 pkg G. Washington's Rich
Brown Seasoning and Broth
14½ oz can stewed tomatoes,
cut into small pieces,
undrained
2¼ cups water

In a large saucepan or stockpot, sauté onion in margarine, about 5 minutes. Cook, rinse, and drain both pastas according to package directions; set aside. Add remaining ingredients to saucepan with onions.

Diet Portion
Remove 1½ cups (348 gm) soup to a smaller saucepan. Add cooked low protein pasta and rewarm over low heat.

Family Portion
Add cooked regular elbow macaroni to remaining soup and rewarm over low heat.

Yield: 2 cups (413 gm) *Diet Portion*, 5 cups *Family Portion*.

	Phenylalanine (mg)	Protein (gm)	Calories
Per diet recipe	100	2.8	228
Per ½ cup (103 gm) serving	25	0.7	57

Pilgrims' Potato Chowder

A delicious, rich soup to take winter's chill away.

¼ cup margarine or butter
1 tablespoon vegetable oil
1 cup (140 gm) chopped onion
½ cup (56 gm) diced celery
1½ cups (256 gm) diced
  potatoes
1 cup (130 gm) sliced carrots
⅓ cup (60 gm) fresh or
  frozen corn
2 pkg G. Washington's Golden
  Seasoning and Broth
  (optional)
4⅔ cups water

¼ cup (8 gm) chopped fresh
  parsley or 1 tablespoon
  dry parsley
½ teaspoon thyme
1½ teaspoons salt
¼ teaspoon pepper
¼ cup cornstarch dissolved in
  ½ cup cold water
½ cup Rich's Coffee Rich (*Diet
  Portion* only)
13 oz can evaporated milk or
  1½ cups cream (*Family
  Portion* only)

Melt margarine with oil in a large saucepan or stockpot. Add onion and celery and cook, stirring occasionally, about 5 minutes. Add potatoes, carrots, corn, broth powder, water, parsley, thyme, salt, and pepper. Simmer until vegetables are tender, 10 to 15 minutes. Add cornstarch-water mixture and cook several minutes until soup is thickened, stirring constantly.

Diet Portion
Remove 1½ cups (345 gm) soup and put in small saucepan. Add ½ cup Coffee Rich and rewarm over low heat.

Family Portion
Blend in evaporated milk or cream with remaining soup; if desired, add crisp-fried bacon bits to soup before serving. Rewarm over low heat.

Yield: 2 cups (457 gm) *Diet Portion,* 7 cups *Family Portion.*

	Phenylalanine (mg)	Protein (gm)	Calories
Per diet recipe	116	2.8	388
Per ½ cup (114 gm) serving	29	0.7	97

Blender Vegetable Soup

A quick soup with three variations that are equally excellent.

1 tablespoon margarine
   or butter
2 cups water
1 pkg G. Washington's
   Seasoning and Broth,
   or extra salt to taste

¼ teaspoon salt
1 tablespoon cornstarch mixed
   with 1 tablespoon water

Choose any of the 3 vegetable options on page 143. Prepare vegetables. In a medium saucepan melt margarine and sauté chosen vegetables a few minutes, until just tender. Add water, broth powder, and salt. Cover. Bring to a boil, then turn down to simmer for 10 minutes. Add cornstarch-water mixture and cook until thickened. Pour entire soup mixture into a blender and blend until smooth.

Yield: 3 cups (680 gm).

Vegetable Option 1

½ cup (62 gm) cut fresh or
  frozen asparagus
½ cup (44 gm) chopped fresh
  or frozen broccoli

½ cup (72 gm) chopped carrots
¼ cup (35 gm) chopped onion

	Phenylalanine (mg)	Protein (gm)	Calories
Per recipe	115	4.2	212
Per ½ cup (113 gm) serving	19	0.7	35

Vegetable Option 2

½ cup (45 gm) chopped fresh
  or frozen cauliflower
½ cup (44 gm) chopped fresh
  or frozen broccoli

½ cup (72 gm) chopped carrots
½ cup (35 gm) chopped onion

	Phenylalanine (mg)	Protein (gm)	Calories
Per recipe	108	3.5	209
Per ½ cup (113 gm) serving	18	0.6	35

Vegetable Option 3

¾ cup (108 gm) chopped
  carrots
¾ cup (66 gm) chopped fresh
  or frozen broccoli

¼ cup (35 gm) chopped onion

	Phenylalanine (mg)	Protein (gm)	Calories
Per recipe	107	3.6	219
Per ½ cup (113 gm) serving	18	0.6	37

Fresh Tomato and Pasta Soup

3 tablespoons (26 gm)
uncooked Aproten Anellini
or Wel-Plan Spaghetti
Ring Style
2 tablespoons (16 gm) diced
green pepper
2 tablespoons (20 gm) minced
onion
1 tablespoon margarine or
butter
½ cup water

1 cup tomato juice
1 pkg G. Washington's Golden
Seasoning and Broth, or
salt to taste
½ cup (96 gm) peeled, seeded,
and chopped fresh tomatoes
2 tablespoons vinegar
1 teaspoon granulated sugar
¼ teaspoon oregano
⅛ teaspoon pepper

Cook, rinse, and drain pasta according to package directions. In a medium saucepan, sauté green pepper and onion in margarine until tender. Add water, tomato juice, broth powder or salt, fresh tomatoes, and vinegar. Bring to a boil; cover, turn down the heat and simmer 5 minutes without stirring. Add sugar, oregano, pepper, and cooked pasta to soup and heat through.

Yield: 2½ cups (580 gm).

Family Portion
Use regular pasta of your choice in place of low protein pasta. Prepare any multiple of the recipe, to suit family needs.

	Phenylalanine (mg)	Protein (gm)	Calories
Per diet recipe	122	5.1	330
Per ½ cup (116 gm) serving	24	1.0	66

Cabbage Soup

1 cup (90 gm) chopped cabbage
⅓ cup (35 gm) chopped celery
⅓ cup (43 gm) chopped red
    or green pepper
¼ cup (35 gm) chopped onion
½ cup (85 gm) diced potatoes
1 cup (120 gm) cut frozen or
    canned green beans

4 pkg G. Washington's Golden
    Seasoning and Broth,
    or salt to taste
¼ teaspoon marjoram
⅛ teaspoon thyme
4 cups water

Put the vegetables, broth powder or salt, herbs, and water in a medium saucepan; bring to a boil. Cover and turn down the heat to simmer for 15 minutes without stirring.

Yield: 5⅓ cups (1253 gm).

	Phenylalanine (mg)	Protein (gm)	Calories
Per recipe	201	5.7	193
Per ½ cup (118 gm) serving	19	0.5	18

Savory Spinach Soup

To be enjoyed by spinach lovers and others alike.

2 tablespoons margarine or
    butter
¼ cup (35 gm) chopped onion
½ of 10 oz pkg (90 gm) frozen
    chopped spinach, thawed
    and moisture squeezed out

¼ cup water
2 pkg G. Washington's Golden
    Seasoning and Broth,
    or salt to taste
½ cup (85 gm) diced potatoes
½ cup Rich's Coffee Rich

In a medium saucepan, melt margarine; sauté onion until golden, about 3 to 5 minutes. Add spinach, water, and broth powder or salt. Cover and cook 2 to 3 minutes. Add potatoes and 3 additional cups water. Cover and cook 10 minutes without stirring, until potatoes are tender. Purée in a blender, leaving some texture. Return to the pan; add Coffee Rich and heat through.

Yield: 2⅔ cups (612 gm).

	Phenylalanine (mg)	Protein (gm)	Calories
Per recipe	470	10.4	525
Per ½ cup (115 gm) serving	88	1.9	98

Cream of Tomato Soup

Very similar to canned cream of tomato soup, but considerably lower in protein.

2 tablespoons margarine
   or butter
2 tablespoons cornstarch
24 oz can tomato juice
   (or four 6 oz cans)

¾ cup water
½ teaspoon salt
2 teaspoons granulated sugar
1 cup Rich's Coffee Rich

In a large saucepan, melt margarine; remove from heat, add cornstarch and mix until smooth. Add about ½ cup tomato juice and stir constantly over medium heat, until mixture thickens. Add remaining tomato juice, water, salt, sugar, and Coffee Rich. Heat through without boiling.

Yield: 4½ cups (1103 gm).

	Phenylalanine (mg)	Protein (gm)	Calories
Per recipe	176	6.5	775
Per ½ cup (123 gm) serving	20	0.7	86

Salads

For recipes using "Prono" low protein gelled desert (Dietary Specialties), "Low Protein Gel" (Kingsmill) could also be used with similar results, although the recipes were developed using Prono.

Other low protein gelled-dessert salads can be created, with the following preparation tips in mind:

- Prepare Prono (or Low Protein Gel) according to package directions, using 2 cups boiling water per package. Stir to dissolve, then let stand at *room temperature.* The gel will become soft-set in approximately 20 minutes, and set in approximately 45 minutes. Refrigerate only after it has set, for firm-setting.
- Do not try to speed the setting process by preparing like Jell-O (using 1 cup boiling water, 1 cup cold water). The low protein gel will become cloudy and will never set firmly.
- Do not add fresh fruit or vegetables, except bananas, for optimal setting. The gel will not become firm, or may "weep" when other fresh fruits or vegetables are added. If you want to add fruit, add well-drained canned fruit such as crushed pineapple, peach slices, or fruit cocktail. Use the full 2 cups of water, or a combination of water and juice from the fruit—never more than 2 cups liquid in total. Heat the fruit along with the water or water/juice and add directly to the gel powder for optimal setting. You may also add cool or cold fruit after the gel has become "soft-set," approximately 20 to 30 minutes after the boiling water has been added, but the gel may not become as firm.
- Whipped non-dairy creamer (such as Rich's Richwhip or Coolwhip) can be folded into the gel after it has "soft-set," for a fluffy dessert-like salad.

Apple Fruit Salad

2½ cups (300 gm) diced
   unpeeled red apples
16 oz can fruit cocktail,
   drained
½ cup (20 gm) mini
   marshmallows

½ cup (80 gm) sliced bananas
4 oz container Coolwhip
   (1¾ cups) or ½ cup liquid
   Rich's Richwhip Topping,
   whipped

Mix all ingredients together in a large bowl. Chill.

Yield: 6 cups (663 gm).

	Phenylalanine (mg)	Protein (gm)	Calories
Using Richwhip			
Per recipe	97	3.0	880
Per ½ cup (55 gm) serving	8	0.3	73
Using Coolwhip			
Per recipe	141	4.8	954
Per ½ cup (55 gm) serving	12	0.4	80

Waldorf Salad

3 cups (360 gm) diced
   unpeeled red apples
½ cup (53 gm) diced celery
¼ cup (40 gm) raisins
½ cup (20 gm) mini
   marshmallows

2 tablespoons Miracle Whip
   Salad Dressing
2 tablespoons Coolwhip

Mix apples, celery, raisins, and marshmallows in a large bowl. Blend together the Miracle Whip and Coolwhip; mix into salad. Chill.

Yield: 4¼ cups (514 gm).

	Phenylalanine (mg)	Protein (gm)	Calories
Per recipe	76	2.9	563
Per ½ cup (60 gm) serving	9	0.3	66

Fruit Salad

1 cup (180 gm) halved green grapes
½ cup (116 gm) pineapple tidbits or cut-up chunks, drained

10 quartered maraschino cherries
¾ cup (51 gm) Coolwhip or whipped liquid Rich's Richwhip Topping

Mix fruits together in a medium bowl. Gently fold whipped topping into the combined fruits. Chill.

Yield: 2 cups (397 gm).

	Phenylalanine (mg)	Protein (gm)	Calories
Using Richwhip			
Per recipe	50	2.0	415
Per ½ cup (99 gm) serving	13	0.5	104
Using Coolwhip			
Per recipe	88	2.7	384
Per ½ cup (99 gm) serving	22	0.7	96

Fresh Fruit Salad

3-inch section (40 gm) banana, sliced
¼ cup (50 gm) cut-up orange segments
¼ cup (35 gm) cut-up unpeeled apple slices

2 quartered maraschino cherries
10 miniature marshmallows or 1 large marshmallow, cut-up

Mix ingredients together in a bowl and serve.

Yield: 1 cup (145 gm).

	Phenylalanine (mg)	Protein (gm)	Calories
Per recipe	30	1.1	100
Per ½ cup (73 gm) serving	15	0.6	50

Fruit Delight Salad

21 oz can Comstock or
   Wilderness Peach Pie Filling
20 oz can chunk pineapple,
   drained

2¼ cup (270 gm) diced
   unpeeled apple
¾ cup (120 gm) sliced banana

Mix all ingredients in a bowl and chill.

Yield: 6 cups (1370 gm).

	Phenylalanine (mg)	Protein (gm)	Calories
Per recipe	151	5.1	1312
Per ½ cup (112 gm) serving	13	0.4	109

Creamy Fruit Salad

Try using fruits packed in their own juice for this light, dessert-like salad.

16 oz can fruit cocktail
8¼ oz can pineapple tidbits
11 oz can mandarin oranges
1 cup (150 gm) sliced fresh
   strawberries
1 pkg (4-serving size) vanilla
   Jell-O Instant Pudding and
   Pie Filling mix

4 oz container Coolwhip
   (1¾ cups) or ½ cup liquid
   Rich's Richwhip Topping,
   whipped

Drain fruit cocktail, pineapple tidbits, and mandarin oranges, reserving the 1½ cups juice which you should have in total. In a medium bowl, beat juice into pudding mix, using no additional liquid, mixing 1 to 2 minutes on low speed with electric mixer or by hand. Add fruits and mix. Add whipped topping. Chill several hours.

Yield: 5¾ cups (1300 gm).

	Phenylalanine (mg)	Protein (gm)	Calories
Using Richwhip			
Per recipe	116	3.9	1332
Per ½ cup (113 gm) serving	10	0.3	116
Using Coolwhip			
Per recipe	200	5.5	1263
Per ½ cup (113 gm) serving	17	0.5	110

Watermelon Boat Salad

Using a watermelon shell as a bowl is a popular and beautiful party-picnic way to serve this salad, but you can make ½ the recipe and serve it in a bowl for a delicious mid-summer "every day" salad, or serve in cut-out cantaloupe shells.

2 cups (320 gm) watermelon
    balls
2 cups (280 gm) cantaloupe
    balls
1 cup (146 gm) green grapes
1 cup (160 gm) fresh
    blueberries

2 cups (300 gm) fresh
    strawberries, halved
2 cups (160 gm)
    peach slices

Cut a small watermelon in half. Scoop watermelon balls from center using a small melon scoop or measuring teaspoon. Reserve 2 cups balls for salad and refrigerate remainder for another use. Cut edges of watermelon "boat" with a knife, zigzag fashion. Mix all fruit ingredients in the "boat" and serve.

Yield: 10 cups (1366 gm).

	Phenylalanine (mg)	Protein (gm)	Calories
Per recipe	259	9.2	541
Per ½ cup (68 gm) serving	13	0.5	27

Blushing Apple Cranberry Salad

Excellent for the fall and early winter cranberry and apple season.

2 cups (200 gm) whole fresh or
frozen cranberries
⅓ cup granulated sugar
2 cups (240 gm) diced, peeled
apples
½ cup (140 gm) crushed
pineapple, drained

½ cup (20 gm) mini
marshmallows
4 oz container Coolwhip (1¾
cups) or ½ cup liquid Rich's
Richwhip Topping, whipped

Chop cranberries in a food processor or put them through a food grinder. Sprinkle the cranberries with sugar; let stand 2 hours or longer. Drain the cranberries, discarding the liquid. In a medium bowl, combine drained cranberries, apples, pineapple, and marshmallows. Chill. Just before serving fold in the whipped topping.

Yield: 4½ cups (781 gm).

	Phenylalanine (mg)	Protein (gm)	Calories
Using Richwhip			
Per recipe	46	1.8	965
Per ½ cup (87 gm) serving	5	0.2	107
Using Coolwhip			
Per recipe	130	3.4	897
Per ½ cup (87 gm) serving	14	0.4	100

Five-Cup Salad

1 cup (187 gm) pineapple
   chunks, drained
1 cup (200 gm) cut-up fresh
   orange sections
1 cup (41 gm) mini
   marshmallows

1 cup (80 gm) shredded
   coconut
1 cup (68 gm) Coolwhip or
   whipped liquid Rich's
   Richwhip Topping

In a medium bowl, mix together pineapple, orange sections, marshmallows, and coconut. Fold in whipped topping. Chill.

Yield: 3 cups (573 gm).

	Phenylalanine (mg)	Protein (gm)	Calories
Using Richwhip			
Per recipe	197	5.4	916
Per ¼ cup (47 gm) serving	16	0.4	76
Using Coolwhip			
Per recipe	248	6.4	875
Per ¼ cup (47 gm) serving	21	0.5	73

Frosted Blueberry Salad

1 pkg (4-serving size) blueberry
or blackberry Jell-O
1 cup boiling water
8 oz can crushed pineapple
1 cup (160 gm) fresh
blueberries, or 1 cup
(170 gm) canned, drained
blueberries

juice from pineapple
2 cups (137 gm) Coolwhip or
whipped liquid Rich's
Richwhip Topping

Dissolve Jell-O in boiling water. Drain pineapple, reserving juice and adding enough water to make a total of 1 cup liquid; stir into Jell-O. Remove 3 tablespoons Jell-O mixture and set aside (do not refrigerate). Add pineapple and blueberries to the remaining Jell-O. Pour into a 9 × 5-inch loaf pan or an 8-inch square pan. Chill several hours until firm. To the whipped topping, mix in the reserved 3 tablespoons liquid Jell-O. Spread this mixture over the top of chilled Jell-O. Cut in 12 pieces.

Yield: 5 cups (1059 gm).

	Phenylalanine (mg)	Protein (gm)	Calories
Using Richwhip			
Per recipe	200	8.8	976
Per serving (106 gm)	20	0.8	98
Using Coolwhip			
Per recipe	302	10.8	893
Per serving (106 gm)	30	1.0	89

Pistachio Fluff Salad

An all-around favorite, also known as "Watergate" salad.

20 oz can crushed pineapple
1 pkg (4-serving size) Jell-O
   Instant Pistachio Pudding
   and Pie Filling mix*
8 oz container (3½ cups)
   Coolwhip or 8 oz carton
   liquid Rich's Richwhip
   Topping, whipped

1 cup (41 gm) mini
   marshmallows

Pour pineapple and its juice into a bowl. Sift nuts out of pudding mix, using a fine-meshed strainer (there will be about 1 tablespoon), then mix with pineapple until dissolved. Mix in whipped topping and marshmallows. Chill. Salad is best after several hours or the next day, after flavors have blended.

Yield: 6 cups (915 gm).

	Phenylalanine (mg)	Protein (gm)	Calories
Using Richwhip			
Per recipe	54	2.0	1448
Per ½ cup (76 gm) serving	4	0.2	121
Using Coolwhip			
Per recipe	222	5.2	1312
Per ½ cup (76 gm) serving	18	0.4	109

*Sift out any nuts.

Orange Tapioca Salad

Kids love it.

1 pkg (4-serving size) orange
   Jell-O or Prono low protein
   gelled dessert mix
1 cup boiling water
1 pkg (4-serving size) tapioca
   Jell-O Pudding and Pie
   Filling mix

1 cup Rich's Coffee Rich
8¼ oz can fruit cocktail
11 oz can mandarin oranges
4 oz container Coolwhip
   (1¾ cups) or ½ cup liquid
   Rich's Richwhip Topping,
   whipped

Dissolve Jell-O or Prono in boilding water. In a saucepan, cook tapioca pudding in Coffee Rich over medium heat, stirring constantly until mixture comes to a full boil. Combine hot gelatin and hot pudding in a bowl, mixing thoroughly. Chill. When slightly thickened, add drained fruit cocktail and drained mandarin oranges. Fold in whipped topping. Chill.

Yield: 5 cups (843 gm).

	Phenylalanine (mg)	Protein (gm)	Calories
Using Prono and Richwhip			
Per recipe	102	2.4	1626
Per ½ cup (84 gm) serving	10	0.2	163
Using Prono and Coolwhip			
Per recipe	186	4.0	1558
Per ½ cup (84 gm) serving	19	0.4	156
Using Jell-O and Richwhip			
Per recipe	250	9.6	1626
Per ½ cup (84 gm) serving	25	1.0	163
Using Jell-O and Coolwhip			
Per recipe	334	11.2	1558
Per ½ cup (84 gm) serving	33	1.1	156

Frozen Lime Mint Salad

Refreshing as a salad, or as a light dessert or snack.

20 oz can crushed pineapple
8 oz can crushed pineapple
1 pkg (4-serving size) lime
    Jell-O or Prono low protein
    gelled dessert mix
3½ cups (143 gm) mini
    marshmallows

1 cup (125 gm) Kraft
    Buttermints, crushed
8 oz container Coolwhip
    (3½ cups) or 8 oz carton
    liquid Rich's Richwhip
    Topping, whipped

In a large mixing bowl, combine undrained pineapple, Jell-O or Prono, marshmallows, and mints. Cover and refrigerate several hours or overnight, until marshmallows soften and mints melt. Fold in whipped topping. Spoon ⅓ cup of mixture into each of 24 muffin cups lined with cupcake liners. Cover and freeze until firm. To serve, peel off paper and place on lettuce-lined plates, or eat as a snack straight from the freezer.

Yield: 8 cups (1096 gm).

	Phenylalanine (mg)	Protein (gm)	Calories
Using Prono and Richwhip			
Per recipe	98	3.8	2413
Per ⅓ cup (46 gm) serving	4	0.2	101
Using Prono and Coolwhip			
Per recipe	266	7.0	2277
Per ⅓ cup (46 gm) serving	11	0.3	95
Using Jell-O and Richwhip			
Per recipe	246	11.0	2413
Per ⅓ cup (46 gm) serving	10	0.5	100
Using Jell-O and Coolwhip			
Per recipe	414	14.2	2277
Per ⅓ cup (46 gm) serving	17	0.6	95

Frozen Strawberry Banana Salad

Also nice as a snack during warm weather.

2 cups (82 gm) mini
  marshmallows
1 cup (186 gm) pineapple
  slices, cut in small pieces
½ cup juice from pineapple

10 oz pkg frozen strawberries,
  thawed, undrained
4 oz container Coolwhip (1¾
  cups) or ½ cup liquid Rich's
  Richwhip Topping, whipped

Mix marshmallows with pineapple and pineapple juice in a large bowl. Refrigerate for several hours or overnight, until marshmallows soften. Mix in strawberries and whipped topping. Spoon ⅓ cup of mixture into each of 18 muffin pans lined with paper baking cups. Cover and freeze until firm. To serve, peel off paper and place on lettuce-lined plates, or eat as a snack straight from the freezer.

Yield: 6 cups (875 gm).

	Phenylalanine (mg)	Protein (gm)	Calories
Using Richwhip			
Per recipe	72	3.2	947
Per ⅓ cup (49 gm) serving	4	0.2	53
Using Coolwhip			
Per recipe	156	4.9	879
Per ⅓ cup (49 gm) serving	9	0.3	49

Strawberry Salad

1 pkg (4-serving size)
  strawberry Jell-O
½ cup (120 gm) applesauce
½ cup water

8 oz can crushed pineapple
10 oz pkg frozen strawberries,
  partially thawed

Put Jell-O powder in a bowl. Mix applesauce and water in a saucepan and bring to a boil; pour over Jell-O and mix until dissolved; add undrained pineapple and undrained strawberries. Pour into a 9 × 5-inch loaf pan. Chill.

Yield: 3¼ cups (828 gm).

	Phenylalanine (mg)	Protein (gm)	Calories
Per recipe	189	9.5	855
Per ½ cup (127 gm) serving	29	1.5	132

158

Low Strawberry Salad

1 pkg strawberry Prono low
  protein gelled dessert mix
8 oz can crushed pineapple

10 oz pkg frozen strawberries,
  thawed

Put Prono powder in a bowl. Place undrained pineapple in a sauce-pan. Drain juice from strawberries and add to saucepan. Heat to just boiling. Stir hot juices into Prono powder and mix until dissolved. Let soft-set 30 minutes at room temperature. Mix in reserved straw-berries. Chill.

Yield: 2 cups (509 gm).

Note
Texture will be more like pudding rather than a firm gel.

	Phenylalanine (mg)	Protein (gm)	Calories
Per recipe	35	2.0	764
Per ½ cup (127 gm) serving	9	0.5	191

Holiday Cranberry Salad

1 pkg (4-serving size)
  strawberry Jell-O
1 cup boiling water
½ cup cold water
1 lb can whole or jellied
  cranberry sauce

½ cup (60 gm) finely diced
  peeled apples
¼ cup (26 gm) finely diced
  celery
1 to 2 teaspoons grated orange
  rind (optional)

Place Jell-O in a large bowl; pour boiling water over and stir until dissolved. Add ½ cup cold water. Chill until slightly thickened. If whole cranberry sauce is used, drain. Mix cranberry sauce, apple, cel-ery, and orange rind into slightly thickened mixture. Pour into a 1-quart mold or 9 × 5-inch loaf pan. Chill until firm.

Yield: 3½ cups (891 gm).

	Phenylalanine (mg)	Protein (gm)	Calories
Per recipe	176	8.5	1063
Per ½ cup (127 gm) serving	25	1.2	152

Orange Applesauce Salad

1 cup (267 gm) applesauce   6 oz 7-Up
¾ cup orange juice
1 pkg (4-serving size) orange
    Jell-O

Heat applesauce and orange juice to boiling in a large saucepan. Pour over Jell-O in a bowl, stirring until dissolved. Add 7-Up. Chill (salad will remain somewhat soft).

Yield: 2½ cups (587 gm).

	Phenylalanine (mg)	Protein (gm)	Calories
Per recipe	184	8.8	679
Per ½ cup (117 gm) serving	37	1.8	136

Low Orange Applesauce Salad

1 cup (267 gm) applesauce   1 pkg orange Prono low protein
1 cup orange juice   gelled dessert mix

Heat applesauce and orange juice to boiling in a saucepan; pour over Prono powder in a bowl, stirring until dissolved. Let soft-set 30 minutes at room temperature. Chill (salad will remain somewhat soft).

Yield: 2 cups (537 gm).

	Phenylalanine (mg)	Protein (gm)	Calories
Per recipe	44	2.0	635
Per ½ cup (134 gm) serving	11	0.5	159

Yum Yum Salad

A sweet and fluffy salad that is more like dessert.

1 pkg (4-serving size) Jell-O or
    Prono low protein gelled
    dessert mix (any flavor)
1 cup boiling water
8 oz can crushed pineapple,
    drained
2 tablespoons sugar

⅔ cup (27 gm) mini
    marshmallows
8 oz container Coolwhip
    (3½ cups) or 8 oz carton
    liquid Rich's Richwhip
    Topping, whipped

Place Jell-O or Prono in a large bowl; pour boiling water over and stir until dissolved. Allow to soft-set (see note, page 147, if using Prono). Mix sugar with the crushed, drained pineapple. Fold in pineapple, marshmallows, and whipped topping. Chill.

Yield: 4 cups (720 gm).

Note

This salad is also good frozen.

	Phenylalanine (mg)	Protein (gm)	Calories
Using Prono and Richwhip			
Per recipe	23	0.9	1322
Per ½ cup (90 gm) serving	3	0.1	165
Using Prono and Coolwhip			
Per recipe	191	4.1	1186
Per ½ cup (90 gm) serving	24	0.5	148
Using Jell-O and Richwhip			
Per recipe	171	8.1	1322
Per ½ cup (90 gm) serving	21	1.0	165
Using Jell-O and Coolwhip			
Per recipe	339	11.3	1186
Per ½ cup (90 gm) serving	42	1.4	148

Brown Rice Salad

Somewhat unusual combination of ingredients makes a slightly sweet, irresistible main-dish salad. For the rest of the family, it is a nice accompaniment to cold chicken or pork on a warm summer day.

1 cup (176 gm) uncooked
   brown rice
¼ teaspoon salt
3 tablespoons lemon juice
¼ cup olive oil or other
   vegetable oil
¼ teaspoon cinnamon

1 tablespoon minced parsley or
   1 teaspoon dry parsley
2 tablespoons (14 gm) chopped
   green onions
1 teaspoon minced fresh mint
   leaves (optional)
¾ cup (150 gm) chopped dates

Add rice to 2 cups boiling salted water; reduce heat and cook on low for 40 to 45 minutes, until water is absorbed and rice is tender. In a small bowl, mix together lemon juice, oil, cinnamon, parsley, green onions, and mint. Pour over slightly cooled rice. Mix in dates. Chill several hours or overnight to blend flavors. Serve garnished with orange slices for a decorative touch. Keeps up to 1 week in refrigerator and also freezes well.

Yield: 4½ cups (822 gm).

	Phenylalanine (mg)	Protein (gm)	Calories
Per recipe	817	17.2	1566
Per ¼ cup (46 gm) serving	45	1.0	87

Curried Fruit and Rice Salad

A colorful, unusual, and delicious salad.

¾ cup (132 gm) uncooked regular white rice

½ cup (72 gm) finely chopped carrots

½ cup (93 gm) pineapple chunks, drained

½ cup (100 gm) cut-up orange sections

¾ cup (90 gm) apple chunks

½ cup (90 gm) halved red or green grapes

¼ cup (40 gm) raisins

1½ teaspoons lemon juice

¼ cup Miracle Whip Salad Dressing

¼ cup juice from pineapple

1½ teaspoons curry powder

Add rice to 1½ cups boiling salted water and cook according to package directions; chill. In a large bowl mix carrots and all the fruits. Sprinkle in the lemon juice and toss. In a small bowl mix the Miracle Whip with the pineapple juice and curry powder; add to the fruit mixture. Mix well. Add the chilled rice and toss again. Chill.

Yield: 4¼ cups (940 gm).

Family Portion
For the rest of the family ⅓ to ½ cup chopped nuts can be added after diet portion is removed.

	Phenylalanine (mg)	Protein (gm)	Calories
Per recipe	620	13.8	1142
Per ¼ cup (55 gm) serving	36	0.8	67

Variation

Low Curried Fruit and Rice Salad

Use ⅓ cup (61 gm) uncooked rice and ¾ cup (86 gm) Aproten Ditalini. Cook rice and Ditalini according to package directions and combine as directed in recipe.

	Phenylalanine (mg)	Protein (gm)	Calories
Per recipe	365	9.1	1188
Per ¼ cup (55 gm) serving	21	0.5	70

Coleslaw

⅓ cup Miracle Whip Salad
    Dressing
1½ teaspoons granulated sugar
1 teaspoon vinegar

3 cups (269 gm) shredded
    cabbage
⅓ cup (38 gm) shredded
    carrots

In a medium bowl, mix together Miracle Whip, sugar, and vinegar. Mix in the shredded cabbage and carrots. Chill.

Yield: 3 cups (392 gm).

	Phenylalanine (mg)	Protein (gm)	Calories
Per recipe	138	3.4	512
Per ½ cup (65 gm) serving	23	0.6	85

German Coleslaw

4 cups (358 gm) finely
    shredded cabbage
¼ cup (32 gm) finely chopped
    green pepper

¼ cup (35 gm) finely chopped
    red or yellow onion

Dressing

1½ tablespoons granulated
    sugar
1½ tablespoons hot water
1½ tablespoons cider vinegar
¼ teaspoon celery seed
    (optional)

¼ teaspoon salt
dash of pepper
2 tablespoons vegetable oil

Place cabbage, green pepper, and onion in a large bowl; toss well to mix. For the dressing, combine sugar and hot water in a small bowl, stirring until sugar dissolves; stir in remainder of dressing ingredients. Pour over slaw and toss well. Toss well before serving.

Yield: 4½ cups (510 gm).

	Phenylalanine (mg)	Protein (gm)	Calories
Per recipe	170	4.4	497
Per ¼ cup (28 gm) serving	9	0.2	28

Carrot Salad

2½ cups (285 gm) shredded carrots
½ cup (80 gm) raisins
½ cup (140 gm) crushed pineapple, drained, or 3 diced pineapple slices

1 cup Miracle Whip Salad Dressing
3 tablespoons juice from pineapple

In a medium bowl, mix carrots, raisins, and pineapple. Blend Miracle Whip with pineapple juice in a small bowl, then add to carrot mixture and mix thoroughly. Chill.

Yield: 3 cups (760 gm).

	Phenylalanine (mg)	Protein (gm)	Calories
Per recipe	210	6.9	1584
Per ¼ cup (63 gm) serving	17	0.6	132

Potato Salad

5 cups (800 gm) cooked, peeled, and cubed potatoes (about 6 medium)
1 cup (105 gm) sliced celery
¼ cup (35 gm) chopped onion
2 tablespoons chopped dill or sweet pickles

¾ cup Miracle Whip Salad Dressing
½ teaspoon prepared (wet) mustard
½ teaspoon salt
1 teaspoon pickle juice, or to taste

In a large bowl, toss prepared potatoes with celery and onions. In a small bowl, mix together Miracle Whip, mustard, salt, and pickle juice; add to potatoes and toss until moistened. Chill.

Yield: 5¼ cups (1122 gm).

	Phenylalanine (mg)	Protein (gm)	Calories
Per recipe	782	17.6	1520
Per ¼ cup (53 gm) serving	37	0.8	72

German Hot Potato Salad

The author's favorite picnic salad.

6 medium potatoes
  (about 2 lbs)
3 tablespoons bacon fat
2 tablespoons vegetable oil
¾ cup (105 gm) chopped or
  thinly sliced onion
1½ tablespoons cornstarch

2 tablespoons granulated sugar
½ teaspoon salt
½ teaspoon celery seed
  (optional)
dash of pepper
¾ cup water
½ cup vinegar

Boil potatoes in skins until tender (20 to 25 minutes). While potatoes are cooling, fry 6 slices of bacon until crisp. Remove bacon and drain on paper toweling. In a large skillet, cook the onion in a mixture of 3 tablespoons strained bacon fat and 2 tablespoons oil for 4 to 5 minutes or until soft. Mix in cornstarch, sugar, salt, celery seed, and pepper. Gradually stir in water and vinegar. Cook, stirring until mixture boils; boil 1 minute. Remove from heat and cover to keep warm.

Peel and thinly slice slightly cooled potatoes (you should have 5 cups, 853 gm). Place in a large bowl and pour hot sauce over. Cover and let stand until ready to serve. Can be reheated over hot water. Serve garnished with minced parsley or chives.

Yield: 5½ cups (1178 gm).

Family Portion
Remove diet portion and add reserved crisp bacon bits just before serving.

	Phenylalanine (mg)	Protein (gm)	Calories
Per diet recipe	820	20.1	1584
Per ¼ cup (53 gm) serving	37	0.9	72

Summer Vegetable Salad

½ cup (75 gm) peeled, seeded, and chopped cucumber
½ cup (70 gm) chopped zucchini squash
¾ cup (144 gm) seeded, chopped, fresh tomatoes

2 tablespoons (18 gm) chopped onion
1 tablespoon vinegar
2 tablespoons vegetable oil
salt and pepper to taste

In a medium bowl, toss the cucumber and zucchini with a generous sprinkling of salt and allow to sit for 30 minutes. Drain off any liquid that collects. Add the tomatoes and onion. Mix together the vinegar and oil; add to the vegetables and toss. Add salt and pepper to taste. Chill.

Yield: 1¾ cups (333 gm).

	Phenylalanine (mg)	Protein (gm)	Calories
Per recipe	81	2.9	306
Per ¼ cup (48 gm) serving	12	0.4	44

Cucumber Salad

⅓ cup granulated sugar
1 cup cider vinegar
1 cup (135 gm) thinly sliced carrots
1 cup (140 gm) thinly sliced onion

1 cup (110 gm) thinly sliced green pepper
1 cup (105 gm) thinly sliced celery
3 cups (415 gm) thinly sliced cucumber

In a large bowl, combine sugar and vinegar; stir to dissolve the sugar. Prepare vegetables in a food processor for greatest convenience. Add all of the sliced vegetables and toss to mix vegetables with vinegar. Cover and refrigerate at least overnight.

Yield: 6 cups (850 gm drained).

Storage Tip
Keeps well in the refrigerator up to 2 weeks, or can be frozen and then thawed in the refrigerator.

	Phenylalanine (mg)	Protein (gm)	Calories
Per recipe	257	8.6	708
Per ¼ cup (35 gm) serving	11	0.4	30

167

Two-Bean Salad

Low protein version of a "classic."

⅔ cup vinegar
⅓ cup granulated sugar
½ cup vegetable oil
½ teaspoon Worcestershire
   sauce
¼ teaspoon garlic powder

16 oz can green beans, drained
16 oz can wax beans, drained
⅔ cup (93 gm) sliced onion
1 cup (105 gm) sliced celery
¼ cup (34 gm) thinly sliced
   carrots

In a large bowl, combine vinegar, sugar, oil, Worcestershire sauce, and garlic powder. Stir until sugar dissolves. Add beans, onion, celery, and carrots and gently toss until beans are well coated with dressing. Cover and refrigerate overnight.

Yield: 5¼ cups (707 gm drained).

	Phenylalanine (mg)	Protein (gm)	Calories
Per recipe	319	10.6	1711
Per ¼ cup (34 gm) serving	15	0.5	81

Potato Green Bean Salad

An excellent summer main-dish salad.

16 oz can whole new potatoes, diced, or 2 cups (300 gm) diced cooked potatoes
16 oz can green beans, or 2 cups (240 gm) cooked fresh or frozen green beans

1 tablespoon (9 gm) minced onion
⅓ cup Italian salad dressing
1 cup (192 gm) seeded, chopped, fresh tomatoes

In a large bowl, mix diced potatoes, green beans, onion, and salad dressing. Cover and chill for at least 1 hour. At serving time toss with chopped tomatoes. Nice served on a bed of fresh garden lettuce, with black olives for a garnish.

Yield: 4¾ cups (811 gm).

Family Portion
For each individual portion, serve a mound of tuna salad next to *Potato Green Bean Salad* for the traditional "Salad Niçoise."

	Phenylalanine (mg)	Protein (gm)	Calories
Per diet recipe	423	11.5	713
Per ¼ cup (43 gm) serving	22	0.6	38

Marinated Mushrooms

Wonderful in a green salad, or just plain.

2½ cups (227 gm) small fresh
   mushrooms (½ lb)
2½ tablespoons white wine
   vinegar or cider vinegar
2½ tablespoons vegetable oil
½ teaspoon prepared (wet)
   mustard
1 tablespoon packed brown
   sugar

¼ cup (35 gm) chopped onion
salt and pepper to taste
¼ to ½ teaspoon dried herb of
   your choice (basil,
   marjoram, thyme, or
   parsley)

Clean mushrooms, leaving whole if quite small, or cutting in half or quarters if larger. Mix remaining ingredients in a medium saucepan and heat to boiling; add mushrooms and cover. Turn heat to low and simmer for 5 minutes. Chill before serving.

Yield: 1½ cups (227 gm drained).

	Phenylalanine (mg)	Protein (gm)	Calories
Per recipe	207	5.9	431
Per ¼ cup (38 gm drained) serving	34	1.0	72

Low Pro Tabouleh

A tasty version of the popular Mid-Eastern salad traditionally made with bulgur wheat. Excellent as a main dish or with a sandwich.

2 Aproten rusks, crushed
⅓ cup (9 gm) chopped fresh parsley
½ small tomato (60 gm), chopped
½ cup (75 gm) chopped cucumber

2 tablespoons olive oil or other vegetable oil
1 tablespoon chopped green onion
salt and a little lemon juice to taste

Toss all ingredients together in a bowl and serve.

Yield: 1½ cups (200 gm).

Note
This salad is especially good when served right away, as the fresh rusks give it a nice crunchiness; rusk crumbs could be added at the last minute if you wish to make the salad in advance.

	Phenylalanine (mg)	Protein (gm)	Calories
Per recipe	52	1.8	343
Per ¼ cup (33 gm) serving	9	0.3	57

171

Jell-O Vegetable Salad

An interesting combination of Jell-O and vegetables.

1 pkg (4-serving size) lime
  Jell-O
1¾ cups boiling water
¼ cup (70 gm) crushed
  pineapple, drained
⅓ cup (23 gm) Coolwhip
¼ cup Miracle Whip Salad
  Dressing

¼ cup (26 gm) chopped celery
¼ cup (32 gm) chopped green
  pepper
¼ cup (28 gm) sliced green
  onions

In a medium bowl, combine Jell-O and boiling water. Stir until dissolved. Allow to cool until just warm. Add crushed pineapple and Coolwhip and stir until Coolwhip is distributed through the Jell-O as small flecks. Pour into an 8-inch square pan or shallow dish. Refrigerate until set. In a small bowl, combine the Miracle Whip with the chopped vegetables and spread on top of the gelled mixture. Chill. Cut in 12 pieces (each piece will be ¼ cup).

Yield: 3 cups (731 gm).

	Phenylalanine (mg)	Protein (gm)	Calories
Per recipe	218	9.0	714
Per ¼ cup (61 gm) serving	18	0.7	60

Apple Macaroni Salad

½ cup (55 gm) uncooked
  Aproten Ditalini, Wel-Plan
  Macaroni, or regular elbow
  macaroni
1 cup (120 gm) diced unpeeled
  apples

2 tablespoons (13 gm) chopped
  celery
2 tablespoons (20 gm) raisins
2 tablespoons Miracle Whip
  Salad Dressing

Cook, rinse, and drain pasta according to package directions. In a medium bowl, combine the cooked pasta with the rest of the ingredients and toss lightly. Chill.

Yield: 2⅓ cups (316 gm).

	Phenylalanine (mg)	Protein (gm)	Calories
Using low protein pasta			
Per recipe	39	1.3	468
Per ½ cup (68 gm) serving	8	0.3	100
Using regular pasta			
Per recipe	373	8.2	393
Per ½ cup (68 gm) serving	79	1.7	84

Summer Pasta Salad

Can be served on lettuce or in a hollowed-out tomato.

¾ cup (69 gm) uncooked
  Aproten Rigatini
2 tablespoons Miracle Whip
  Salad Dressing
1½ teaspoons vinegar

1 tablespoon (9 gm) minced
  onion
⅓ cup (35 gm) chopped celery
¼ cup (38 gm) diced unpeeled
  cucumber

Cook, rinse, and drain Rigatini according to package directions. Allow to cool. In a medium bowl, mix together salad dressing and vinegar; add the onion, celery, cucumber, and Rigatini. Mix well. Cover and chill at least one hour before serving.

Yield: 1⅔ cups (295 gm).

Family Portion
Prepare any multiple of the recipe, to suit family needs, using regular elbow macaroni or ziti.

	Phenylalanine (mg)	Protein (gm)	Calories
Per diet recipe	38	1.0	401
Per ½ cup (91 gm) serving	11	0.3	120

Low Pro Macaroni Salad

¾ cup (69 gm) uncooked
   Aproten Rigatini
2 tablespoons Rich's Coffee
   Rich
2 teaspoons Miracle Whip
   Salad Dressing

¼ cup (29 gm) shredded
   carrots
⅓ cup (35 gm) thinly sliced
   celery

Cook, rinse, and drain Rigatini according to package directions. Allow to cool. In a medium bowl, stir together Coffee Rich and Miracle Whip until smooth. Add grated carrot, celery, and Rigatini and toss to combine. Chill.

Yield: 1¾ cups (279 gm).

Family Portion
Prepare any multiple of the recipe, to suit family needs, using regular macaroni or ziti.

	Phenylalanine (mg)	Protein (gm)	Calories
Per diet recipe	42	1.0	446
Per ½ cup (80 gm) serving	12	0.3	127

Macaroni Pea Salad

½ cup (55 gm) uncooked
   Aproten Ditalini, Wel-Plan
   Macaroni, or regular elbow
   macaroni
2 tablespoons (24 gm) canned
   or frozen cooked peas

2 tablespoons (25 gm) diced
   sweet or dill pickles
3 tablespoons Miracle Whip
   Salad Dressing
2 teaspoons pickle juice

Cook, rinse, and drain pasta according to package instructions. Mix in peas and diced pickle. Mix Miracle Whip with pickle juice until smooth; pour over pasta and mix well. Chill.

Yield: 1¼ cups (240 gm).

	Phenylalanine (mg)	Protein (gm)	Calories
Using low protein pasta			
Per recipe	72	1.7	430
Per ¼ cup (48 gm) serving	14	0.3	86
Using regular pasta			
Per recipe	406	8.6	355
Per ¼ cup (48 gm) serving	81	1.7	71

Mixed Vegetables and Pasta Salad

½ cup (55 gm) Aproten
Ditalini, Wel-Plan Macaroni,
or regular elbow macaroni
1½ cups (132 gm) fresh
broccoli, cut in small
flowerets
1¼ cups (150 gm) cut fresh
green beans

¼ cup (35 gm) thinly sliced red
onion
½ cup (75 gm) small cherry
tomatoes, halved
½ cup *Simple Vinaigrette
Dressing* or bottled Italian
dressing
salt and pepper to taste

To Make Diet Portion Only

Cook, rinse, and drain pasta according to package directions. Cook broccoli and green beans until crisp-tender. Drain; cool to room temperature. In a bowl, combine broccoli, beans, onion, cherry tomatoes, dressing, and cooked pasta. Mix well. Cover and chill several hours before serving.

To Make Diet Portion plus Family Portion

For each ½ cup diet serving, mix 6 tablespoons vegetable mixture with 2 tablespoons cooked low protein pasta. Add dressing as desired. For family portion, mix regular cooked macaroni with remainder of vegetables and dressing.

Yield: 4½ cups (655 gm).

	Phenylalanine (mg)	Protein (gm)	Calories
Using low protein pasta			
Per recipe	221	7.8	809
Per ½ cup (73 gm) serving	25	0.9	90
Using regular pasta			
Per recipe	555	14.7	734
Per ½ cup (73 gm) serving	62	1.6	82

Olive Rigatini Salad

¾ cup (69 gm) uncooked
  Aproten Rigatini
⅓ cup (35 gm) sliced celery
¼ cup (34 gm) thinly sliced
  carrots
1 tablespoon chopped black
  olives (2 large)

1 tablespoon chopped green
  olives (3 small)
¼ cup Miracle Whip Salad
  Dressing

Cook, rinse, and drain Rigatini according to package directions. When Rigatini is cooled, in a small bowl mix together Rigatini, celery, carrot, olives, and Miracle Whip. Chill.

Yield: 2 cups (321 gm).

Family Portion
Prepare any multiple of the recipe, to suit family needs, using regular elbow macaroni or ziti. A nice addition is slivered or diced mild cheese such as Jack or Muenster (approximately ½ cup per recipe).

	Phenylalanine (mg)	Protein (gm)	Calories
Per diet recipe	50	1.2	561
Per ½ cup (80 gm) serving	12	0.3	140

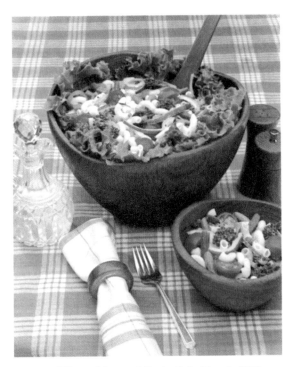

Mixed Vegetables and Pasta Salad (page 177)
Simple Vinaigrette Dressing (page 55)

Creamy Tomato and Carrot Soup (page 136); Low Pro Croutons (page 98)

179

Waffles (page 116)

Cinnamon Rolls (page 78)

Soft Pretzels (page 92); Cinnamon Graham Crackers (page 106)
Breadsticks (page 92); Crispy Chips (page 112); Snack Crackers (page 104)

Best White Bread (page 72); Best Homestyle Bread (page 74)

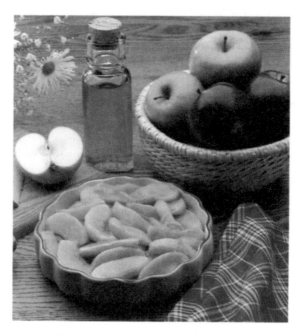

Honey Glazed Apple Slices (page 315)

Basic Cut-Out Cookies (page 354); Oatmeal Raisin Cookies (page 349)
Brownies (page 370); Neapolitan Cookies (page 359)
Chocolate Chip Cookies (page 363); Crackly Molasses Cookies (page 364)
Peanut Butter Cookies (page 373)

Chocolate Bon Bons, Pastel Bon Bons (pages 436–37)
Million Dollar Candy Bars (page 439)

Fresh Peach Ice Cream (churned) (page 455)
Vanilla Ice Cream (churned) (page 453)
with Microwave Hot Fudge Sauce (page 61)
Ice Cream Sandwiches (strawberry, mint chocolate chip, and
pineapple variations of Vanilla Ice Cream [churned]) (page 458)

Vegetable Stew (page 240)

Mushroom Burgers (page 234); Burger Buns (page 89)

Taco Chips (page 110); Salsa Fresca (page 60); Guacamole (page 59)
Burritos (page 262); Mexican Rice (page 264)

Mock Egg Rolls (page 258); Sweet and Sour Sauce (page 60)
Chinese Fried Rice (page 261)
Chinese Sweet and Sour Vegetables (page 260)

Thick Crust Pizza (page 269)

Strawberry Orange Freeze (page 48); Pineapple Smoothie (page 53)
Chocolate Shake (page 49); Frosted Orange Creme (page 47)

Main Dishes and Vegetables

All of the recipes in this section are designed for use by the whole family, or give instructions for modifications to suit non-diet needs. Many are simple recipes; others take more time.

The recipes were chosen for their diversity, versatility, and appeal. Some may be easily modified to suit individual taste preferences, by replacing one vegetable with another. To change a vegetable ingredient, consult *The Low Protein Food List for PKU* and use the method described on page 23 to refigure nutrient content.

Special Tips

All of the recipes in this section freeze well, except for those containing pasta or potatoes. The pasta or potatoes will become a little mushy, but many people are not bothered by this. See *Food Freezing Tips* (pages 532–34) for advice about freezing foods.

The portion size for most of the recipes in this section is ¼ cup (or in a few cases, 2 tablespoons or ⅓ cup). This size serving was chosen to suit the appetites of younger children, to provide a portion that is relatively low in phenylalanine/protein, and to provide a "base" from which nutrient content for multiples of ¼ cup could easily be calculated.

Many of the recipes use fresh vegetables, for optimal flavor and texture and maximal nutritional value. Canned or frozen vegetables are often given as options, however, and can certainly be used satisfactorily in the recipes where they are suggested as alternatives. When canned or frozen options are not given, usually the recipe works best with the fresh ingredients (for example, in *Broccoli Burgers*, or *Mushroom Burgers*, only fresh vegetables will work well). It is a good idea to get into the habit of using fresh produce for your whole family whenever possible.

Preparation of the vegetables in the recipes may be done in several different ways, even though usually only one method is indicated. For maximum convenience and retention of nutrients, using a microwave oven is optimal. Using a metal vegetable steamer fitted into a large saucepan with a small amount of water is also a good way of cooking vegetables to retain nutrients. The least desirable method of vegetable cooking is boiling the vegetables in water, as many nutrients can boil away in the liquid. If you do use the boiling method, use a minimum amount of water and cook vegetables until crisp-tender to preserve the most nutrients.

Some of the recipes call for fresh tomatoes which have been "peeled, seeded, and chopped." To peel a tomato most conveniently, there are two methods:

1. Drop whole tomato into boiling water and let cook only 10 seconds for ripe tomatoes, 15 to 30 seconds for firmer tomatoes. Remove from water with a slotted ladle or spoon and put under cold water.

When cool enough to handle, pull skin off with a small paring knife.

2. Tomatoes may also be put in a microwave oven on High 15 to 30 seconds to loosen the skin. Peel as in 1.

To seed a tomato conveniently, halve it (parallel to stem ends) and gently squeeze out the jelly-like juice and seeds. The flesh that remains is the "meat" of the tomato.

For recipes which call for low protein pasta, options of using products from either Wel-Plan pastas or Aproten pastas are given when they are essentially interchangeable. Some recipes call for a particular brand when a particular shape is desired; however, even in these recipes, alternatives could be used.

All of the pasta-containing recipes indicate the dry measure and weight of pasta to be used, so that you make just the amount of cooked pasta needed. If you happen to have cooked pasta on hand, approximately 1 cup can be used in recipes calling for ½ cup dry pasta.

Cooking low protein pastas in a microwave oven does not work well.

For the casserole recipes using pasta and condensed soup for a sauce, you may increase the portion size for the phenylalanine/protein content given in the recipe by using up to 50% more low protein pasta and diluting the amount of soup called for with water. By "extending" the casserole with additional low protein pasta and water, the portion size will be larger but the phenylalanine/protein content will remain the same or essentially the same.

With a little experience many of the recipes, including the pasta-based casseroles, can easily be adapted for microwave cookery.

Any of the pasta-based casseroles can be finished with a crumb topping, which will be attractive and add a delicious flavor. Some suggestions:

● Crushed Aproten Rusk crumbs dribbled with melted margarine.
● Dry low protein bread crumbs dribbled with melted margarine.
● Crushed *Snack Crackers*
● Crushed saltines*
● French's canned French Fried Onions*
● Crushed Pringle's Potato Chips*

A quantity of fine dry bread crumbs can be made by drying low protein bread slices in the oven at 200° until crisp, then breaking them into pieces and whirling in a food processor or blender until crumbs are fine.

---

* See *The Low Protein Food List for PKU* for nutrient content.

Many of the casserole recipes can be conveniently portioned into individual-size casserole dishes or other small containers that can be baked in a conventional oven or microwave oven. For conventional oven baking, "E-Z Foil Cupcake Cups" available in many grocery stores and some hardware stores are a perfect size for a ¼ to ½ cup serving portion. These are also great for freezing, when stored in an airtight plastic container or plastic freezer bags. Although the metal makes them unsuitable for reheating in most microwave ovens, they are still inexpensive and convenient for freezing individual portions; just remove to a microwave-suitable casserole or other dish to heat.

Another handy "casserole dish" for individual portions is a small size margarine tub, suitable for baking in a microwave oven and for freezing, although the plastic will not hold up for repeated use in a microwave oven.

There are many other individual casserole containers available, such as tiny individual white ceramic ramekins (from a kitchen housewares store) or individual soufflé dishes that are very attractive and can be used for both conventional and microwave cooking. More individual microwave cookware pieces are also becoming available.

Glazed Carrots

2½ cups (360 gm) carrots, cut in thin 2-inch lengthwise strips
¼ cup packed brown sugar
¼ teaspoon salt
¼ to ½ teaspoon grated fresh orange or lemon rind
1½ tablespoons margarine or butter

In a saucepan, cook carrots in a small amount of water or in a vegetable steamer for 18 to 20 minutes or until tender. Cook and stir brown sugar, salt, orange peel, and margarine in a skillet until bubbly. Add carrots to skillet; cook over medium heat, stirring occasionally, until carrots are glazed and heated through, about 5 to 8 minutes.

Yield: 1¾ cups (332 gm).

	Phenylalanine (mg)	Protein (gm)	Calories
Per recipe	125	3.8	512
Per ¼ cup (47 gm) serving	18	0.5	73

Butter Steamed Carrots

3 tablespoons margarine or butter
3 tablespoons water
3½ cups (473 gm) thinly sliced carrots
⅛ teaspoon salt
¼ cup light Karo corn syrup

Melt margarine in a large skillet or electric frying pan set at medium heat. Add water, then carrots. Stir to coat carrots. Cover and cook over medium heat, stirring several times, 15 to 20 minutes or until carrots are very tender and most liquid is gone. Some of the carrots may become lightly browned. Add salt. Mix in syrup to glaze.

Yield: 2¼ cups (370 gm).

	Phenylalanine (mg)	Protein (gm)	Calories
Per recipe	170	5.1	734
Per ¼ cup (41 gm) serving	19	0.6	82

Sunshine Carrots

The sauce is a subtle, tangy-sweet addition to everyday cooked carrots.

2 cups (270 gm) thinly sliced
    carrots
3 tablespoons orange juice
½ teaspoon cornstarch

⅛ teaspoon ground ginger or
    cinnamon
⅛ teaspoon salt

In a saucepan, in a small amount of boiling water, or using a vegetable steamer, cook carrots 12 to 15 minutes or until tender. Meanwhile, combine remaining ingredients in a small saucepan and cook over medium heat, stirring, for several minutes or until bubbly and thickened. Put carrots in a serving bowl and pour sauce over.

Yield: 2 cups (305 gm).

	Phenylalanine (mg)	Protein (gm)	Calories
Per recipe	93	3.0	144
Per ¼ cup (38 gm) serving	12	0.4	18

Carrots and Cranberries

A colorful fall dish that is "not like eating vegetables."

2 cups (228 gm) shredded
    carrots
1¼ cups (150 gm) shredded
    apple (about 1 medium)
½ cup (50 gm) fresh or frozen
    whole cranberries
2 to 4 tablespoons packed
    brown sugar

¼ cup apple cider or apple
    juice
½ teaspoon salt
1 tablespoon margarine or
    butter

Combine shredded carrots and apples, cranberries, sugar, cider or juice, and salt in a greased 1½-quart casserole with cover. Dot with margarine. Cover and bake at 350° for 40 to 45 minutes.

Yield: 2 cups (490 gm).

	Phenylalanine (mg)	Protein (gm)	Calories
Per recipe	90	2.8	550
Per ¼ cup (61 gm) serving	11	0.4	69

Baked Apples and Carrots

A child-appealing combination.

1 cup (135 gm) carrots, cut in
   ½-inch chunks
1¼ cups (150 gm) apple, cut in
   ½-inch chunks
2 tablespoons granulated sugar
   mixed with ¼ teaspoon
   cinnamon

1 tablespoon margarine or
   butter

In a saucepan, in a small amount of boiling water or a vegetable steamer, cook carrots 12 to 15 minutes or until tender. Combine carrots and apples in a 1-quart casserole. Sprinkle with cinnamon-sugar mixture; dot with margarine. Bake at 375° for 20 to 25 minutes. Sprinkle with a little chopped parsley for a decorative touch, if desired.

Yield: 1½ cups (250 gm).

	Phenylalanine (mg)	Protein (gm)	Calories
Per recipe	57	1.8	345
Per ¼ cup (42 gm) serving	9	0.3	57

Parsnips and Pears

A delicious combination of flavors.

2 tablespoons margarine or
    butter
3⅔ cups (380 gm) parsnips,
    pared and sliced in strips
    (from approximately 1 lb
    parsnips)
1½ cups (250 gm) fresh pears,
    peeled and sliced

⅔ cup orange juice
2 tablespoons packed brown
    sugar
½ teaspoon cinnamon
½ teaspoon grated orange peel
½ teaspoon salt
1 tablespoon chopped parsley

Melt margarine in a large skillet over high heat. Add parsnips and cook, stirring until crisp-tender, about 5 to 7 minutes. Add pears, orange juice, brown sugar, cinnamon, grated orange peel, and salt. Cover and cook over medium heat until pears are tender, about 3 minutes. Remove parsnips and pears to a heated serving dish. Boil orange juice mixture until reduced to a few tablespoons, or until thickened slightly. Pour over parsnips and mix in. Sprinkle with parsley before serving.

Yield: 3 cups (625 gm).

	Phenylalanine (mg)	Protein (gm)	Calories
Per recipe	291	8.1	898
Per ¼ cup (52 gm) serving	24	0.7	75

Harvard Beets

3 tablespoons beet juice (from can or cooking water)
2 tablespoons vinegar
2 teaspoons granulated sugar
2 teaspoons cornstarch

⅛ teaspoon salt
1½ teaspoons margarine or butter
1 cup (160 gm) cubed or sliced cooked beets

Mix beet juice, vinegar, sugar, cornstarch, and salt in a saucepan and cook several minutes over medium heat until sauce is thickened. Add margarine and stir until melted. Mix in beets. Heat through.

Yield: 1 cup (235 gm).

	Phenylalanine (mg)	Protein (gm)	Calories
Per recipe	80	2.8	170
Per ¼ cup (59 gm) serving	20	0.7	42

Apple Beets

The apples turn bright red and add a delicious flavor.

2 cups (320 gm) diced cooked beets
1¼ cups (150 gm) chopped tart apples
¼ cup (35 gm) chopped onion

1 tablespoon packed brown sugar
¼ teaspoon salt
2 tablespoons margarine or butter

Combine all ingredients except margarine in a 1- to 1½-quart casserole. Dot with pieces of margarine. Cover and bake at 375° for 30 minutes.

Yield: 3 cups (500 gm).

	Phenylalanine (mg)	Protein (gm)	Calories
Per recipe	184	6.4	489
Per ¼ cup (42 gm) serving	15	0.5	41

Green Beans Supreme

2 cups (240 gm) cut fresh or
    canned green beans
1 cup (75 gm) sliced fresh
    mushrooms
2 tablespoons (14 gm) sliced
    green onions
1 tablespoon margarine or
    butter

3 tablespoons condensed
    Campbell's Cream of
    Mushroom Soup
3 tablespoons water
2 tablespoons (8 gm) French's
    French Fried Onions

If using fresh green beans, cook in a small amount of water, covered, until barely tender, about 4 minutes. Meanwhile, in a skillet sauté mushrooms and onion in margarine for several minutes. Measure soup into a small saucepan and gradually add the water. Stir to remove most of the lumps. Add undiluted soup and water mixture to the mushrooms and onion and heat and stir until no lumps remain. Mix soup mixture and green beans in a 1-quart casserole. Top with French Fried Onions. Bake at 350°, uncovered, for 20 minutes.

Yield: 2¼ cups (370 gm).

	Phenylalanine (mg)	Protein (gm)	Calories
Per recipe	267	7.8	319
Per ¼ cup (41 gm) serving	30	0.9	35

Green Beans Polynesian

2 tablespoons (18 gm) chopped onion
1 tablespoon vegetable oil
2 cups (240 gm) fresh or frozen cut green beans
¾ cup (140 gm) canned pineapple tidbits, drained
3 tablespoons juice from pineapple
1½ teaspoons cornstarch
2 tablespoons granulated sugar
½ teaspoon dry mustard
1 tablespoon vinegar
1½ teaspoons soy sauce

In a medium saucepan, sauté onion in hot oil until onion is tender, about 5 minutes. Add green beans. Cover and keep heat high until steam comes from the edge of the pan lid, then immediately turn heat down to low and cook without lifting the lid for 5 to 8 minutes. After cooking, beans should remain bright green and slightly crunchy. Add pineapple tidbits. Mix pineapple juice with cornstarch and sugar until smooth and add to the beans and pineapple with the rest of the seasonings. Stir and cook over medium heat until sauce is thickened and mixture is heated through.

Yield: 2¼ cups (500 gm).

	Phenylalanine (mg)	Protein (gm)	Calories
Per recipe	149	5.1	447
Per ¼ cup (56 gm) serving	17	0.6	50

Stir-Fried Green Beans

2 tablespoons vegetable oil
2 cups (240 gm) cut fresh or
  frozen green beans
¾ cup (56 gm) sliced fresh
  mushrooms, or ¼ cup
  (44 gm) canned sliced
  mushrooms
¼ cup (24 gm) sliced green
  onions

¼ cup (30 gm) sliced canned
  water chestnuts
½ teaspoon chopped fresh
  ginger (optional)
1 teaspoon cornstarch
½ teaspoon granulated sugar
3 tablespoons water
1½ teaspoons soy sauce

Heat oil in a heavy skillet or wok. Add green beans, mushrooms, onion, water chestnuts, and ginger. Stir to coat with oil and cook, stirring a few minutes. Turn heat down to low and cook without lifting the lid for 5 to 8 minutes. After cooking, beans should remain bright green and slightly crunchy. In a small bowl mix cornstarch and sugar with water and soy sauce until smooth. Add to bean and mushroom mixture. Stir and cook over medium heat until sauce is thickened and mixture is heated through.

Yield: 2 cups (353 gm).

	Phenylalanine (mg)	Protein (gm)	Calories
Per recipe	197	6.1	405
Per ¼ cup (44 gm) serving	25	0.8	51

Cauliflower with Beans and Tomatoes

¾ cup (173 gm) stewed
   tomatoes
1 cup (120 gm) cut fresh or
   frozen green beans
2 cups (181 gm) cauliflower,
   cut into small flowerets

½ teaspoon cornstarch
1 tablespoon water
salt to taste

Combine tomatoes and green beans in a small saucepan. Cover and cook over medium heat, about 5 minutes. Add cauliflower; cover and cook an additional 5 minutes. Mix cornstarch with water to a smooth paste and add to cauliflower and beans. Cook and stir until juices thicken, a minute or so. Add salt to taste.

Yield: 2¼ cups (360 gm).

	Phenylalanine (mg)	Protein (gm)	Calories
Per recipe	207	6.4	141
Per ¼ cup (40 gm) serving	23	0.7	16

Potato Apple Skillet

An interesting flavor combination. Leave potato and apple skins on for nice color and extra nutrition.

1 tablespoon vegetable oil
2 cups (243 gm) potatoes, cut
    in ¼-inch strips
salt and pepper to taste
1¼ cups (150 gm) apple, cut in
    chunks

¼ cup (35 gm) chopped onion
3 tablespons (20 gm) sliced
    celery

Heat oil in a skillet with cover. Sprinkle potatoes generously with salt and pepper; add to skillet with apple, onion, and celery. Stir to coat with oil. Cover and cook over low heat until potatoes are tender, about 20 minutes. (To retain more shape to soft apples, wait until potatoes have cooked for 5 to 10 minutes before adding).

Yield: 2½ cups (410 gm).

Family Portion
Remove diet portion. Sprinkle ½ cup shredded cheddar cheese over top of family portion before serving.

	Phenylalanine (mg)	Protein (gm)	Calories
Per diet recipe	244	6.2	417
Per ¼ cup (41 gm) serving	24	0.6	42

Twice-Baked Potatoes

Excellent for the whole family. They freeze well and can conveniently be made in quantity.

For each serving:

1 medium potato (about 130 gm)	salt and pepper to taste
	paprika (optional)
1 teaspoon margarine or butter	
1 teaspoon water, or enough to moisten potatoes as desired	

Scrub potato and use fork tines to prick into the potato several times. Bake at 425° for 40 to 45 minutes or until done. Cut a lengthwise slice from top of long side of potato. Discard skin from the slice. Preserving ¼ inch potato around shell, scoop out inside of potato with a spoon and add to potato portion from top slice.

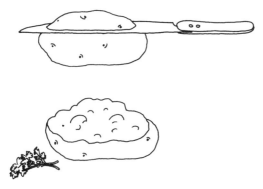

Weigh or measure amount of potato scooped out, to equal 6 tablespoons (60 gm). Mash, then add margarine and water. Season to taste with salt and pepper. Stir in desired stuffing (see *Stuffing Options*). Pile mashed potato mixture into potato shell. Sprinkle with paprika. Place in a baking dish and return to 425° oven for 20 to 25 minutes. The potato can also be stuffed in advance, covered loosely for up to 24 hours, or frozen and reheated.

Yield: 1 serving.

Microwave Instructions

Prick washed potato with fork tines. Microwave on High for 3 to 5 minutes for one potato, or according to oven manufacturer's directions. Stuff potato, then return to microwave for 15 seconds, or if it has been refrigerated prior to serving, microwave for 45 seconds to 1 minute.

Stuffing Options

Carrot Stuffing

2½ tablespoons (18 gm) grated   1 teaspoon margarine or butter
   carrots

Sauté carrots in margarine for 2 to 3 minutes until tender.

	Phenylalanine (mg)	Protein (gm)	Calories
Per potato (not including potato shell)	65	1.6	123

Mushroom Stuffing

2 tablespoons (22 gm) finely   1 teaspoon margarine
   chopped canned
   mushrooms or
   2½ tablespoons (13 gm)
   chopped raw mushrooms

Sauté mushrooms in margarine for 1 minute or until tender.

	Phenylalanine (mg)	Protein (gm)	Calories
Per potato (not including potato shell)	69	1.7	119

Broccoli Stuffing

2 tablespoons (11 gm) finely   1 tablespoon (9 gm) finely
   chopped fresh or frozen   chopped onion
   broccoli   1 teaspoon margarine or butter

Sauté vegetables in margarine for 2 to 3 minutes or until tender.

	Phenylalanine (mg)	Protein (gm)	Calories
Per potato (not including potato shell)	71	1.8	122

Curried Cauliflower Stuffing

2 tablespoons (11 gm) finely
    chopped fresh or frozen
    cauliflower
1 tablespoon (9 gm) finely
    chopped onion

1 teaspoon margarine or butter
¼ teaspoon curry powder
¼ teaspoon dried parsley

Sauté vegetables in margarine for 2 to 3 minutes or until tender.

	Phenylalanine (mg)	Protein (gm)	Calories
Per potato (not including potato shell)	69	1.7	122

Potato Zucchini Curry

An instant hit with cookbook taste-testers.

2 tablespoons margarine or
    butter
1 teaspoon curry powder
2 cups (320 gm) raw potatoes,
    cut in ¾-inch cubes
2 cups (266 gm) zucchini
    squash, ¼-inch slices cut
    in half

½ cup (96 gm) seeded,
    chopped, fresh tomatoes
salt to taste
crushed red pepper (optional)

Melt margarine in a large skillet which has a tightly fitting lid. Stir in curry powder and cook over medium-low heat a few minutes. Add cubed potatoes and stir so that all potatoes are covered with curry. Cover tightly. Increase heat to high; leave heat on high only until a good head of steam has built up under the lid, then immediately turn heat down to medium-low and cook 10 to 15 minutes without lifting the lid. Potatoes will be not quite tender. Add zucchini; stir to coat with curry. Cover and cook about 6 minutes or until zucchini is tender. Stir in tomatoes; replace cover and heat through several minutes. Sprinkle with salt and crushed red pepper as desired.

Yield: 4 cups (690 gm).

	Phenylalanine (mg)	Protein (gm)	Calories
Per recipe	423	11.1	397
Per ¼ cup (43 gm) serving	26	0.7	25

Herb Fried Potatoes

Excellent variation on plain fried potatoes.

3 tablespoons margarine or
butter
3 cups (510 gm) thinly sliced
potatoes
2 tablespoons (18 gm) chopped
onion

2 tablespoons (13 gm) chopped
celery
½ teaspoon oregano
salt and pepper to taste

Melt margarine in a large heavy skillet. Add potatoes and cook over medium high heat, about 15 to 20 minutes, turning carefully until browned. During the last five minutes of cooking mix in the chopped onion, celery, and oregano. Season with salt and pepper before serving.

Yield: 2 cups (346 gm).

	Phenylalanine (mg)	Protein (gm)	Calories
Per recipe	492	11.8	718
Per ¼ cup (38 gm) serving	62	1.5	90

Onion Potatoes

Excellent for the grill.

3 cups (620 gm) peeled,
quartered potatoes
(6 medium potatoes)

¼ cup margarine or butter
1 pkg Knorr French Onion
Soup Mix

Place cut potatoes on a sheet of heavy duty aluminum foil or in a shallow pan which can be covered. Drizzle melted margarine over potatoes, then sprinkle on onion soup mix. Enclose potatoes in aluminum foil and fold edges securely, or cover baking pan with a lid or foil. Bake in an oven at 375° for 45 minutes or on a grill over hot coals for 45 minutes to 1 hour, until potatoes are fork tender.

Yield: 4 cups (660 gm).

	Phenylalanine (mg)	Protein (gm)	Calories
Per recipe	741	17.4	1033
Per ¼ cup (41 gm) serving	46	1.1	65

Potato Onion Bake

Good for grilling, or in the oven.

½ teaspoon celery seed
½ teaspoon garlic salt
½ teaspoon seasoned salt
4 cups (683 gm) peeled, thinly
   sliced potatoes (6 medium
   potatoes)

1 cup (140 gm) thinly sliced
   onion
¼ cup margarine or butter

Combine the dry seasonings in a small bowl. Place one third of the sliced potatoes on a sheet of heavy duty aluminum foil or in a shallow pan that can be covered. Top the potatoes with ⅓ of the onion slices and a sprinkling of ⅓ of the seasonings. Dot with some of the margarine. Repeat the layers twice more. Seal package of foil securely or cover pan tightly. Bake at 375° for 30 minutes, or grill over hot coals for 30 to 35 minutes.

Yield: 4 cups (700 gm).

	Phenylalanine (mg)	Protein (gm)	Calories
Per recipe	696	17.3	1005
Per ¼ cup (44 gm) serving	43	1.1	63

Scalloped Potatoes

Scalloped potato flavor without the cheese or milk.

4 cups (683 gm) peeled, thinly
   sliced potatoes (6 medium)
½ cup (70 gm) minced onion
1 tablespoon minced fresh
   parsley

¾ teaspoon salt
pepper to taste
¼ cup margarine or butter
¾ cup boiling water

In a shallow baking dish, spread potatoes, onion, and parsley. Sprinkle with salt and pepper and dot with margarine. Pour boiling water over all. Bake at 400° for 30 to 40 minutes, until brown and crusty on top and water is absorbed.

Yield: 3 cups (710 gm).

	Phenylalanine (mg)	Protein (gm)	Calories
Per recipe	671	16.4	976
Per ¼ cup (59 gm) serving	56	1.4	81

Hash Browns

For each hash brown patty:

2 tablespoons (33 gm) grated
   raw potatoes
1 teaspoon minced onion

1 tablespoon margarine
   or butter
salt and pepper to taste

After potato is grated, cover it with cold water to rinse off the excess starch; then drain, squeeze out extra water, and pat dry on a paper towel or dish towel until thoroughly dry. Two tablespoons of raw grated potato (33 gm) will make 2 tablespoons (22 gm) grated potato after it has been dried in this manner. To the dry grated potato add 1 teaspoon of minced onion and mix.

Melt margarine in a heavy skillet. Add grated potato and onion to pan. Flatten and spread to about 3 inches in diameter. Add salt and pepper to taste. Cook over medium high heat to brown on both sides, about 5 minutes each side.

Yield: 1 hash brown patty.

	Phenylalanine (mg)	Protein (gm)	Calories
Per patty	37	0.9	129

Potato Pancakes

A German tradition. Serve with hot applesauce sprinkled with cinnamon and sugar.

1 cup (260 gm) grated raw potatoes	½ teaspoon salt
½ cup (70 gm) minced onion	⅛ teaspoon pepper
1 tablespoon cornstarch	2 tablespoons vegetable oil

Combine all ingredients except oil in a bowl; toss to mix thoroughly. Divide mixture into 6 equal portions (55 gm each). Heat the oil in a skillet or on a griddle. Spread potato mixture, flattening into six 3-inch circles. Over medium-high heat, brown on both sides, several minutes.

Yield: 6 pancakes (330 gm).

Family Portion
Top pancakes with sour cream if desired, and serve with sausage.

	Phenylalanine (mg)	Protein (gm)	Calories
Per diet recipe	258	6.5	508
Per pancake (55 gm)	43	1.1	85

Apple-Filled Sweet Potatoes

Almost like dessert.

1½ cups (320 gm) mashed
    sweet potatoes (from canned
    or fresh potato)
2 tablespoons margarine or
    butter
1 tablespoon packed brown
    sugar

½ teaspoon vanilla
¼ teaspoon nutmeg
2½ cups (300 gm) apples,
    peeled and cut into ½-inch
    chunks
1 tablespoon granulated sugar
¼ teaspoon cinnamon

To mashed sweet potato, add margarine, brown sugar, vanilla, and nutmeg in a mixing bowl. Blend on medium speed of electric mixer until mixture is light and fluffy. In a small saucepan over medium heat, bring apples and water to boiling; cover and simmer 8 to 10 minutes, until apples are tender but not mushy. Drain. Sprinkle with sugar and cinnamon mixed together. Spoon sweet potato mixture into a 1-quart casserole. With a spoon, make an indentation in center of sweet potatoes; place apples in indentation. Bake at 400° for 15 minutes.

Yield: 1¾ cups (665 gm).

	Phenylalanine (mg)	Protein (gm)	Calories
Per recipe	394	6.2	812
Per 2 tablespoons (48 gm) serving	28	0.4	58

Candied Sweets

½ cup packed brown sugar
¼ cup unsweetened pineapple
   juice or orange juice
¼ teaspoon ground cinnamon
⅛ teaspoon nutmeg

17 oz can sweet potatoes,
   drained
1 tablespoon margarine
   or butter

In a bowl, combine sugar, pineapple juice or orange juice, cinnamon, and nutmeg. Slice sweet potatoes in half, then cut each piece in half again. Place potatoes in a 1-quart casserole or baking pan. Pour liquid over top. Dot with margarine. Bake, uncovered, at 350° for 40 to 45 minutes or until potatoes are nicely glazed and most of the liquid is absorbed. While potatoes are baking, spoon glaze over top several times.

Yield: 3 cups (630 gm).

	Phenylalanine (mg)	Protein (gm)	Calories
Per recipe	498	7.4	979
Per ¼ cup (53 gm) serving	41	0.6	82

Candied Sweet Potatoes

¼ cup margarine or butter
¼ cup packed brown sugar
¼ cup water

17 oz can sweet potatoes,
   drained

Combine margarine, brown sugar, and water in a medium skillet. When margarine is melted and mixture is bubbly, add sweet potatoes. In a large skillet cook over low heat, turning potatoes occasionally, for about 10 to 15 minutes or until sugar-margarine mixture is reduced to a thick glaze.

Yield: 3 cups (463 gm).

	Phenylalanine (mg)	Protein (gm)	Calories
Per recipe	508	7.4	1049
Per ¼ cup (39 gm) serving	42	0.6	87

Spicy Candied Yams

17 oz can yams or sweet
  potatoes, drained
3 tablespoons packed brown
  sugar
2 tablespoons margarine or
  butter, cut in pieces

½ cup Rich's Coffee Rich
½ teaspoon cinnamon
¼ teaspoon ginger
¼ teaspoon cloves
⅔ cup (26 gm) mini
  marshmallows

Mash sweet potatoes or yams in a 1-quart casserole. Stir in brown sugar, margarine, Rich's Coffee Rich, and spices. Top with marshmallows. Bake at 350°, uncovered, for 15 minutes; or microwave on 70% power for 5 minutes.

Yield: 2⅔ cups (670 gm).

	Phenylalanine (mg)	Protein (gm)	Calories
Per recipe	528	7.9	1049
Per 2 tablespoons (31 gm) serving	25	0.4	49

Sweet Shepherd's Pie

1 cup (88 gm) chopped fresh or
   frozen broccoli
2 tablespoons (18 gm) chopped
   onion
2 teaspoons vegetable oil
¾ cup (101 gm) sliced carrots

¼ cup water
3 tablespoons tomato sauce
⅔ cup (142 gm) mashed fresh
   or canned sweet potatoes
1 tablespoon water

Cut broccoli into flowerets and stems into thin slices. In a skillet, sauté onion in oil for 1 to 2 minutes until soft. Add broccoli, carrots, and water. Bring to a boil, cover, and turn heat to low. Simmer 10 to 15 minutes, until vegetables are just tender. Stir in tomato sauce. Put into a 1-quart casserole, or individual casseroles. Mix sweet potato with water. Spread potato over top of vegetables. Bake at 350° for 15 minutes. Shake cinnamon or paprika over top before serving, if desired.

Yield: 2 cups plus 2 tablespoons (420 gm).

	Phenylalanine (mg)	Protein (gm)	Calories
Per recipe	293	6.9	316
Per ¼ cup (49 gm) serving	34	0.8	37

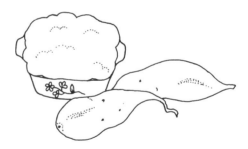

The Great Stuffed Pumpkin

Children will love to help with this at Halloween time. The combination of ingredients will surprise you but the flavor is rich and so fitting with the pumpkin. You could make up other combinations for the filling that would also work well.

1⅓ cups (180 gm) sliced
   carrots
¼ cup (35 gm) chopped onion
½ cup (85 gm) diced potatoes
1 medium tomato (180 gm),
   diced
8 dried apricots
¼ cup (40 gm) raisins
2 tablespoons margarine or
   butter, cut up

¼ teaspoon cinnamon
⅛ teaspoon nutmeg
¼ teaspoon dried thyme
   (optional)
1 pkg G. Washington's Golden
   Seasoning and Broth, or
   salt to taste
1 cup boiling water
one 3 to 5 lb pumpkin
   (preferably pie-type)

Prepare vegetables. Mix all ingredients, except pumpkin, together in a bowl. Cut off pumpkin top. Scoop out seeds and stringy pulp. Rub inside of pumpkin with a little salt. Fill pumpkin with vegetable-fruit-margarine-spice mixture (if you have too much for the pumpkin, bake in a separate casserole for 1 hour, or until vegetables are tender). Bake at 375° for 1½ to 2 hours or until pumpkin tests tender with a fork. Serve pumpkin filling directly from pumpkin. Scrape out pumpkin with a spoon in portions desired, serving plain or mixed with filling (1 or 2 tablespoons pumpkin would be a reasonable child's portion).

Yield: 3⅓ cups stuffing (650 gm).

Note
Do not omit apricots; they add a delicious flavor.

	Phenylalanine (mg)	Protein (gm)	Calories
Per recipe	266	8.3	592
Per ¼ cup (49 gm) serving stuffing	20	0.6	44
Per 1 tablespoon (13 gm) pumpkin	5	0.1	4

Simple Squash

Very similar in taste to sweet potatoes but lower in protein.

¼ cup (60 gm) cooked
  butternut squash
2 teaspoons packed brown
  sugar
½ teaspoon margarine or
  butter

dash of salt
dash of cinnamon
5 mini marshmallows

Peel a butternut squash with a potato peeler; cut into small cubes. In a medium saucepan, add water just enough to cover squash. Cook over medium heat for 20 to 25 minutes, or until squash is very tender. Remove from heat; pour off excess water. Mash squash.

For a convenient premeasured diet portion, measure ¼ cup (60 gm) mashed squash. Place in an individual casserole or on a double layer of aluminum foil. Mix in brown sugar, margarine, salt, and cinnamon; top with marshmallows. Heat at 350° for a few minutes, until marshmallows melt.

Yield: 1 serving.

Family Portion

Measure remaining mashed squash. Follow recipe for each ¼ cup squash. Put desired portion in an individual casserole or small baking dish.

	Phenylalanine (mg)	Protein (gm)	Calories
Per ¼ cup (78 gm) serving	37	0.9	83

Squash and Apple Casserole

A tasty dish which is appealing to even the youngest child.

1¼ cups (300 gm) mashed or
  puréed acorn squash
½ cup (120 gm) applesauce
1 tablespoon packed brown
  sugar

1 tablespoon margarine
  or butter
¼ teaspoon salt
½ teaspoon cinnamon
dash of nutmeg

Cut a medium to large squash in half, remove seeds, and bake at 350° for 1 hour or until tender. While squash is baking, cook one apple cut in six slices in 2 tablespoons water in a saucepan, for 5 to 10 minutes or until very soft. Purée as for making applesauce, in food mill or blender, measuring ½ cup (120 gm).

When squash is tender, cut cooked halves into sixths and remove skins with a knife. Mash or purée and measure 1¼ cups (306 gm). Mix squash and applesauce together. Add sugar, margarine, salt, cinnamon, and nutmeg; mix well.

Diet Portion

Remove diet portion, placing in a small individual casserole. Sprinkle with 1 tablespoon dry low protein bread or Aproten Rusk crumbs mixed with 1 teaspoon melted margarine. Bake at 425° for 15 to 20 minutes or microwave on High for 1 minute.

Family Portion

To remainder of squash, add a mixture of ¼ cup chopped pecans or walnuts. Sprinkle ¼ cup dry bread crumbs mixed with 2 teaspoons of melted margarine over casserole before baking. Bake at 425° for 20 to 30 minutes or microwave on High for 2 to 3 minutes.

Yield: 1¾ cups (466 gm).

Note

½ cup commercially prepared applesauce could be substituted for homemade; or ½ cup pear sauce, made from puréeing about 1½ fresh cooked pears, is a delicious substitute for applesauce. Nutrient values will remain approximately the same.

	Phenylalanine (mg)	Protein (gm)	Calories
Per diet recipe	193	4.8	467
Per ¼ cup (66 gm) serving	28	0.7	67

Glazed Acorn Rings

2 medium acorn squash
  (about 1 lb each)
⅓ cup orange juice
⅓ cup packed brown sugar
3 tablespoons light Karo corn
  syrup or honey

3 tablespoons margarine
  or butter
½ teaspoon cinnamon
2 teaspoons grated fresh
  orange rind (optional)
⅛ teaspoon salt

Cut off ends of squash and discard. Cut each squash crosswise, into 3 rings (total of 6 rings). Remove seeds with a spoon. Place squash rings in a single layer in a 13 × 9-inch baking pan. Pour in orange juice. Cover and bake at 350° for 30 to 40 minutes, or until tender.

Combine brown sugar, syrup or honey, margarine, cinnamon, orange rind, and salt in a small saucepan; simmer 5 minutes over low heat. Pour over squash rings and bake uncovered, 15 minutes longer, basting 1 or 2 times. To serve, spoon remaining sauce over squash rings.

Yield: 6 squash rings.

Note

Nutrient calculations are based on an estimate that from an average squash slice (110 to 120 gm before baking) you will get approximately 2½ tablespoons (40 gm) of cooked squash.

	Phenylalanine (mg)	Protein (gm)	Calories
Per recipe	167	4.3	906
Per squash ring	28	0.7	151

Zucchini Dinner

This is a bright and colorful dish, especially nice for summer.

2 cups (266 gm) zucchini
    squash, ⅜-inch thick slices
⅔ cup (50 gm) sliced fresh
    mushrooms
2 tablespoons (14 gm) sliced
    green onion
½ clove garlic, minced

2 teaspoons vegetable oil
3 tablespoons tomato sauce
½ cup (96 gm) diced fresh
    tomatoes
1 tablespoon chopped fresh
    parsley or basil
salt and pepper to taste

Cook zucchini in a small amount of water or in vegetable steamer 6 to 7 minutes, until just tender. Meanwhile, in a skillet sauté mushrooms, onion, and garlic in oil for 1 to 2 minutes. In a 1-quart casserole, mix together zucchini and sautéed vegetables. Mix in tomato sauce and fresh tomatoes. Add salt and pepper to taste. Bake, uncovered, at 350° for 10 to 15 minutes.

Yield: 2½ cups (413 gm).

Family Portion

Remove diet portion. Sprinkle grated parmesan cheese on top of family portion, or add ½ lb browned ground beef or sausage for use as a vegetable spaghetti sauce.

	Phenylalanine (mg)	Protein (gm)	Calories
Per diet recipe	197	6.1	188
Per ¼ cup (40 gm) serving	20	0.6	19

Zucchini Stuffing Casserole

1 cup (134 gm) sliced zucchini
squash
3 tablespoons (25 gm)
shredded or grated carrots
1 tablespoon (20 gm) chopped
onion
1 tablespoon margarine or
butter

3 tablespoons condensed
Campbell's Cream of
Mushroom Soup
1 tablespoon water
¼ teaspoon salt
¼ teaspoon sage or other
herb seasoning
½ cup *Low Pro Croutons*

Cook zucchini in a small amount of water, or steam until tender; drain. Grate carrot and onion (in a blender with a small amount of water makes it easy; drain). Sauté carrot and onion in margarine for 2 minutes; remove from heat. Stir in undiluted soup and water. Mix in zucchini, seasonings, and croutons. Put mixture into a greased 2-cup casserole or into individual casseroles. Bake at 350° for 20 minutes, or microwave on High for 2 to 3 minutes.

Yield: 1¼ cups (220 gm).

Family Portion
Prepare any multiple of the basic diet recipe, using seasoned bread stuffing cubes in place of low protein croutons. Add 1 to 2 tablespoons sour cream in place of water. Sprinkle top of casserole with grated parmesan cheese if desired.

	Phenylalanine (mg)	Protein (gm)	Calories
Per diet recipe	125	3.5	261
Per ¼ cup (44 gm) serving	25	0.7	52

Zucchini Sauté

2 tablespoons vegetable oil
⅓ cup (47 gm) chopped onion
1 large clove garlic, minced
2 cups (267 gm) sliced
    zucchini squash

¾ cup (144 gm) seeded,
    chopped, fresh tomatoes
¼ teaspoon basil
¼ teaspoon salt

Heat oil in a small skillet. Sauté onion and garlic in oil until onion is tender, about 5 minutes. Add zucchini, tomatoes, and seasonings. Cook, uncovered, over medium heat until vegetables are tender and liquid thickened, about 10 minutes.

Yield: 1⅔ cups (365 gm).

	Phenylalanine (mg)	Protein (gm)	Calories
Per recipe	148	4.8	341
Per ¼ cup (55 gm) serving	22	0.7	51

Mediterranean Vegetable Casserole

A tasty version of the traditional Italian "ratatouille."

3 cups (260 gm) eggplant
    (approximately 1 medium),
    peeled and cut into ¾-inch
    chunks
½ cup (70 gm) chopped onion
1 clove garlic, minced
2 tablespoons vegetable oil

1½ cups (200 gm) sliced
    zucchini squash
¾ cup (96 gm) chopped
    green pepper
1 teaspoon dried basil
6 tablespoons tomato paste
salt and pepper to taste

In a medium skillet, sauté eggplant, onion, and garlic in 1 tablespoon of the oil until vegetables are tender, about 5 minutes. Add zucchini, green pepper, and basil to the skillet and continue cooking 2 minutes. Combine tomato paste with remaining 1 tablespoon oil and add to skillet, mixing well. Cover tightly and cook on medium heat 10 minutes to heat through. Add salt and pepper to taste.

Yield: 3 cups (535 gm).

	Phenylalanine (mg)	Protein (gm)	Calories
Per recipe	330	10.1	458
Per ¼ cup (45 gm) serving	28	0.8	38

Spanish Eggplant

Also good as a taco or burrito filling.

2 tablespoons vegetable oil
1 cup (120 gm) peeled
 eggplant, cut in ½-inch
 cubes
½ cup (64 gm) green pepper,
 cut in short strips

½ cup (53 gm) chopped celery
¼ cup (35 gm) chopped onion
½ cup tomato juice or
 6 tablespoons tomato sauce
 plus 2 tablespoons water
salt and pepper to taste

Heat oil in a medium skillet. Sauté eggplant, green pepper, celery, and onion in oil until vegetables are tender, about 8 to 10 minutes. Add tomato juice, or sauce and water, and cook on medium heat until slightly thickened. Season with salt and pepper.

Yield: 1 cup plus 2 tablespoons (276 gm).

	Phenylalanine (mg)	Protein (gm)	Calories
Per recipe	127	3.8	336
Per ¼ cup (64 gm) serving	30	0.9	78

Oven-Fried Eggplant

Irresistibly delicious way to fix eggplant that kids like too. Zucchini squash pieces could be prepared in the same manner.

1 cup (87 gm) peeled eggplant,
   cut in ⅜-inch-wide strips
¼ cup margarine or butter
⅓ cup (30 gm) fine dry low
   protein bread crumbs or
   crushed Aproten rusks

¼ teaspoon salt

Preheat oven to 375°. Cut eggplant in strips as for french fries. Melt margarine. Mix crumbs and salt. Dig eggplant strips in melted margarine; roll in crumbs. Place on an ungreased cookie sheet in a single layer. Bake for 15 to 20 minutes, until light golden brown.

Yield: 24 strips.

Family Portion
Use the same technique as for diet portion, using regular cracker or bread crumbs to coat eggplant.

	Phenylalanine (mg)	Protein (gm)	Calories
Per diet recipe	69	1.5	553
Per ¼ recipe (6 strips)	17	0.4	138

Stuffed Cabbage Rolls

1 medium head of cabbage
½ cup (88 gm) uncooked
   regular rice
¼ cup (35 gm) chopped onion
¼ cup (26 gm) chopped celery

½ cup (68 gm) chopped carrots
2 tablespoons vegetable oil
1 teaspoon cinnamon
2 cups tomato sauce

Blanch the cabbage. Remove outer damaged leaves from cabbage and core with a sharp knife. Place head of cabbage in a large saucepan with ½ cup water and cover. Bring to a boil over high heat until steam is escaping from the edge of the pan lid. Immediately turn down to low and cook for 5 minutes. Remove cabbage from the pan to drain and cool.

When cabbage is cool enough to handle carefully, remove the best 16 leaves. If the inner section is not cooked enough to be pliable, repeat the 5-minute cooking process on the inner section. Leaves used should be approximately the same size (30 to 40 gm). Two smaller leaves can be overlapped to be used as one, as necessary. Trim the thick stem part of the leaf to be thin so the leaves will roll easily. Chop enough of the remaining center of cabbage to equal 1 cup.

Place rice in a saucepan with 1 cup salted water. Bring to a simmer on high, then cover and turn down to simmer 15 minutes. Sauté onion, celery, and carrot in oil about 5 minutes. In a medium bowl mix cooked rice, sautéed vegetables, 1 cup of chopped cabbage, cinnamon, and ½ cup tomato sauce.

Place 3 tablespoons of filling on the edge of each cabbage leaf. Fold over the ribbed end of the leaf, then fold over the two sides and roll

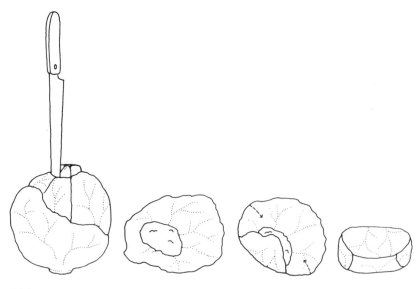

up. Place rolls in a shallow baking dish, flap side down. Pour the remainder of the tomato sauce over the rolls. Cover the dish and bake at 350° for 40 minutes.

Yield: 16 cabbage rolls.

Family Portion

Prepare recipe as is, then remove diet portion desired. For family portion, add ¼ to ½ lb cooked ground beef to the remaining filling. Identify the diet cabbage rolls with a toothpick.

	Phenylalanine (mg)	Protein (gm)	Calories
Per diet recipe	675	16.3	836
Per cabbage roll	42	1.0	52

Sweet and Tangy Cabbage

Apple flavor predominates in this delicious way to prepare cabbage.

¼ cup (35 gm) chopped onion
1 tablespoon vegetable oil
3 cups (269 gm) shredded
   cabbage
1½ cups (180 gm) coarsely
   chopped, unpeeled apples

½ cup water
1 tablespoon vinegar
1½ teaspoons cornstarch
1½ teaspoons packed brown
   sugar
½ teaspoon salt

In a large saucepan with a tight fitting lid, sauté onion in oil until soft, about 5 minutes. Add cabbage, apple, and ¼ cup of the water. Cover tightly. Cook on high heat just until steam is escaping from the edge of the lid, then turn down to low and cook 5 minutes. In a small bowl or jar mix together the remaining ¼ cup of water, vinegar, cornstarch, brown sugar, and salt. Add to cabbage mixture after the 5 minutes of cooking and cook, stirring until thickened, about 5 minutes.

Yield: 2⅓ cups (524 gm).

	Phenylalanine (mg)	Protein (gm)	Calories
Per recipe	127	3.5	365
Per ¼ cup (56 gm) serving	14	0.4	39

Fried Okra

The okra retains a lovely bright green color and is not at all gummy.

1½ cups (128 gm) sliced fresh
    okra
1 to 2 tablespoons cornstarch
2 tablespoons margarine or
    butter

½ cup (96 gm) seeded,
    chopped, fresh tomatoes
¼ cup (35 gm) chopped onion

Sprinkle cornstarch over sliced okra. Mix until coated. Set aside. Melt margarine in a medium skillet. Add tomatoes and onion and cook several minutes until tender. Add okra; fry a few minutes until crisp-tender.

Yield: 1⅓ cups (205 gm).

	Phenylalanine (mg)	Protein (gm)	Calories
Per recipe	119	3.7	310
Per ¼ cup (38 gm) serving	22	0.7	58

Steamed Okra

A flavorful way to "fix-up" okra.

¼ cup (35 gm) chopped onion
1 tablespoon vegetable oil
⅓ cup tomato sauce
⅓ cup water
½ teaspoon garlic salt
salt and pepper to taste

½ teaspoon Worcestershire
    sauce
¼ teaspoon oregano
¼ teaspoon granulated sugar
1½ cups (128 gm) sliced okra

In a medium skillet, sauté onion in oil until tender, several minutes. Add tomato sauce, water, seasonings, and sugar. Cook a few minutes over low heat. Add okra, stirring to blend. Cover and cook 10 minutes over low heat, or until okra is tender.

Yield: 1⅓ cups (196 gm).

	Phenylalanine (mg)	Protein (gm)	Calories
Per recipe	120	4.0	198
Per ¼ cup (37 gm) serving	23	0.8	37

Creamed Spinach

1 teaspoon margarine or butter   ¼ cup Rich's Coffee Rich
1 teaspoon wheat starch or
   Wel-Plan Baking Mix
¼ cup (45 gm) chopped,
   cooked, fresh or frozen
   spinach

Melt margarine in a small saucepan. Blend in wheat starch or Baking Mix and cook a few minutes. Add Coffee Rich and cook, stirring until thickened. Mix in spinach and cook until heated through.

Yield: ⅓ cup (90 gm).

Note
This recipe makes two servings. The second portion can be frozen and reheated in a microwave oven on High until heated through (about 30 to 45 seconds).

	Phenylalanine (mg)	Protein (gm)	Calories
Per recipe	75	1.6	140
Per 2½ tablespoons (45 gm) serving	37	0.8	70

Stroganoff

Wine imparts a delicious flavor that masks the slight sweetness of Coffee Rich. Alcohol from the wine evaporates in cooking.

2 teaspoons margarine or
   butter
2 tablespoons (18 gm) chopped
   onion
⅔ cup (50 gm) sliced fresh
   mushrooms

2 teaspoons cornstarch
¼ cup dry white wine or water
¼ cup Rich's Coffee Rich
salt and pepper to taste

Melt margarine in a small skillet; sauté onion and mushrooms in margarine over medium heat until tender. Sprinkle in cornstarch and stir to coat vegetables. Stir in wine or water and Coffee Rich and bring to a boil. Cook and stir until thickened. Season with salt and pepper to taste. Serve over rice or low protein pasta.

Yield: ⅔ cup (145 gm).

	Phenylalanine (mg)	Protein (gm)	Calories
Per recipe	60	1.5	185
Per ⅓ cup (72 gm) serving (not including rice or pasta)	30	0.7	93

Lasagna Swirls

Nice to serve when others have lasagna, or serve these for the whole family as a side or main dish.

3 regular lasagna noodles
  (76 gm dry, 180 gm cooked)
6 tablespoons (80 gm)
  chopped, cooked, and
  squeezed fresh or frozen
  spinach
3 tablespoons (45 gm)
  condensed Campbell's
  Cream of Mushroom Soup

⅛ teaspoon nutmeg (optional)
dash of salt
6 tablespoons tomato sauce or
  Easy Spaghetti Sauce
6 tablespoons water

Cook lasagna noodles according to package directions, until tender but not overcooked. Rinse with cold water and drain. Stretch out flat. Mix spinach, soup, and nutmeg in a bowl. Add a dash of salt. Cut cooked lasagna noodles in half crosswise so you have 6 noodles (30 gm) each. Spread 1½ tablespoons (20 gm) of spinach mixture thinly on each of the noodles, leaving the last ½ inch without spinach.

Roll up noodles, as for a jellyroll, and place rolls in a greased casserole or baking dish, seam side down. Mix tomato sauce and water together. Put 2 tablespoons diluted tomato sauce or spaghetti sauce over the top of each roll. Cover and bake 20 minutes at 350°.

Yield: 6 lasagna swirls.

Storage Tip
These can be made in advance and refrigerated, or frozen and thawed; bake an extra 5 minutes.

Family Portion
Make any multiple of the recipe, to suit family needs. Add 1 tablespoon ricotta cheese to each 1 tablespoon mixture for a main dish serving and/or add 1 tablespoon cooked hamburger to each 3 tablespoons sauce.

	Phenylalanine (mg)	Protein (gm)	Calories
Per diet recipe	895	19.6	211
Per lasagna swirl	149	3.2	35

Mushroom Stew

A nice, filling meal served over (or with) *Biscuit Topper.*

2 tablespoons margarine or
   butter
2 tablespoons vegetable oil
2 cups (150 gm) sliced fresh
   mushrooms
1 bay leaf
½ clove garlic, minced
½ cup (70 gm) chopped onion
½ teaspoon basil
½ teaspoon thyme

1 pkg G. Washington's Rich
   Brown or Golden Seasoning
   and Broth, or salt to taste
½ cup water mixed with
   2 teaspoons cornstarch
1 cup (230 gm) canned
   tomatoes, cut in small
   pieces
½ cup tomato juice from
   tomatoes

In a medium skillet, melt 1 tablespoon margarine with 1 table-spoon oil. Sauté mushrooms over high heat several minutes, stirring often; remove to a dish. Add remaining margarine and oil to skillet along with remaining ingredients. Return mushrooms to skillet. Simmer over medium-low heat for about 20 minutes. Remove bay leaf.

Yield: 1½ cups (275 gm).

Family Portion
Remove diet portion. Add ¾ to 1 lb of cooked ground meat or stew meat. Serve the stew over or with regular baking powder–type biscuits.

	Phenylalanine (mg)	Protein (gm)	Calories
Per diet recipe	182	5.2	584
Per ¼ cup (46 gm) serving	30	0.9	97

Rice and Mushrooms

½ cup (88 gm) uncooked
  regular rice
2⅔ cups (200 gm) sliced fresh
  mushrooms
¼ cup (35 gm) chopped onion
½ cup (96 gm) seeded, chopped,
  fresh tomatoes
3 tablespoons vegetable oil

1 pkg G. Washington's Golden
  Seasoning and Broth, or
  extra salt and seasoning of
  your choice
1 cup water
¼ cup white wine or water
¼ teaspoon salt
dash pepper

In a large skillet, sauté rice, mushrooms, and onion in hot oil until onion is tender, about 8 minutes, stirring occasionally. Dissolve broth powder in 1 cup boiling water. Add broth, wine or additional water, salt, and pepper to skillet; mix well. Bring to a boil, cover, and reduce heat to low, simmering 20 minutes. Mix in tomatoes and heat through. Add salt and pepper.

Yield: 2⅓ cups (530 gm).

	Phenylalanine (mg)	Protein (gm)	Calories
Per recipe	528	11.7	770
Per ¼ cup (57 gm) serving	57	1.3	83

Variation

Low Rice and Mushrooms

Use ⅓ cup (44 gm) uncooked regular rice and ¼ cup (38 gm) uncooked Aproten Ditalini in place of the ½ cup regular rice.

Yield: 2⅓ cups (583 gm).

	Phenylalanine (mg)	Protein (gm)	Calories
Per recipe	367	8.7	745
Per ¼ cup (57 gm) serving	39	0.9	80

Family Portion plus Low Rice and Mushrooms

Follow the original *Rice and Mushrooms* recipe as is. While it is cooking, cook, rinse, and drain 2 tablespoons Aproten Ditalini according to package directions. When rice is ready, mix ¼ cup of it with the ¼ cup cooked low protein pasta to make ½ cup. Nutrient content will be the same per serving as *Low Rice and Mushrooms*.

Stuffed Mushrooms

A treat for mushroom lovers.

4 large fresh mushrooms, approximately 2 inches in diameter (about 25 gm each)
2 teaspoons margarine or butter
2 teaspoons (6 gm) finely chopped onion
1 tablespoon (7 gm) finely chopped celery

2 teaspoons fine dry low protein bread crumbs or Aproten Rusk crumbs
1 teaspoon water
⅛ teaspoon salt
⅛ teaspoon thyme
⅛ teaspoon sage
⅛ teaspoon parsley flakes

Wash mushrooms; pat dry. Remove stems by breaking them off so that they leave a cavity to stuff. Finely chop enough of the stems to make 1 tablespoon. Discard remainder.

Melt margarine in a medium skillet and add mushroom caps, cavity side up. Cover and cook over medium heat about 5 minutes, until liquid appears inside the caps. Turn caps over; cover and cook an additional 4 to 5 minutes. Remove caps to a small shallow baking pan. To the liquid and margarine left in the pan add the onion, celery, and chopped mushrooms. Cook over medium heat an additional 5 minutes, until vegetables are tender. Add crumbs, water, and seasoning. Let stand a few minutes so crumbs absorb moisture. Divide stuffing equally among the 4 mushroom caps. Bake at 350° for 15 minutes.

Yield: 4 stuffed mushrooms.

Family Portion
Prepare any multiple of the diet recipe, to suit family needs, using regular bread crumbs. Add chopped nuts and/or parmesan cheese to filling if desired. Allow 4 mushrooms per person for a filling side dish.

	Phenylalanine (mg)	Protein (gm)	Calories
Per diet recipe	67	2.2	120
Per mushroom	17	0.6	30

Veggie Spaghetti

This sauce makes the perfect base for a meatless meal for the whole family.

2 tablespoons vegetable oil	½ cup (70 gm) chopped onion
2 cups (267 gm) sliced zucchini squash	1 garlic clove, minced
1 cup (75 gm) sliced fresh mushrooms	1 cup *Best Homemade Tomato Sauce,* or 1 cup canned tomato sauce
½ cup (64 gm) sliced green pepper	

Heat oil in a medium skillet. Sauté zucchini, mushrooms, green pepper, onion, and garlic in oil until tender, about 8 minutes. Mix tomato sauce into the vegetables. Cover and cook over medium heat a few minutes to heat through. Serve over low protein pasta.

Yield: 3⅓ cups (751 gm).

Family Portion
Serve sauce over regular cooked spaghetti. Top each serving with parmesan cheese.

	Phenylalanine (mg)	Protein (gm)	Calories
Using canned tomato sauce			
Per diet recipe	300	9.7	430
Per ¼ cup (50 gm) serving (not including pasta)	20	0.6	29
Using Best Homemade Tomato Sauce			
Per diet recipe	303	10.0	500
Per ¼ cup (56 gm) serving (not including pasta)	20	0.7	33

Mushroom Burgers

These tasty "burgers" can be served plain or in a *Burger Bun.*

3 cups (225 gm) very finely
    chopped fresh mushrooms
    (do not use canned
    mushrooms)
¾ cup (105 gm) finely chopped
    onion
⅔ cup (50 gm) fine dry low
    protein bread crumbs or
    crushed Aproten rusks

¼ teaspoon salt
1 medium egg, beaten
2 tablespoons catsup
1 tablespoon Wel-Plan
    Baking Mix
vegetable oil for frying

Combine all ingredients in a bowl and mix thoroughly. With hands, press mixture into 9 patties, about ⅜-inch thick. Heat vegetable oil in a skillet, using an ample quantity to prevent sticking. Brown patties on both sides over medium heat, 1½ to 2 minutes per side.

Yield: 9 burgers.

Note

Mushroom Burgers can conveniently be made using a food processor (a blender will not satisfactorily chop mushrooms). Using the steel blade, make fine bread crumbs first; remove to a bowl. Next, chop onions; remove to the bowl. Finally, chop mushrooms. Be careful not to overprocess or mushrooms will become mushy; pulse, with the steel blade in, just a few times. Remove steel blade and mix in remaining ingredients by hand so that mushrooms are not overprocessed.

Storage Tip

Uncooked patties may also be frozen. Stack with wax paper between each one in an airtight container. Remove òne at a time as needed, thaw and fry.

	Phenylalanine (mg)	Protein (gm)	Calories
Per recipe	539	12.4	779
Per burger	60	1.4	87

Low Mushroom Burgers

These are somewhat fragile but are very tasty, and with care will hold together.

1 cup (75 gm) very finely
  chopped fresh mushrooms
  (do not use canned
  mushrooms)
¼ cup (35 gm) finely chopped
  onion

3 tablespoons (15 gm) fine dry
  low protein bread crumbs or
  crushed Aproten rusks
⅛ teaspoon salt
1 tablespoon catsup
1 teaspoon water
vegetable oil for frying

Follow directions for *Mushroom Burgers*, forming mixture into 3 patties.

Yield: 3 burgers.

	Phenylalanine (mg)	Protein (gm)	Calories
Per recipe	81	2.3	224
Per burger	27	0.8	75

Broccoli Burgers

An appealing way to serve a vegetable. Serve plain, with catsup, or in a *Burger Bun*.

1 cup (110 gm) very finely
    chopped fresh broccoli
¼ cup (35 gm) finely chopped
    onion
½ cup (45 gm) fine dry low
    protein bread crumbs or
    crushed Aproten rusks

¼ teaspoon salt
1½ tablespoons catsup
1 tablespoon water
vegetable oil for frying

Combine all ingredients in a bowl and mix thoroughly. With hands, press mixture into 6 patties. Heat vegetable oil in a skillet, using an ample quantity to prevent sticking. Brown patties on both sides over medium heat, 1½ to 2 minutes per side.

Yield: 6 burgers.

Note

Broccoli Burgers can conveniently be made using a blender, or better, using a food processor. Using the steel blade of food processor, make the bread crumbs first; remove to a bowl, then chop broccoli and onion using steel blade of food processor. Return crumbs and mix in remaining ingredients with a few pulses.

Storage Tip

Uncooked patties may be frozen. Stack with wax paper between each one in an airtight container. Remove one at a time as needed, thaw and fry.

	Phenylalanine (mg)	Protein (gm)	Calories
Per recipe	127	4.5	484
Per burger	21	0.7	81

Crepes

A fun way to serve vegetables and definitely worth the effort if you freeze extras for a later time. Excellent flavor and texture, surprisingly like the "regular" version.

7 tablespoons (48 gm) Wel-Plan
    Baking Mix
1½ tablespoons (13 gm)
    Softasilk cake flour (do not
    use regular flour)
1 teaspoon baking powder
¼ teaspoon salt

2 teaspoons granulated sugar
1 tablespoon plus 1 teaspoon
    vegetable oil
¾ cup water with 1 drop yellow
    food coloring
3 tablespoons margarine or
    butter

Combine Baking Mix, cake flour, baking powder, salt, and sugar. In a measuring cup, combine vegetable oil and water mixed with food coloring. Add to dry ingredients and mix until smooth.

For each crepe, in a 7- to 8-inch skillet or crepe pan, melt 1 teaspoon margarine over medium-high heat. When margarine begins to bubble, pour in about 2 tablespoons batter and quickly swirl pan in a circular motion to allow batter to spread in an even layer (don't worry about ragged edges). Cook for 45 seconds to 1 minute on first side (until batter looks set), then carefully turn over with a spatula (crepe should be lightly browned). Cook second side for about 30 seconds. Remove to a plate by turning pan upside down on top of plate.

Continue cooking each crepe in the same manner, stacking crepes with wax paper or paper toweling in between as they are finished. Put desired filling down the center of each crepe and roll up. Place seam side down in a lightly greased baking dish. Bake at 350° for 12 to 15 minutes.

Yield: 9 crepes.

Storage Tip

Baked crepes freeze well, either filled or unfilled. If unfilled, stack with wax paper between each crepe and place on a paper plate to provide stability. Before filling, thaw and heat slightly in a toaster oven, in a skillet or in microwave oven to facilitate rolling.

	Phenylalanine (mg)	Protein (gm)	Calories
Per recipe	71	1.6	696
Per crepe	8	0.2	77

Asparagus Crepes

A "low" and satisfying main dish which can be frozen for convenient use.

¾ cup (93 gm) fresh or frozen asparagus, cut in small pieces

¼ cup (57 gm) condensed Campbell's Cream of Mushroom Soup

9 prepared *Crepes*

Cook fresh asparagus for 5 to 6 minutes, or frozen asparagus according to package directions. Mix undiluted soup with drained vegetables. Spread 1½ tablespoons of this mixture down center of each crepe. Fold sides over each other. Place the crepes you wish to serve right away in a lightly greased baking dish. Bake at 350° for 10 to 15 minutes, covered, to thoroughly heat. Wrap and freeze unbaked crepes. If desired, for each 2 crepes you wish to bake, mix 1 tablespoon cream of mushroom soup with 1 tablespoon water and spoon over crepes before baking.

Yield: filling for 9 crepes (¾ cup plus 2 tablespoons).

Family Portion

Prepare a regular crepe batter and make 6-inch diameter for adult size. Make vegetable filling recipe as is, or add ¼ cup cooked chicken cut in small pieces to each 1 cup vegetable-soup mixture for a main dish crepe. Use 2 tablespoons filling for each crepe. Serve 2 to 3 crepes per person for a main dish and 1 to 2 crepes for a side dish.

	Phenylalanine (mg)	Protein (gm)	Calories
Per diet recipe	189	5.5	761
Per crepe (including filling)	21	0.6	85
Per crepe plus 1 tablespoon sauce	27	0.7	91

Broccoli Crepes

¾ cup (83 gm) fresh or frozen broccoli, cut in very small pieces

¼ cup (57 gm) condensed Campbell's Cream of Mushroom Soup

9 prepared *Crepes*

Cook fresh broccoli for 5 to 7 minutes, or frozen broccoli according to package directions. Mix undiluted soup with drained vegetables. Spread 1½ tablespoons of this mixture down center of each crepe. Fold sides over each other. Place the crepes you wish to serve right away in a lightly greased baking dish. Bake at 350° for 10 to 15 minutes, covered, to thoroughly heat. Wrap and freeze unbaked crepes. If desired, for each 2 crepes you wish to bake, mix 1 tablespoon cream of mushroom soup with 1 tablespoon water and spoon over crepes before serving.

Yield: filling for 9 crepes (¾ cup plus 2 tablespoons).

Family Portion
Prepare a regular crepe batter and make 6-inch diameter for adult-size. Make vegetable filling recipe as is, or add ¼ cup cooked chicken cut in small pieces to each 1 cup vegetable-soup mixture for a main dish crepe. Use 2 tablespoons filling for each crepe. Serve 2 to 3 crepes per person for a main dish and 1 to 2 crepes for a side dish.

	Phenylalanine (mg)	Protein (gm)	Calories
Per diet recipe	202	5.6	762
Per crepe (including filling)	22	0.6	85
Per crepe plus 1 tablespoon sauce	28	0.7	91

Vegetable Stew

1 cup (135 gm) sliced carrots
½ cup (53 gm) sliced celery
½ cup (70 gm) chopped onion
1 cup (160 gm) cubed potatoes
1 cup (120 gm) fresh, frozen,
or canned cut green beans
1 cup (135 gm) cubed rutabaga
or turnip
½ cup tomato sauce

1½ cups water
2 pkg G. Washington's Rich
Brown Seasoning and
Broth, or salt to taste
dried or chopped fresh herbs
as desired (optional)
2 tablespoons cornstarch
dissolved in ⅓ cup cold
water

Mix all ingredients except cornstarch-water mixture in a large pot and cook over medium heat until the potatoes are tender, about 10 to 15 minutes. Mix cornstarch-water mixture into the pot. Cook for several minutes, until thickened.

Yield: 5 cups (1200 gm).

Note
A very nice way to serve the stew is with a baked round of *Biscuit Topper;* or place desired portion in an individual casserole, top with unbaked *Biscuit Topper,* and bake at 425° for 12 to 15 minutes.

Storage Tip
Individual portions of stew topped with unbaked *Biscuit Topper* can be frozen and later thawed and baked for a convenient and satisfying meal.

	Phenylalanine (mg)	Protein (gm)	Calories
Per recipe	372	11.6	440
Per ¼ cup (60 gm) serving	19	0.6	22

Vegetable Stir-Frying

Sauce

2 teaspoons G. Washington's
  Rich Brown or Golden
  Seasoning and Broth, or
  salt and seasonings of your
  choice
1 tablespoon water or dry
  sherry
½ teaspoon cornstarch

2 tablespoons vegetable oil
¼ teaspoon minced garlic or
  a little garlic powder or
  garlic salt
½ teaspoon fresh minced
  gingerroot or a little
  powdered ginger (optional)

Vegetable Options (choose one)

1. ¾ cup (93 gm) fresh or frozen cut asparagus
   1 cup (75 gm) sliced fresh mushrooms
   ¼ cup (28 gm) sliced green onions

Yield: 1¼ cups (201 gm).

2. ¼ cup (35 gm) chopped onion
   2 cups (179 gm) shredded cabbage
   1 cup (75 gm) sliced fresh mushrooms

Yield: 1 cup (143 gm).

3. ¾ cup (101 gm) thinly sliced carrots
   1 cup (88 gm) coarsely chopped cauliflower
   ¼ cup (32 gm) chopped green pepper

Yield: 1 cup (125 gm).

4. ½ cup (54 gm) fresh pea pods, cut in half (about 13 pods)
   1 cup (88 gm) coarsely chopped cauliflower
   ½ cup (96 gm) seeded, chopped fresh tomatoes

Yield: 1⅓ cups (210 gm).

5. 1 cup (133 gm) sliced zucchini squash
   ¾ cup (65 gm) eggplant cut in ½-inch strips
   ¼ cup (49 gm) seeded, chopped, fresh tomatoes

Yield: ⅔ cup (135 gm).

For *Sauce*, in a small bowl, mix broth (or seasonings) and sherry or water. Mix in cornstarch and set aside. Heat oil to very hot in a skillet or wok. Stir in ginger and garlic and toss for 30 seconds. Add the first vegetable in the *Vegetable Option* you choose (this is the one with the firmest texture) and cook, stirring for 1 minute. Add the next two vegetables (except tomato in options 4 and 5) and cook and stir for 2 additional minutes. If tomato is used in the option you are making, add it at the end of frying and toss lightly to mix; heat through. Add the sauce ingredients and stir until thickened. Serve over rice or low protein pasta.

Family Portion

Make any multiple of the recipe, to suit family needs. For each single recipe, first stir-fry ½ cup chopped raw breast of chicken, ¼ lb raw shelled shrimp, or ½ cup thinly sliced raw beef in hot oil in wok or skillet until opaque. Remove from pan. Stir-fry your choice of vegetables. Add sauce ingredients. Remove diet serving, then return cooked chicken, shrimp, or beef to the remaining vegetables and heat through.

	Phenylalanine (mg)	Protein (gm)	Calories
Stir-Fry #1			
Per diet recipe	136	4.5	295
Per ¼ cup (40 gm) serving			
(not including rice or pasta)	27	1.0	59
Stir-Fry #2			
Per diet recipe	142	3.8	331
Per ¼ cup (36 gm) serving			
(not including rice or pasta)	35	0.9	83
Stir-Fry #3			
Per diet recipe	103	3.0	318
Per ¼ cup (32 gm) serving			
(not including rice or pasta)	26	0.8	82
Stir-fry #4			
Per diet recipe	129	4.0	309
Per ¼ cup (39 gm) serving			
(not including rice or pasta)	24	0.7	57
Stir-Fry #5			
Per diet recipe	90	2.6	299
Per ¼ cup (51 gm) serving			
(not including rice or pasta)	35	1.0	115

Hamburgerless Pie

⅓ cup (57 gm) diced raw
  potato
1 tablespoon potato water
2 tablespoons condensed
  Campbell's Tomato Soup

⅓ cup (40 gm) frozen or
  canned cut green beans
1 teaspoon margarine or butter
salt, pepper, and paprika to
  taste

Boil potato and mash with potato water. Divide tomato soup and green beans equally between 2 individual casseroles. Mix mashed potato with margarine and salt to taste; spread over top of beans and soup. Sprinkle potatoes with pepper and paprika. Bake, covered, at 350° for 15 to 20 minutes or until heated through.

Yield: 2 pies (⅔ cup, 160gm).

Note
You may substitute 4½ tablespoons dehydrated potato flakes reconstituted with ⅓ cup water for the raw potato.

Family Portion
Make any multiple of recipe to suit family needs. Remove diet portion. Add cooked hamburger as desired to filling for family portion.

	Phenylalanine (mg)	Protein (gm)	Calories
Per diet recipe	85	2.3	119
Per pie (⅓ cup, 80 gm)	42	1.1	60

Shepherd's Pie

An excellent way to use leftover potatoes and carrots. Or improvise your own "pie"—any vegetables could be used in place of peas, carrots, and mushrooms.

⅔ cup (155 gm) mashed
   potatoes
½ teaspoon margarine
   or butter
3 tablespoons Rich's Coffee
   Rich or water
1 tablespoon (9 gm) chopped
   onion

3 tablespoons (36 gm) frozen peas
½ cup (60 gm) sliced
   cooked carrots
¼ cup (45 gm) sliced canned
   mushrooms (½ of a 4 oz can)
¼ cup water
2 teaspoons (5 gm) Schilling
   Brown Gravy Mix

Mash potatoes with margarine and Coffee Rich or water. Place ½ of potatoes in bottom of a small greased casserole. Top with onion, peas, carrots, and mushrooms. Add water to gravy mix in a small saucepan and bring to a simmer. Pour over vegetables in casserole. Top with remaining potatoes. Bake, covered, at 400° for 20 to 25 minutes, or microwave on High for 2 to 3 minutes.

Yield: 2 cups (375 gm).

Note
You may substitute 9 tablespoons dehydrated potato flakes reconstituted with ⅔ cup water for the mashed potato.

Family Portion
Prepare any multiple of the basic diet recipe, adding ¼ cup cooked ground beef along with vegetables for each single recipe. Add additional Brown Gravy Mix to moisten as desired.

	Phenylalanine (mg)	Protein (gm)	Calories
Per diet recipe	306	7.4	291
Per ¼ cup (47 gm) serving	38	0.9	37

Shish Kabob

A nice late-summer meal when garden vegetables are abundant.

For each shish kabob:

2 large, fresh mushrooms
(30 gm)
2 cherry tomatoes (28 gm)
two 1-inch chunks green
pepper (16 gm)

two ½-inch slices from a small
zucchini squash (32 gm)
⅓ cup Italian salad dressing
(bottled or your own
homemade)

Twenty to 30 minutes before serving, toss vegetables with dressing; cover. Drain vegetables, reserving dressing for another use. On a 14-inch metal skewer, alternately thread vegetables.

To Grill

Place skewer on grill over medium-hot coals; grill about 20 minutes or until vegetables are tender, occasionally turning skewers.

To Broil

Place skewer on broiler pan. Broil (550°) in oven for 15 to 20 minutes or until tender, occasionally turning.

Yield: 1 shish kabob.

Note

Other shish kabob ideas include cauliflower flowerets, pearl onions, whole water chestnuts, unpeeled orange wedges, and eggplant chunks.

Family Portion

For rest of family, marinate additional vegetables and 1-inch chunks of beef, lamb, pork, or chicken. Thread vegetables alternately with meat.

	Phenylalanine (mg)	Protein (gm)	Calories
Per diet shish kabob	47	1.4	100

Little Vegetable Tarts

Freeze unbaked pie crusts for convenience, then bake fresh for use in this delicious and attractive little main dish pie.

baked low protein pie crust of your choice, using either a 4-inch pie pan or 3-inch tart pan
½ cup (68 gm) thickly sliced carrot, slices halved
1 cup (91 gm) cauliflower, cut into small flowerets

2 tablespoons (18 gm) frozen peas
1 cup (75 gm) quartered fresh mushrooms
2 tablespoons (18 gm) sliced onion or green onions
1 tablespoon margarine or butter

Mushroom Sauce

⅔ cup (152 gm) condensed Campbell's Cream of Mushroom Soup (½ can)

⅓ cup water

Prepare pastry. Put carrots in a small amount of water in a saucepan, or in a vegetable steamer. Cook and steam 5 minutes over medium heat. Add cauliflower and cook another 5 to 8 minutes until both carrots and cauliflower are barely tender. Add peas and cook another 2 minutes. While cauliflower, carrots, and peas are steaming, in a skillet sauté mushrooms and onions in margarine about 2 minutes or until just tender. Mix all vegetables together. For *Mushroom Sauce* mix soup with water and heat, mixing until smooth.

For a 3-inch tart pan, use ¼ cup vegetable mixture and spoon 2 tablespoons *Mushroom Sauce* over top. For a 4-inch pie pan, put ½ cup vegetable mixture into baked crust and spoon ¼ cup sauce over top. Bake at 375° for 15 to 20 minutes.

Yield: 2 cups (155 gm) vegetables plus 1 cup sauce, for eight 3-inch tarts or four 4-inch tarts.

Note
A 4-inch pie pan is a generous portion for an adult. A 3-inch tart pan is a very nice size for a child. Purchase both in the kitchen supplies section of a department store or at a kitchen or housewares specialty store. You could also use an E-Z Foil Cupcake Cup, obtainable in grocery stores.

Other combinations of vegetables can be used. A casserole rather than a tart can also be made, adding cooked low protein pasta in amount desired and turning into a small casserole.

Family Portion

Add 2 tablespoons or more cooked chicken pieces per 4-inch pie and top with grated parmesan cheese, using a regular pie crust.

	Phenylalanine (mg)	Protein (gm)	Calories
Per diet recipe	361	9.3	309
Per ¼ cup vegetables (20 gm) plus 2 tablespoons sauce (not including crust)	45	1.2	39
Per ½ cup vegetables (39 gm) plus ¼ cup sauce (not including crust)	90	2.3	77

French Fried Veggies

Crisp and golden brown, these veggies could be enjoyed by the whole family. This batter rated higher than a regular batter among taste-testers!

Batter

6 tablespoons (41 gm) Wel-Plan Baking Mix

2 tablespoons (18 gm) Softasilk cake flour (do not use regular flour)

⅛ to ¼ teaspoon salt

2 teaspoons vegetable oil

¼ cup Rich's Coffee Rich

¼ cup water mixed with 1 scant drop yellow food coloring

In a small bowl, mix Baking Mix, cake flour, and salt together. Add oil, Coffee Rich, and colored water; mix until no lumps remain. Dip vegetables of your choice in batter. Deep-fry in hot vegetable oil (375°), several at a time, for 3 to 4 minutes or until light golden brown. Remove to a paper towel to absorb any excess oil, then serve while hot.

Note

These do not freeze and reheat well, since they lose their crispness. If the whole family is not partaking of them, making ½ the recipe may be advisable, as the whole recipe coats more than would be normally eaten for one meal. Do not make less than ½ the recipe, even if you do not want to use it all, as it becomes too difficult to coat the vegetables.

The batter is also good for making apple fritters. Sprinkle apple chunks with cinnamon and sugar to taste, then dip in batter and fry until golden brown.

	Phenylalanine (mg)	Protein (gm)	Calories
Per recipe batter	66	1.2	359

Makes enough batter for one of the following:

1. Onion Rings

1 medium onion (110 gm) or 110 gm of rings from any size onion. Cut onion into ¼-inch-thick slices after removing skin. Separate into rings.

	Phenylalanine (mg)	Protein (gm)	Calories
Per recipe with batter	114	3.0	409
Per ¼ total number of rings with batter	29	0.8	102

2. Cauliflower

1 cup (75 gm) cauliflower flowerets. Cut cauliflower into small flowerets.

	Phenylalanine (mg)	Protein (gm)	Calories
Per recipe with batter	135	3.3	386
Per ¼ cup flowerets with batter	34	0.8	97

3. Mushrooms

9 medium fresh mushrooms (75 gm). Cut mushrooms in half.

	Phenylalanine (mg)	Protein (gm)	Calories
Per recipe with batter	143	3.3	386
Per ½ mushroom with batter	8	0.2	21

Note

Other vegetables such as broccoli, green beans, eggplant, green peppers, and aparagus could also be french fried.

Garden Fresh Casserole

2 tablespoons margarine
  or butter
¾ cup (105 gm) sliced onion
2 tablespoons (16 gm) chopped
  green pepper
1 cup (120 gm) fresh or canned
  green beans
¾ cup (101 gm) carrots, cut
  in thin 1-inch strips

1 cup (192 gm) chopped fresh
  tomatoes or 1 cup (230 gm)
  chopped canned tomatoes
1 cup (105 gm) celery, cut
  in thin 1-inch strips
½ teaspoon granulated sugar
½ teaspoon salt

Melt margarine in a skillet or saucepan which has a tight fitting lid. Sauté onion and green pepper in hot margarine until tender, about 5 minutes. Add the green beans, carrots, tomatoes, celery, sugar, and salt. Cover tightly and heat on high until steam is escaping from the edge of the lid. Immediately turn down to low heat and cook for 10 to 15 minutes or until tender.

Yield: 2½ cups (408 gm).

	Phenylalanine (mg)	Protein (gm)	Calories
Per recipe	202	6.8	409
Per ¼ cup (41 gm) serving	20	0.7	41

Grated Vegetable Pancakes

½ cup (90 gm) grated raw
zucchini squash
½ teaspoon salt
½ cup (130 gm) grated raw
potatoes

1 tablespoon (9 gm) finely
chopped onion
1 tablespoon (8 gm) finely
chopped green pepper
1 tablespoon cornstarch
2 tablespoons vegetable oil

Place zucchini in a colander or small bowl; sprinkle with salt and let stand 30 minutes, then squeeze out the excess water using a paper towel. Place grated potato in a small bowl and cover with cold water to rinse off the excess starch, then drain. Squeeze out extra water and pat thoroughly dry on a paper towel.

In a medium bowl, mix the dried zucchini, dried potato, onion, pepper, and cornstarch. Divide the mixture into 8 portions (22 gm each). Heat the oil in a skillet; drop individual portions onto the pan and spread around with a spoon or spatula to make a 2-inch pancake. Brown on both sides over medium heat, several minutes per side.

Yield: 8 pancakes (176 gm).

Storage Tip

Stack pancakes between waxed paper; freeze in an airtight container and remove 1 or 2 at a time as needed, thaw and fry.

	Phenylalanine (mg)	Protein (gm)	Calories
Per recipe	159	4.1	402
Per pancake (22 gm)	20	0.5	50

251

Supper Shortcake

Low protein version of creamed tuna with peas on biscuits.

2½ tablespoons (36 gm)
    condensed Campbell's
    Cream of Mushroom Soup
1 tablespoon water
1 tablespoon (9 gm)
    frozen peas

1 Pillsbury Buttermilk Biscuit
    (21 gm) or 1 low protein
    biscuit (*Biscuit Topper*)

Mix all ingredients in a saucepan and heat through. Serve over biscuit which has been baked according to package or recipe directions.

Yield: ¼ cup (64 gm) sauce, for 1 biscuit.

Family Portion
Prepare your favorite creamed tuna with peas recipe and serve over Pillsbury biscuits or homemade biscuits.

	Phenylalanine (mg)	Protein (gm)	Calories
Per low protein biscuit with ¼ cup sauce	58	1.4	143
Per Pillsbury biscuit with ¼ cup sauce	128	2.8	85

Pot Pie Dough

This makes pastry that is not as "short" as the other low protein pastry recipes.

1⅓ cups (146 gm) wheat starch
½ teaspoon salt
½ cup yellow vegetable
    shortening (such as Fluffo
    or Butter-Flavored Crisco)

1 tablespoon water
2½ tablespoons light Karo
    corn syrup

Combine wheat starch and salt in a mixing bowl. Cut in shortening with a pastry blender, fork, or 2 knives, until mixture resembles coarse bread crumbs; sprinkle water over and blend with a fork. Dribble syrup over and continue mixing with a fork. Dough will be moist. Gather dough into a ball, adding wheat starch to your hands if sticky. Roll out on surface dusted with wheat starch, or pat out into desired shape.

Makes enough dough for one of the following:

    10 pot pies (using about 25 gm each)
    8 small turnovers (using about 30 gm each)
    4 large turnovers (using about 60 gm each)
    four 4-inch diameter pie pans (using about 60 gm each)

Storage Tip
    The dough freezes well when kept in an airtight container. Cut off portion desired, without first thawing. Baked rounds of dough on pot pies also freeze well for up to several months.

	Phenylalanine (mg)	Protein (gm)	Calories
Per recipe	15	0.4	1721
Per pot pie	1	trace	172
Per small turnover	2	trace	215
Per large turnover or 4-inch pie pan	4	0.1	430

Vegetable Pot Pie

An excellent do-ahead main dish.

Pot Pie Dough or low protein pie crust dough of your choice

Basic Vegetable Mixture

1 cup (170 gm) diced potatoes
1 cup (135 gm) diced or sliced
   carrots

¼ cup (35 gm) chopped onion

Vegetable Option 1

1 cup (75 gm) quartered fresh
   mushrooms or ½ cup
   (86 gm) sliced canned
   mushrooms

2 tablespoons (18 gm)
   frozen peas

Vegetable Option 2

1 cup (120 gm) fresh or frozen
   cut green beans

⅓ cup (35 gm) chopped celery

Gravy

2 tablespoons cornstarch
1 pkg G. Washington's Golden
   Seasoning and Broth, or
   seasonings of your choice

1¾ cups water

Prepare pastry and set aside. Prepare vegetables from *Basic Vegetable Mixture*, then prepare vegetables from either of the two vegetable options. As all vegetables are prepared, divide equally among 8 individual casserole dishes. Sprinkle with salt and pepper as desired.

To prepare *Gravy*, in a small saucepan mix cornstarch and broth powder. Add a few tablespoons of the water and mix to a paste, then add remainder of water; bring to a boil, stirring constantly until thickened. Pour 3 tablespoons gravy over vegetables in each casserole, just enough to cover the vegetables. Cut pastry into rounds to fit casserole dish; place a round of pastry on each pie. Bake at 400° for 12 to 15 minutes.

Yield: 8 pot pies.

Storage Tip
Pot pies freeze well, either baked or unbaked, for up to several months. Thaw and reheat in microwave oven, or bake as directed.

	Phenylalanine (mg)	Protein (gm)	Calories
Using Vegetable Option 1			
Per recipe	305	7.9	315
Per pot pie (not including crust)	38	1.0	39
Using Vegetable Option 2			
Per recipe	274	7.7	340
Per pot pie (not including crust)	34	1.0	42

Quickie Vegetable Pot Pie

3 cups (384 gm) Vege-All
    canned mixed vegetables or
    frozen mixed vegetables
    (remove lima beans)
salt and pepper to taste
2 tablespoons cornstarch
1 pkg G. Washington's Golden
    Seasoning and Broth
    (optional)

1¾ cups water
Pot Pie Dough, or low protein
    pie crust dough of your
    choice

Follow instructions for *Vegetable Pot Pie*, ignoring instructions for vegetable preparation.

Yield: 8 pot pies.

Storage Tip
Pot pies freeze well, either baked or unbaked, for up to several months. Thaw and reheat in microwave oven, or bake as directed.

	Phenylalanine (mg)	Protein (gm)	Calories
Per recipe	372	9.6	242
Per pot pie (not including crust)	47	1.2	30

Chop Suey

½ cup (70 gm) chopped onion
⅔ cup (70 gm) chopped celery
1½ tablespoons vegetable oil
⅔ cup (152 gm) condensed
   Campbell's Cream of
   Mushroom Soup (½ can)

6 tablespoons water
⅔ cup (75 gm) sliced water
   chestnuts (½ of 8 oz can)
⅔ cup (117 gm) sliced canned
   mushrooms (4 oz can)

In a skillet, sauté onion and celery in hot oil several minutes, until tender. Mix in remainder of ingredients and heat through. Serve over low protein pasta, rice, or chow mein noodles.

Yield: 2 cups (500 gm).

	Phenylalanine (mg)	Protein (gm)	Calories
Per recipe	312	8.0	394
Per ¼ cup (63 gm) serving (not including pasta, rice, or noodles)	39	1.0	49

Chow Mein

Comparable to chow mein found in any American-Chinese restaurant.

2 tablespoons vegetable oil
¾ cup (105 gm) sliced onion
2 cups (210 gm) sliced celery
1 tablespoon cornstarch
1 cup water
1 tablespoon soy sauce
1 pkg G. Washington's Golden
   Seasoning and Broth, or
   salt to taste

1 cup (75 gm) sliced fresh
   mushrooms or ¼ cup
   (45 gm) sliced canned
   mushrooms
½ cup (64 gm) sliced or
   chopped green pepper
¾ cup (90 gm) sliced canned
   water chestnuts

Heat oil in a large skillet. Sauté onion and celery in oil about 2 minutes. Meanwhile measure cornstarch into a 1-cup measuring cup and mix a little bit of the water in to make a smooth thin paste; add the remainder of the water to make 1 cup. Add the soy sauce and the broth powder or salt to this liquid. Add the mushrooms, green pepper, and water chestnuts to the vegetables and continue to cook another 3 to 4 minutes, until vegetables are crisp-tender. Add cornstarch mixture; cook and stir until liquid is thickened and mixture is heated through. Serve over low protein pasta, rice, or chow mein noodles.

Yield: 3 cups (553 gm).

Family Portion
   Remove diet portion. Add 2 cups of cooked pieces of chicken or turkey or 2 cups of tiny beef meatballs to remainder of vegetables.

	Phenylalanine (mg)	Protein (gm)	Calories
Per diet recipe	210	6.1	433
Per ¼ cup (46 gm) serving (not including pasta, rice, or noodles)	17	0.5	36

Mock Egg Rolls

The individual vegetables create a delicious flavor blend, not unlike "authentic" egg rolls. They are worth the time and patience required!

¼ cup (28 gm) shredded
   carrots
½ cup (45 gm) shredded
   cabbage
⅓ cup (25 gm) finely chopped
   fresh mushrooms or ¼ cup
   (44 gm) chopped canned
   mushrooms

2 tablespoons (17 gm) finely
   chopped onion
1 tablespoon vegetable oil
salt to taste
½ recipe *Tortillas* dough
vegetable oil for deep-frying

In a skillet, fry all vegetables in oil until crisp-tender, about 2 minutes. Add salt to taste. Set aside to cool completely.

Prepare *Tortillas* dough, making sure that it is not at all dry. Divide dough into 6 pieces (about 25 gm dough each). Form each piece into a small flat disk and roll out to a 6-inch circle on a surface dusted with Wel-Plan Baking Mix or wheat starch (using a pastry cloth or wooden surface works best). The dough will be very thin. Stack the dough circles as you roll them, placing a piece of waxed paper on top of each one to keep them from sticking together.

Put 2 tablespoons vegetable filling in center of each dough circle. Carefully fold one side to just cover the filling. Moisten remaining edge with fingers dipped in water, then fold in the two ends. Fold remaining edge over and press lightly to seal. If any cracking of the dough occurs while folding, gently push it together with a finger moistened with water. Do not let filled rolls stand for more than 1 hour before deep-frying.

Fry egg rolls in 1 or more inches of hot oil (375°) for about 4 minutes, until golden and crispy. Drain on paper towels. Serve with *Sweet and Sour Sauce* or catsup (not included in nutrient analysis).

Yield: ¾ cup (110 gm) filling, for 6 egg rolls.

Storage Tip

For convenience, make rolls in advance and reheat in oven at 350° for about 10 minutes (they must be deep-fried before storing). They also freeze well, when already deep-fried (do not freeze unfried rolls).

	Phenylalanine (mg)	Protein (gm)	Calories
Per recipe	63	2.1	1272
Per egg roll (including tortilla)	11	0.4	212

Chinese Sweet-Sour Vegetables

Like a sweet-sour dish you would find in any American-Chinese restaurant.
Serve over low protein pasta, rice, or chow mein noodles.

¾ cup (90 gm) sliced water
   chestnuts
24 fresh or frozen snow
   peapods, 3 inches long
   (90 gm)
2 teaspoons soy sauce
½ cup juice from pineapple
1 teaspoon vinegar
1 tablespoon cornstarch
¼ teaspoon ground ginger or
   a small piece of fresh
   minced ginger root

3 tablespoons vegetable oil
2½ tablespoons (18 gm) sliced
   green onions
1⅓ cups (100 gm) sliced fresh
   mushrooms
¾ cup (140 gm) pineapple
   chunks
salt to taste

Cut water chestnut slices in half crosswise. If using fresh peapods, wash and remove ends and strings. If using frozen peapods, thaw and dry on paper towel. Cut pods in half if desired. Combine soy sauce, pineapple juice, vinegar, cornstarch, and ginger in a small bowl. Heat oil in a large skillet or wok. Add water chestnuts, peapods, green onions, and mushrooms, stirring several minutes until soft. Add pineapple and quickly heat through. Salt to taste. To retain bright green color of the peapods, serve immediately, over low protein pasta, rice, or chow mein noodles.

Yield: 3 cups (590 gm).

Family Portion
Sauté or stir-fry ½ to ¾ lb boned chicken or turkey breast meat, or shrimp, in a little oil for 3 to 6 minutes (until opaque). Remove to a dish. Proceed with recipe. Remove diet portion. Return the cooked chicken, turkey, or shrimp for rest of family, heating briefly before serving.

	Phenylalanine (mg)	Protein (gm)	Calories
Per diet recipe	233	6.6	559
Per ¼ cup (49 gm) serving (not including pasta, rice, or noodles)	19	0.6	47

Chinese Fried Rice

¼ cup vegetable oil
¾ cup (165 gm) uncooked
   regular white rice

⅓ cup (30 gm) chopped green
   onion
1 teaspoon La Choy soy sauce

Cook rice according to directions. Heat vegetable oil in a large skillet. Add cooked rice and heat through. Add scallions and soy sauce and mix well. Serve immediately.

Yield: 3 cups (506 gm).

Family Portion

Remove diet portion. Make a nest in rice; break 2 whole eggs into nest, exposing eggs to surface of skillet. Over medium heat, scramble eggs slightly and when they are partially cooked, mix in with rest of rice and continue cooking for several minutes.

	Phenylalanine (mg)	*Protein (gm)*	*Calories*
Per diet recipe	693	12.6	1106
Per ¼ cup (42 gm) serving	58	1.0	92

Burritos

The filling is also good plain, as a vegetable dish.

1 cup (140 gm) chopped
   zucchini squash
¼ cup (45 gm) fresh or
   frozen corn
¼ cup (35 gm) chopped onion
½ clove garlic, minced
1 teaspoon vegetable oil
⅔ cup (128 gm) seeded,
   chopped, fresh tomatoes or
   canned tomatoes

¼ teaspoon dried oregano
¼ teaspoon thyme
¼ teaspoon salt
2 teaspoons cornstarch
   dissolved in 2 tablespoons
   cold water
pre-baked *Tortillas*
taco sauce (any brand)

Cook zucchini and corn in a saucepan, in a small amount of boiling water or using a vegetable steamer, about 10 minutes or until tender. Meanwhile, sauté onions and garlic in hot oil in a skillet for 1 to 2 minutes; add zucchini, corn, and remaining ingredients to skillet and heat through, until sauce is slightly thickened. Put 3 tablespoons vegetable mixture in middle of each warmed tortilla. Dribble on 2 teaspoons taco sauce; roll up and serve immediately.

Yield: 1⅔ cups (320 gm) filling.

Family Portion
Remove diet portion. Add ½ to ¾ lb of cooked hamburger or small chunks of beef to the vegetables. Use regular flour tortilla and sprinkle each burrito with shredded cheese before rolling up.

	Phenylalanine (mg)	Protein (gm)	Calories
Per diet recipe filling	146	4.0	165
Per 3 tablespoons (36 gm) filling	17	0.5	19
Per burrito (including tortilla and taco sauce)	27	0.8	126

Tacos

1 pre-baked *Tortilla*
½ cup (28 gm) shredded lettuce
3 tablespoons (35 gm) chopped
    fresh tomatoes

2 teaspoons taco sauce (any
    brand)

Prepare a crisp taco shell, according to *Tortillas* recipe directions. When tortilla has cooled slightly and holds its taco shape, fill with lettuce, then tomato. Spoon taco sauce over top.

Yield: 1 serving.

	Phenylalanine (mg)	Protein (gm)	Calories
Per taco (including tortilla and sauce)	23	0.7	117

Other Taco Filling Ideas

	Phenylalanine (mg)	Protein (gm)	Calories
chopped olives, 1 tablespoon (8 gm)	3	0.1	15
sliced mushrooms, 1 tablespoon (5 gm)	3	0.2	2
chopped onions, 1 tablespoon (11 gm)	3	0.1	3
chopped green peppers, 1 tablespoon (10 gm)	3	0.1	2

Mexican Rice

Like "fast-food" Mexican rice—only better!

½ cup (88 gm) uncooked
   regular white rice
¼ cup (35 gm) chopped onion
½ clove garlic, minced
1 tablespoon vegetable oil
½ cup (96 gm) seeded,
   chopped, fresh tomatoes or
   canned tomatoes

½ teaspoon chili powder or
   2 tablespoons diced green
   chilies
½ teaspoon salt
1 pkg G. Washington's Rich
   Brown Seasoning and Broth
   (optional)
1 cup water

In a skillet, sauté rice, onion, and garlic in oil for several minutes until rice is crackly and lightly golden. Stir in remaining ingredients. Bring to a simmer; cover and cook over low heat for 20 to 30 minutes or until rice is tender. Fluff with a fork before serving.

Yield: 2 cups (280 gm).

	Phenylalanine (mg)	Protein (gm)	Calories
Per recipe	396	8.3	484
Per ¼ cup (35 gm) serving	49	1.0	60

Spanish Rice

2 tablespoons vegetable oil
¾ cup (105 gm) chopped onion
¼ cup (32 gm) chopped green
   pepper
1 garlic clove, minced
   (½ teaspoon)

½ cup (88 gm) uncooked
   regular white rice
1 cup tomato juice
½ cup water
½ teaspoon paprika
½ teaspoon salt

Heat oil in medium saucepan or skillet which has a tightly fitting lid. Sauté onion, green pepper, and garlic in oil until onion is tender, about 5 minutes. Add rice, tomato juice, water, and seasonings. Bring to a boil then cover; turn heat to low and cook 20 minutes. Fluff with a fork before serving.

Yield: 2¼ cups (500 gm).

	Phenylalanine (mg)	Protein (gm)	Calories
Per recipe	416	9.6	651
Per ¼ cup (56 gm) serving	46	1.1	72

Variation

Low Spanish Rice

Add ¼ cup (44 gm) regular white rice and ¼ cup (38 gm) uncooked Aproten Anellini or Aproten Imitation Rice in place of the ½ cup regular rice.

Yield: 2 cups plus 2 tablespoons (520 gm).

	Phenylalanine (mg)	Protein (gm)	Calories
Per recipe	255	6.6	625
Per ¼ cup (61 gm) serving	28	0.7	69

Orange Rice

⅓ cup (35 gm) chopped celery
2 tablespoons (14 gm) chopped
   green onions, including
   green top
½ cup (88 gm) uncooked
   regular white rice

2 tablespoons margarine
   or butter
½ cup orange juice
½ cup water
½ teaspoon salt

In a medium saucepan, sauté celery, onions, and rice in hot margarine until onions are tender and rice is lightly browned, about 8 minutes. Stir in orange juice, water, and salt. Heat to a boil, cover, and reduce heat to low; simmer 20 minutes.

Yield: 2¼ cups (400 gm).

	Phenylalanine (mg)	Protein (gm)	Calories
Per recipe	381	7.8	591
Per ¼ cup (44 gm) serving	42	0.9	66

Rice and 'Roni

½ cup (55 gm) uncooked Aproten Ditalini, Wel-Plan Macaroni, or regular elbow macaroni
½ cup (48 gm) uncooked instant rice
⅔ cup (152 gm) condensed Campbell's Cream of Mushroom Soup (½ can)

1 pkg G. Washington's Rich Brown Seasoning and Broth, or salt and seasoning of your choice
⅔ cup (75 gm) sliced water chestnuts (½ of 8 oz can)
¼ cup (36 gm) frozen peas
1¼ cups water
chopped pimento (optional)

To Make Diet Portion Only

Mix all ingredients in a bowl. Pour into a 1½-quart casserole or baking dish, or put desired portion in individual casseroles. Cover. Bake large casserole for 35 to 40 minutes or individual casserole for 30 to 35 minutes or until rice and pasta are tender; refrigerate or freeze remainder for a later time.

Yield: 2⅓ cups (475 gm).

To Make Diet Portion plus Family Portion

Mix together all ingredients except pasta in a bowl. For a ½ cup *Diet Portion,* mix ½ cup plus 1 tablespoon of the liquid mixture with 2 tablespoons uncooked low protein or regular pasta in an individual casserole.

For rest of family, to remaining liquid mixture, add ½ cup uncooked elbow macaroni and 1 cup of cooked chicken cut in pieces or 1 cup of cooked hamburger. Pour into a 2-quart casserole or baking dish. Cover and bake side by side with small diet casserole, but for 35 to 40 minutes instead of 30 to 35 minutes.

	Phenylalanine (mg)	Protein (gm)	Calories
Using low protein pasta			
Per diet recipe	465	10.2	563
Per ¼ cup (63 gm) serving	62	1.4	75
Using regular pasta			
Per diet recipe	799	17.1	488
Per ¼ cup (63 gm) serving	106	2.3	65

Traditional Pizza Crust

½ pkg (1⅛ teaspoons) active
 dry yeast
½ teaspoon granulated sugar
1 cup warm water (105° to
 115°) with 3 drops yellow
 food coloring

2 tablespoons vegetable oil
3 cups plus 3 tablespoons
 (351 gm) Wel-Plan
 Baking Mix
½ teaspoon salt

In a medium bowl, mix yeast with sugar; add warm water and let
stand 5 minutes. Add vegetable oil. Mix in Baking Mix and salt and
stir to form a soft dough. Knead dough briefly on a surface dusted
with Baking Mix until smooth, adding a little Baking Mix as needed
to prevent sticking.

Divide dough into 4 parts. On a cookie sheet, pat out two pieces
of dough into 6½- to 7-inch circles. Pat out remaining dough into
circles on another cookie sheet. Let dough stand at room temperature
for 20 to 30 minutes, then spread with sauce and toppings of your
choice. Bake in an oven preheated to 425° for 15 to 20 minutes.

Yield: four pizzas.

Storage Tip

Freeze partially baked crusts (bake for only 9 to 10 minutes) or
freeze fully or partially baked pizzas complete with sauce and topping. To reheat a fully baked pizza with sauce and topping, use a
regular oven or toaster oven to retain a crisp crust, or use a microwave oven for a soft crust.

	Phenylalanine (mg)	Protein (gm)	Calories
Per recipe	89	2.3	1479
Per pizza crust (not including sauce or topping)	22	0.6	370

Thick Crust Pizza

1 recipe *Best White Bread*
melted margarine or butter
sauce and topping of choice

Prepare dough for *Best White Bread.* After the 30-minute rising, knead for 1 to 2 minutes. Divide dough into 3 parts (about 230 gm each) for making 10-inch pizzas, or in 9 parts (about 75 gm each) for making 6-inch pizzas. Pat dough out to desired size on lightly greased pizza pans or cookie sheets. Let rise for 15 minutes at room temperature.

Meanwhile, preheat oven to 425°. After dough has risen, brush lightly with melted margarine. Bake for 10 minutes, then put on sauce and toppings desired and bake an additional 10 to 12 minutes until crust is nicely browned. Freeze extra pizzas or pizza slices for a later time.

If you do not want to bake all pizzas right away, dough may be frozen in bulk or shaped into desired size crust and frozen with plastic wrap between each one for easy removal. Before baking, thaw frozen dough (either on lowest setting of microwave oven or at room temperature), let rise and bake as directed.

Yield: three 10-inch pizzas or nine 6-inch pizzas.

	Phenylalanine (mg)	Protein (gm)	Calories
Per recipe	170	3.7	1435
Per 10-inch pizza (not including sauce and toppings)	57	1.2	478
Per 6-inch pizza (not including sauce and toppings)	19	0.4	159

Pizza Sauce

1 cup (8 oz can) tomato sauce,
   or 1 cup pizza sauce
   (without meat or cheese),
   or ½ cup catsup mixed with
   ½ cup water
¼ cup catsup
¼ cup (33 gm) chopped green
   pepper
½ cup (86 gm) sliced
   canned mushrooms or
   ⅔ cup (50 gm) sliced
   fresh mushrooms

⅓ cup (47 gm) chopped
   onion or 1½ tablespoons
   onion flakes
salt, pepper, garlic salt or
   powder to taste
6 chopped black olives

Mix all ingredients in a small bowl. Use 7 tablespoons sauce for a
6- to 7-inch pizza, 9 tablespoons for an 8-inch pizza (*Quick Pizza
Crust*, page 307), 12 tablespoons for a 10-inch pizza.

Yield: 1¾ cups.

	Phenylalanine (mg)	Protein (gm)	Calories
Per recipe	195	6.6	182
Per 7 tablespoons	49	1.7	46
Per 9 tablespoons	63	2.1	59
Per 12 tablespoons	85	2.9	79

Other Pizza Sauce and Topping Ideas

Sauce

Use plain tomato sauce, "Pizza Quick" sauce, or Ragu Meatless Spaghetti Sauce (3 tablespoons = 15 mg phenylalanine, 0.6 gm protein, 60 calories).

Toppings

	Phenylalanine (mg)	Protein (gm)	Calories
Chopped olives, 1 tablespoon (8 gm)	3	0.1	15
Sliced mushrooms, 1 tablespoon (5 gm)	3	0.2	2
Sliced carrots, 1 tablespoon (8 gm)	3	0.1	3
Chopped onion, 1 tablespoon (11 gm)	3	0.1	3
Chopped green or red pepper, 1 tablespoon (10 gm)	3	0.1	2
Crushed Nabisco Cheese Nips, 3 nips	16	0.3	5
Sprinkling of parmesan cheese, 1 level teaspoon	26	0.5	4

Easy Tomato Sauce

1 tablespoon vegetable oil
2 tablespoons (18 gm) finely
  chopped onion
2 tablespoons (16 gm) finely
  chopped green pepper

8 oz can tomato sauce
½ teaspoon Italian seasoning
  or dried basil

Heat oil in a small saucepan. Add onion and green pepper and sauté until vegetables are tender, about 5 minutes. Add tomato sauce and seasonings and simmer 5 minutes to blend flavors.

Yield: 1 cup (238 gm).

	Phenylalanine (mg)	Protein (gm)	Calories
Per recipe	106	3.9	205
Per ¼ cup (60 gm) serving	26	1.0	51

Best Homemade Tomato Sauce

2 tablespoons vegetable oil
1½ cups (210 gm) chopped
  onion
2 large garlic cloves, minced
1 lb 14 oz can (3½ cups)
  tomatoes, undrained

6 oz can tomato paste
1 cup water
½ teaspoon basil
½ teaspoon thyme
½ teaspoon salt
¼ teaspoon pepper
red pepper to taste

In a large saucepan heat oil; sauté onions and garlic until soft, about 5 minutes. Cut tomatoes into smaller pieces; add to onion and garlic and bring to a boil. Turn heat down and simmer, uncovered, for 20 minutes, stirring occasionally. Add tomato paste, water, and seasonings. Continue to cook until heated through.

Yield: 4⅔ cups (1140 gm).

	Phenylalanine (mg)	Protein (gm)	Calories
Per recipe	461	17.9	675
Per ¼ cup (61 gm) serving	25	1.0	36

Basic Turnover Preparation Instructions

Favorite Pie Crust is recommended for the pastry. Use 2 cups (210 gm) Wel-Plan Baking Mix and no wheat starch for an exceptionally sturdy crust.

- Roll out pie crust dough to approximately a 4½- to 5-inch circle for a small turnover or 5½- to 6-inch circle for a large turnover. (For a 5-inch circle, a lid from a small margarine tub can be conveniently used to cut out dough with a nice even edge.)
- Spoon filling on ½ of the dough circle (1 tablespoon filling for small turnover, or 2 tablespoons filling for large turnover) leaving a ½-inch border around edges.
- Wet finger with water and run it along edge on side which has been filled. Fold dough over and gently press with fingers to seal.
- Press all along edge with fork tines to further seal and add a decorative touch.
- Trim any ragged dough edges using a sharp knife.
- Prick top of turnover several times with fork tines for steam to escape.
- Transfer turnovers to an ungreased baking sheet.
- Bake in preheated 400° oven for 12 to 18 minutes, until light golden brown on edges.
- Remove from oven and let cool slightly on baking pan, then serve; or remove to wire rack and cool thoroughly, wrap in foil, and place in plastic container for freezing. To use a frozen turnover, remove directly from freezer and bake at 350° for 10 to 15 minutes, or thaw and bake at 350° for 7 to 8 minutes.

Family Portion

Prepare a double recipe (or more) of any of the filling recipes, to suit family needs. Add diced cooked beef, pork, or chicken to any of the fillings. As a guideline, ⅓ cup diced meat could be added per cup of filling. The turnovers freeze very well and can be made in quantity for a convenient meal later.

Use your own favorite pie crust recipe. Using approximately 2 cups of flour, you will be able to get 6 to 7 turnovers (5-inch diameter circle) for using as a side dish. For a substantial main dish serving, this amount will make approximately 4 to 5 turnovers (7-inch diameter circle) which will hold about ½ to ¾ cup filling each.

Beefy Turnover

Like a "cornish pasty," the wonderful, hearty main dish turnover carried by the Cornish miners for lunch at the turn of the century.

2 teaspoons (5 gm) Schilling
    Brown Gravy Mix
    (¼ pkg)
3 tablespoons water
½ cup (80 gm) potatoes, cut
    in ¼-inch cubes
2 tablespoons (24 gm)
    rutabaga or turnip, cut
    in ¼-inch cubes

2 tablespoons (16 gm) finely
    chopped green pepper
3 tablespoons (25 gm) thinly
    sliced carrots, slices cut
    in half
salt and pepper to taste
your choice of low protein
    pie crust dough

Blend gravy mix with water in a small saucepan. Cook several minutes over medium heat, stirring until thickened. Mix gravy with vegetables. Season with salt and pepper to taste. Roll out pie crust dough and fill according to *Basic Turnover Preparation Instructions*, using 2 tablespoons filling for a large turnover and 1 tablespoon for a small turnover.

Yield: 1 cup (190 gm) filling, for 16 small turnovers or 8 large turnovers.

Note
Other vegetable combinations could be used in place of those indicated.

	Phenylalanine (mg)	Protein (gm)	Calories
Per recipe	120	3.0	104
Per 1 tablespoon (12 gm) filling (not including crust)	8	0.2	6
Per 2 tablespoons (24 gm) filling (not including crust)	15	0.4	13

Supper in a Turnover

A good recipe for using leftover mashed potatoes.

¼ cup (35 gm) finely chopped
   onion
2 teaspoons vegetable oil
½ cup (120 gm) mashed
   potatoes
2 tablespoons water
3 tablespoons (36 gm)
   frozen peas

¼ cup (36 gm) chopped
   cooked carrots
1 teaspoon lemon juice
½ teaspoon salt
your choice of low protein
   pie crust dough

In a skillet, sauté onion in vegetable oil until soft. Mix potato with water. Mix all remaining ingredients together in the skillet. Roll out pie crust dough and fill according to *Basic Turnover Preparation Instructions,* using 2 tablespoons filling for a large turnover and 1 tablespoon for a small turnover.

Yield: 1 cup (250 gm) filling, for 16 small turnovers or 8 large turnovers.

Note

You may substitute 7 tablespoons dehydrated potato flakes reconstituted with ½ cup water for the mashed potatoes.

	Phenylalanine (mg)	Protein (gm)	Calories
Per recipe	203	5.2	234
Per 1 tablespoon (16 gm) filling (not including crust)	13	0.3	15
Per 2 tablespoons (31 gm) filling (not including crust)	25	0.6	29

Cabbage-Patch Turnover with Apples

1 cup (90 gm) shredded or
  chopped cabbage
½ cup (67 gm) diced apples
½ cup (70 gm) chopped onion
2 tablespoons vegetable oil
2 teaspoons (5 gm) Schilling
  Brown Gravy Mix
  (¼ pkg)

3 tablespoons water
¼ teaspoon thyme
salt and pepper to taste
your choice of low protein
  pie crust dough

In a skillet, cook cabbage, apples, and onion in vegetable oil for 3 minutes or until soft; remove to a bowl. In the same skillet, combine gravy mix, water, thyme, salt, and pepper. Cook several minutes, stirring, until just thickened. Mix gravy with vegetables. Roll out pie crust dough and fill according to *Basic Turnover Preparation Instructions*, using 2 tablespoons filling for a large turnover and 1 tablespoon for a small turnover.

Yield: 1 cup (210 gm) filling, for 16 small turnovers or 8 large turnovers.

	Phenylalanine (mg)	Protein (gm)	Calories
Per recipe	86	2.4	350
Per 1 tablespoon (13 gm) filling (not including crust)	5	0.1	22
Per 2 tablespoons (26 gm) filling (not including crust)	11	0.3	44

Cabbage-Patch Turnover with Raisins

These have a delicious flavor, "not like cabbage."

2 tablespoons bacon drippings
2 tablespoons water
1 tablespoon vinegar
2 teaspoons packed brown
   sugar
1¾ cups (157 gm) shredded
   or chopped cabbage

2 tablespoons (20 gm) raisins
1½ teaspoons water
1 teaspoon cornstarch
your choice of low protein
   pie crust dough

Stir water, vinegar, and sugar into bacon drippings in a skillet. Add cabbage and raisins, stirring enough to coat. Cover and cook over low heat for about 10 minutes or until cabbage is tender, stirring occasionally. Combine 1½ teaspoons water and cornstarch; stir into skillet mixture. Cook and stir until cabbage is well coated and sauce is slightly thickened. Roll out pie crust dough and fill according to *Basic Turnover Preparation Instructions,* using 2 tablespoons filling for a large turnover and 1 tablespoon for a small turnover.

Yield: 1 cup (215 gm) filling, for 16 small turnovers or 8 large turnovers.

	Phenylalanine (mg)	Protein (gm)	Calories
Per recipe	76	2.2	413
Per 1 tablespoon (13 gm) filling (not including crust)	5	0.1	26
Per 2 tablespoons (27 gm) filling (not including crust)	10	0.3	52

Quickie Vegetable Turnover

2 teaspoons (5 gm) Schilling
  Brown Gravy Mix
  (¼ pkg)
3 tablespoons water
1 cup (128 gm) canned Vege-all
  or frozen mixed vegetables
  (remove lima beans)

your choice of low protein pie
  crust dough

Blend gravy mix with water in a small saucepan. Cook several minutes over medium heat, stirring until thickened. Mix vegetables with gravy. Roll out pie crust dough and fill according to *Basic Turnover Preparation Instructions,* using 2 tablespoons filling for a large turnover and 1 tablespoon for a small turnover.

Yield: 1 cup (165 gm) filling, for 16 small turnovers or 8 large turnovers.

	Phenylalanine (mg)	Protein (gm)	Calories
Per recipe	151	3.7	73
Per 1 tablespoon (10 gm) filling (not including crust)	9	0.2	5
Per 2 tablespoons (21 gm) filling (not including crust)	19	0.5	9

Macaroni Mulligan

An excellent combination of flavors and ease of preparation make this a winning meal.

½ cup (55 gm) uncooked Aproten Ditalini, Wel-Plan Macaroni, or regular elbow macaroni
¼ cup (35 gm) chopped onion
1 tablespoon margarine or butter
⅔ cup (149 gm) condensed Campbell's Vegetarian Vegetable Soup (½ can)

¾ cup (205 gm) stewed tomatoes (½ of 14½ oz can), cut in small pieces
¼ teaspoon salt
¼ teaspoon garlic salt
1 pkg G. Washington's Rich Brown Seasoning and Broth (optional)
¼ teaspoon chili powder (optional)

To Make Diet Portion Only
Cook, rinse, and drain pasta according to package directions. While pasta is cooking, in a skillet sauté onion in margarine for about 2 to 3 minutes or until tender. Mix in remaining ingredients and heat through.

Yield: 2½ cups (530 gm).

To Make Diet Portion plus Family Portion
Follow above method, but mix together all ingredients except pasta. For a ½ cup diet portion, mix ⅓ cup liquid mixture with ¼ cup cooked pasta in a small saucepan. Heat through.

For the family portion, to the remaining liquid mixture, add ⅔ to 1 cup (½ lb) cooked hamburger or sausage and 1 cup cooked regular elbow macaroni. Heat through.

	Phenylalanine (mg)	Protein (gm)	Calories
Using low protein pasta			
Per diet portion	228	6.0	508
Per ¼ cup (53 gm) serving	23	0.6	51
Per ½ cup (106 gm) serving	46	1.2	102
Using regular pasta			
Per diet portion	562	12.9	433
Per ¼ cup (53 gm) serving	56	1.3	43
Per ½ cup (106 gm) serving	112	2.6	87

Best Hot Dish

¾ cup (83 gm) uncooked
Aproten Ditalini, Wel-Plan
Macaroni, or regular elbow
macaroni
½ cup (53 gm) chopped celery
¼ cup (35 gm) chopped onion
1 tablespoon vegetable oil

½ cup (120 gm) cream-style
corn
⅔ cup (152 gm) condensed
Campbell's Cream of
Mushroom Soup (½ can)
¼ cup water
½ teaspoon salt

To Make Diet Portion Only

Cook, rinse, and drain pasta according to package directions. While pasta is cooking, in a skillet sauté celery and onion in vegetable oil for about 5 minutes or until celery is tender; mix in corn, soup mixed with water, and salt. Divide mixture into individual casseroles. Bake one casserole at 350° for 15 minutes; refrigerate or freeze remainder for a later time.

Yield: 2¾ cups (572 gm).

To Make Diet Portion plus Family Portion

Mix together all ingredients except pasta. For a ½ cup diet portion, mix 4½ tablespoons soup-vegetable mixture with ⅓ cup cooked low protein or regular pasta in an individual casserole.

For rest of family, to remaining soup-vegetable mixture, add ⅔ to 1 cup cooked chicken or hamburger pieces and 1 cup cooked elbow macaroni. Put into a 1½-quart casserole or baking dish. Cover; bake side by side with small diet casserole, but 25 to 30 minutes instead of 15 minutes.

	Phenylalanine (mg)	Protein (gm)	Calories
Using low protein pasta			
Per diet recipe	297	7.1	637
Per ¼ cup (52 gm) serving	27	0.6	58
Per ½ cup (104 gm) serving	54	1.3	116
Using regular pasta			
Per diet recipe	801	17.5	525
Per ¼ cup (52 gm) serving	73	1.6	48
Per ½ cup (104 gm) serving	146	3.2	95

Macaroni and Carrots Casserole

½ cup (55 gm) uncooked
  Aproten Ditalini, Wel-Plan
  Macaroni, or regular elbow
  macaroni
1⅓ cups (180 gm) thinly sliced
  carrots, slices cut in half
¼ cup (35 gm) chopped onion

1 teaspoon vegetable oil
⅔ cup (152 gm) condensed
  Campbell's Cream of
  Mushroom Soup (½ can)
¼ cup water
¼ teaspoon salt

To Make Diet Portion Only

Cook, rinse, and drain pasta according to package directions. While pasta is cooking, in a small amount of boiling water or in a vegetable steamer, cook carrots 7 to 8 minutes or until tender. In a skillet, sauté onion in oil for 1 to 2 minutes or until tender. Mix soup with water in a bowl; mix in cooked pasta, carrots, onion, and salt. Divide mixture into individual casseroles. Cover and bake one casserole at 350° for 15 minutes; refrigerate or freeze remainder for a later time.

Yield: 2½ cups (495 gm).

To Make Diet Portion plus Family Portion

Mix together all ingredients except pasta. For a ½ cup diet portion, mix ½ cup soup-vegetable mixture with ¼ cup cooked low protein or regular pasta in an individual casserole.

For rest of family, to remaining soup-vegetable mixture add ⅔ to 1 cup cooked ground beef (½ lb), 2 oz shredded cheddar cheese, and 1 cup cooked elbow macaroni. Put into a 1½-quart casserole or baking dish. Cover and bake side by side with small diet casserole, but 25 to 30 minutes instead of 15 minutes.

	Phenylalanine (mg)	Protein (gm)	Calories
Using low protein pasta			
Per diet recipe	240	6.3	440
Per ¼ cup (50 gm) serving	27	0.7	49
Per ½ cup (99 gm) serving	53	1.4	98
Using regular pasta			
Per diet recipe	574	13.2	366
Per ¼ cup (50 gm) serving	64	1.5	41
Per ½ cup (99 gm) serving	128	2.9	81

Macaroni and Peas Casserole

½ cup (55 gm) uncooked
  Aproten Ditalini, Wel-Plan
  Macaroni, or regular elbow
  macaroni
⅔ cup (152 gm) condensed
  Campbell's Cream of
  Mushroom Soup (½ can)

¼ cup water
¼ cup (36 gm) frozen peas
¼ teaspoon salt

To Make Diet Portion Only

Cook, rinse, and drain pasta according to package directions. Mix soup with water in a bowl; mix in cooked pasta, peas, and salt. Put desired portion into individual casseroles. Cover and bake one casserole at 350° for 15 minutes; refrigerate or freeze remainder for a later time.

Yield: 1⅔ cups (393 gm).

To Make Diet Portion plus Family Portion

Mix together all ingredients except pasta. For a ½ cup diet portion, mix ⅓ cup soup-vegetable mixture with ⅓ cup cooked low protein or regular pasta in an individual casserole.

For rest of family, to remaining soup-vegetable mixture add ½ of a 4½ oz can tuna (drained) and 1 cup cooked elbow macaroni. Put into a 1½-quart casserole or baking dish. Cover and bake side by side with small diet casserole, but 25 to 30 minutes instead of 15 minutes.

	Phenylalanine (mg)	Protein (gm)	Calories
Using low protein pasta			
Per diet recipe	244	5.9	339
Per ¼ cup (59 gm) serving	36	0.9	51
Per ½ cup (118 gm) serving	73	1.8	102
Using regular pasta			
Per diet recipe	578	12.8	265
Per ¼ cup (59 gm) serving	86	1.9	39
Per ½ cup (118 gm) serving	174	3.8	79

Macaroni and Broccoli Casserole

½ cup (55 gm) uncooked
    Ditalini, Wel-Plan Macaroni,
    or regular elbow macaroni
1 cup plus 2 tablespoons
    (140 gm) fresh or frozen
    chopped broccoli (½ of
    10 oz pkg)

⅔ cup (152 gm) condensed
    Campbell's Cream of
    Mushroom Soup (½ can)
¼ cup water
¼ teaspoon salt

To Make Diet Portion Only

Cook, rinse, and drain pasta according to package directions. While pasta is cooking, cut broccoli into small pieces. In a small amount of boiling water or in a vegetable steamer, cook frozen broccoli 5 minutes or fresh broccoli 7 to 10 minutes. Mix soup with water in a bowl; mix in cooked pasta, broccoli, and salt. Divide mixture into individual casseroles. Cover and bake one casserole at 350° for 15 minutes; refrigerate or freeze remainder for a later time.

Yield: 2 cups plus 2 tablespoons (493 gm).

To Make Diet Portion Plus Family Portion

Mix together all ingredients except pasta. For a ½ cup diet portion, mix ⅓ cup soup-vegetable mixture with ¼ cup low protein or regular pasta in an individual casserole.

For rest of family, to remaining soup-vegetable mixture add ⅔ to 1 cup cooked chicken pieces, 2 oz shredded cheddar cheese, and 1 cup cooked elbow macaroni. Put into a 1½-quart casserole or baking dish. Cover and bake side by side with small diet casserole, but 25 to 30 minutes instead of 15 minutes.

	Phenylalanine (mg)	Protein (gm)	Calories
Using low protein pasta			
Per diet recipe	291	8.4	349
Per ¼ cup (58 gm) serving	34	1.0	41
Per ½ cup (116 gm) serving	68	2.0	82
Using regular pasta			
Per diet recipe	625	15.3	274
Per ¼ cup (58 gm) serving	74	1.8	32
Per ½ cup (116 gm) serving	147	3.6	64

Golden Mushroom Casserole

½ cup (55 gm) uncooked
 Aproten Ditalini, Wel-Plan
 Macaroni, or regular elbow
 macaroni
4 oz can whole mushrooms,
 cut in pieces
¼ cup (35 gm) chopped onion
1 teaspoon vegetable oil

⅔ cup (152 gm) condensed
 Campbell's Cream of
 Mushroom Soup (¼ can)
¼ cup water
¼ teaspoon salt

To Make Diet Portion Only

Cook, rinse, and drain pasta according to package directions. While pasta is cooking, in a skillet sauté mushrooms and onion in vegetable oil 1 to 2 minutes or until onions are tender. Mix soup with water in a bowl; mix in cooked pasta, mushrooms, onions, and salt. Divide mixture into individual casseroles. Cover and bake one casserole at 350° for 15 minutes; refrigerate or freeze remainder for a later time.

Yield: 2¼ cups (477 gm).

To Make Diet Portion plus Family Portion

Mix together all ingredients except pasta. For a ½ cup diet portion mix ⅓ cup soup-vegetable mixture with ¼ cup cooked low protein or regular pasta in an individual casserole.

For rest of family, to remaining soup-vegetable mixture, add ⅔ to 1 cup (½ lb) cooked sirloin steak or beef cut in small pieces and 1 cup cooked elbow macaroni. Put into a 1½-quart casserole or baking dish. Cover and bake side by side with small diet casserole, but 25 to 30 minutes instead of 15 minutes.

	Phenylalanine (mg)	Protein (gm)	Calories
Using low protein pasta			
Per diet recipe	188	4.7	333
Per ¼ cup (53 gm) serving	21	0.5	37
Per ½ cup (106 gm) serving	42	1.0	74
Using regular pasta			
Per diet recipe	522	11.6	259
Per ¼ cup (53 gm) serving	58	1.3	29
Per ½ cup (106 gm) serving	116	2.6	57

Macaroni and Asparagus Casserole

½ cup (55 gm) uncooked
  Aproten Ditalini, Wel-Plan
  Macaroni, or regular elbow
  macaroni
1 cup plus 2 tablespoons
  (140 gm) fresh or frozen
  asparagus (½ of 10 oz pkg)

⅔ cup (152 gm) condensed
  Campbell's Cream of
  Asparagus Soup (½ can)
¼ cup water
¼ teaspoon salt

To Make Diet Portion Only
Cook, rinse, and drain pasta according to package directions. While pasta is cooking, cut asparagus into small pieces; if frozen asparagus is used, cook 3 minutes in a small amount of boiling water or in a vegetable steamer. If fresh asparagus is used, cook 4 to 6 minutes or until tender. Mix soup with water in a bowl; mix in cooked pasta, asparagus, and salt. Divide mixture into individual casseroles. Cover and bake one casserole at 350° for 15 minutes; refrigerate or freeze remainder for a later time.

Yield: 2¼ cups (493 gm).

To Make Diet Portion plus Family Portion
Mix together all ingredients except pasta. For a ½ cup diet portion mix ½ cup soup-vegetable mixture with ¼ cup cooked low protein or regular pasta in an individual casserole.

For rest of family, to remaining soup-vegetable mixture add ⅔ to 1 cup diced cooked chicken and 1 cup cooked elbow macaroni. If desired, add 2 oz shredded cheese or ½ cup sour cream. Put into a 1½-quart casserole or baking dish. Cover and bake side by side with small diet casserole, but 25 to 30 minutes instead of 15 minutes.

	Phenylalanine (mg)	Protein (gm)	Calories
Using low protein pasta			
Per diet recipe	258	7.8	342
Per ¼ cup (55 gm) serving	29	0.9	38
Per ½ cup (110 gm) serving	57	1.7	76
Using regular pasta			
Per diet recipe	593	14.6	267
Per ¼ cup (55 gm) serving	66	1.6	30
Per ½ cup (110 gm) serving	132	3.3	59

Pasta with Peas and Tomatoes

2 tablespoons (14 gm)
uncooked Aproten Ditalini
or Wel-Plan Macaroni
1 teaspoon vegetable oil
1 tablespoon (9 gm) chopped
onion
1½ tablespoons (14 gm) frozen
peas

1½ tablespoons (18 gm)
seeded, chopped, fresh or
canned tomatoes, drained
⅛ teaspoon basil
⅛ teaspoon salt

Cook, rinse, and drain pasta according to package directions. In a small saucepan heat oil and sauté onion until tender. Stir in peas; cover and cook over moderate heat 5 minutes. Add tomatoes, basil, and salt. Cook, stirring 2 minutes longer until mixture is bubbling. Add cooked pasta and heat through.

Yield: ½ cup (89 gm).

Family Portion
Prepare any multiple of the recipe to suit family needs, replacing low protein pasta with regular elbow macaroni. Add 2 to 3 tablespoons cooked, diced chicken for each ½ cup vegetable-pasta mixture.

	Phenylalanine (mg)	Protein (gm)	Calories
Per ½ cup (89 gm) diet serving	37	1.0	108

Vegetable Medley Skillet Supper

½ cup (46 gm) uncooked
  Aproten Rigatini
⅓ cup (45 gm) thinly sliced
  carrots
⅓ cup (35 gm) sliced celery
1½ teaspoons dried onion
  flakes or 2 tablespoons
  (18 gm) chopped onion

1 tablespoon vegetable oil
⅓ cup (57 gm) sliced canned
  mushrooms (2 oz can)
3 tablespoons tomato sauce
½ teaspoon salt

Cook, rinse, and drain Rigatini according to package directions. In a skillet, sauté carrots, celery, and onion in vegetable oil for about 5 minutes or until vegetables are tender. Mix in mushrooms, tomato sauce, cooked Rigatini, and salt. Heat through.

*Yield:*1¾ cups (276 gm).

	Phenylalanine (mg)	Protein (gm)	Calories
Per recipe	97	2.8	343
Per ½ cup (79 gm) serving	28	0.8	98

Mock Baked Beans

Baked bean flavor without the protein.

½ cup (55 gm) uncooked
  Aproten Ditalini or Wel-Plan
  Macaroni
2 tablespoons (18 gm) finely
  chopped onion or
  1½ teaspoons dry onion
  flakes moistened with
  2 teaspoons water

2 tablespoons catsup
2 teaspoons molasses
2 tablespoons packed brown
  sugar
¼ teaspoon dry mustard
¼ teaspoon salt
1 tablespoon water

Cook, rinse, and drain pasta according to package directions. Mix the cooked pasta with the remainder of the ingredients in a small casserole. Cover and bake at 325° for 20 minutes, until heated through. If mixture appears dry after baking, mix in a little extra water to moisten.

Yield: 1⅓ cups (235 gm).

	Phenylalanine (mg)	Protein (gm)	Calories
Per recipe	30	0.9	313
Per ¼ cup (45 gm) serving	6	0.2	60

Quick and Easy

This section contains a collection of simple recipes, tips for easy meal preparation, and quick-to-fix food ideas. The recipes are especially for when you are "too busy to cook" or for those who do not enjoy spending time in the kitchen.

The recipes—for main dishes, salads, and desserts—require few ingredients and take little preparation time. Many are suitable for the whole family, either "as is" or with suggested modifications. There are numbers of other recipes in the book which might have been included here, but these recipes were chosen to give a sampling of simple dinner, or perhaps lunch, ideas. Most of the recipes also would be suitable for an older child or for a teenager to prepare.

General Tips for Easy Meal Preparation

Whenever possible, freeze food . . . everything from casseroles to cookies. If you are preparing a recipe your child really likes, double the amount and freeze meal-size portions in plastic containers, plastic freezer bags, or seal-a-meal bags labeled for future use.

Several times a year, bulk order low protein products, especially Wel-Plan Baking Mix, wheat starch, and pastas, so that you always have a supply on hand.

Plan meals a few days or a week in advance. Set aside a routine time for doing this. Purchase necessary ingredients and/or make some items ahead of time either partially or completely, so there is a minimum to do at the last minute.

Plan a "bake day" at intervals of weeks or a few months. When possible let your child participate in the activities of these days; and for older children encourage involvement in recipe choices. One "bake day" might be devoted to preparation of bread, cookies, cupcakes, crackers, or other baked goods; the next might be devoted to casseroles, vegetables, soups. For convenience, consider making multiple variations from a basic recipe (for example, *Basic Cookies*, page 345). Well before the planned day, make sure you have all special ingredients on hand.

Consider purchasing a microwave oven. Reheating small diet portions will be greatly facilitated, and older children can learn to do this independently. There are also a number of recipes in the book which give microwave instructions and many others which can easily be adapted to microwave cookery with a little experience.

Make "dry mixes" for frequently used items such as pizza dough, pot pie dough, pie crust dough, biscuits, waffles, and pancakes (see *Master Mix Pancakes* recipe, page 298). Mix all of the dry ingredients together, store in an airtight plastic container labeled with recipe name, date, and page in cookbook (or brief instructions for completing). Add remaining ingredients when needed.

Make "T.V. dinners." Buy divided plastic plates suitable for a microwave oven. Fill the sections with a prepared vegetable and a casserole or other main dish item. Label with date, food items, and phenylalanine/protein content of each. Freeze, then reheat in microwave oven.

To satisfy restless and hungry young children while you are preparing dinner, take a few minutes to cut up an apple—it's low in phenylalanine/protein, good nutritionally, and keeps them busy while you're cooking.

Quick-to-Fix Food Ideas

—use *The Low Protein Food List for PKU* to calculate nutrient content.

Main Dishes and Vegetables

- Pre-package frozen french fries, weighed or counted into appropriate portion sizes, in plastic freezer bags. They are ready for the deep fryer, oven, or microwave whenever needed.
- "Scalloped potatoes" make a quick and filling meal. Pare, slice, and measure a medium size raw potato. Put in a small casserole dish along with about 1 tablespoon diced onion, 2 to 3 tablespoons condensed Campbell's Cream of Mushroom Soup, and salt/pepper to taste. Cover and microwave on High for about 8 to 10 minutes, stirring twice while cooking and adding a little water during cooking if potatoes seem too dry.
- Freeze unbaked or partially baked low protein pizza complete with sauce and toppings in a plastic freezer bag or freezer container. Bake in toaster oven (or in microwave oven if a crisp crust is not important).
- For a jiffy pizza, put 1 to 2 tablespoons catsup, 1 teaspoon of minced onion, and a little oregano on a slice of low protein bread. Broil 1 to 2 minutes
- Top cooked low protein pasta (any variety) with sautéed fresh vegetables. Use vegetables with a lot of color contrast to make an attractive meal (in general, always keep a large supply of fresh fruits and vegetables on hand for the whole family).
- Keep a box of instant white rice on hand, and a jar of meatless spaghetti sauce. A tasty supper can be concocted in a jiffy with these.
- Add a few peas and a tablespoon of condensed or slightly diluted Campbell's Cream of Mushroom Soup to cooked rice in a small casserole. Heat through.
- Schilling or French's Gravy mixes are tasty and quickly made in a microwave oven. Use not only on potatoes, but also on cooked low protein pasta, rice, or vegetables.
- For a quick soup, add 1 tablespoon dry instant white rice to 1 cup boiling water and a chicken bouillon cube or package of G. Wash-

ington's Seasoning and Broth mix; simmer for a few minutes until rice is tender. This is also good for traveling and camping.

- Package diluted Campbell's Vegetarian Vegetable Soup or other soup favorites in seal-a-meal bags. Freeze. The pouches are all ready to be boiled and are hot in a minute or two.
- Use the quick soup ideas in the *Soups* section of this book.
- Make "fry bread." Spread margarine on both sides of a slice of low protein bread, then fry both sides in margarine, as for a grilled sandwich. Serve with confectioner's sugar, homemade jelly, or maple syrup for breakfast or a light supper.
- For a "no-bacon, lettuce, and tomato sandwich," toast low protein bread, spread with mayonnaise or Miracle Whip, and add a lettuce leaf and a tomato slice.
- Top cooked low protein pasta with tomato sauce, or sprinkle with a little dry G. Washington's Seasoning and Broth powder or seasoned salt for extra flavor.
- For infants, cook vegetables, purée, then measure 2 or 3 tablespoons into ice cube tray slots. When cubes are frozen, put into labeled plastic freezer bags and take out when needed. Heat in a microwave oven using a baby dish or egg poacher.

Low Protein Bread

- Toast bread. Spread generously with protein-free or regular margarine and a mixture of cinnamon and sugar.
- Toast bread. Spread with a small amount of applesauce and sprinkle with a mixture of cinnamon and sugar. Broil until applesauce bubbles.
- Toast bread. Spread with protein-free or regular margarine and pour about 1 tablespoon of maple or maple-flavored syrup on top.
- Spread bread generously with protein-free or regular margarine and sprinkle on garlic salt or other seasonings. Broil for a minute or two.
- Spread Aproten Rusks generously with protein-free or regular margarine. Sprinkle with garlic salt. Broil, microwave, or bake in 300° oven until bubbly.
- Cut up toasted bread into bite-sized pieces in a dish. Sprinkle with a mixture of cinnamon and sugar. Pour hot Rich's Coffee Rich diluted one to one with water over bread for a delicious breakfast treat.
- See recipes in the *Breads* section on pages 64–132.

Snacks/Desserts

- Spoon Hunt's Lemon Snack Pak Pudding into a comet cone for a quick dessert or snack. The pudding is "free" but often hard to find, so stock up if you locate a source.

- Spoon whipped Rich's Richwhip Topping or Coolwhip into a comet cone for a quick "ice cream" cone.
- Make a "free" or very "low" sundae by freezing whipped Rich's Richwhip Topping or Coolwhip, and topping with Smucker's Strawberry Topping or canned cherry or strawberry pie filling.
- Sprinkle whipped Rich's Richwhip Topping or Coolwhip with colored sugar or colored candy sprinkles.
- For a young child, divide Jell-O instant pudding powder into ¼-package amounts and put into junior baby food jars, labeling with instructions. A small portion of pudding can then easily be made by adding 3 tablespoons liquid Rich's Richwhip Topping and 3 tablespoons water and shaking for a minute or two. This is handy both at home and away.
- Sprinkle crushed *Cinnamon Graham Cracker* crumbs over whipped Rich's Richwhip Topping or Coolwhip that has been mixed with a little drained, crushed, pineapple.
- Baskin-Robbins ice cream parlors sell fruit ices that are "free." Buy them by the pint or quart for desserts at home as well as for a cone in the store. Dole Fruit Sorbets are fruit ices which are found in many grocery stores in one-pint containers (½ cup = 15 mg phenylalanine, 0.3 gm protein).

Soup in a Minute

½ cup (40 gm) uncooked Wel-
    Plan Short Cut Spaghetti
⅓ cup (45 gm) thinly sliced or
    diced carrots
1 pkg G. Washington's Golden
    Seasoning and Broth or
    1 teaspoon Wyler's Chicken
    bouillon granules

2 cups water
1 teaspoon dried parsley flakes
½ teaspoon salt
dash of dried herbs of your
    choice

Mix all ingredients together, including uncooked pasta, in a medium saucepan. Cover and bring to a boil over high heat. Turn heat down to low; cover and let simmer 12 minutes, or until all ingredients are very tender.

Yield: 2 cups.

	Phenylalanine (mg)	Protein (gm)	Calories
Using G. Washington's Broth			
Per recipe	19	0.6	170
Per ½ cup serving	5	0.2	43
Using bouillon			
Per recipe	51	1.2	194
Per ½ cup serving	13	0.3	49

Fruit Cocktail Salad

16 oz can fruit cocktail,
   drained
4 oz container Coolwhip
   (1¾ cups) or ½ cup liquid
   Rich's Richwhip Topping,
   whipped

¼ cup (10 gm) flaked coconut

Mix all ingredients together in a medium bowl. Chill.

Yield: 2½ cups (414 gm).

	Phenylalanine (mg)	Protein (gm)	Calories
Using Richwhip			
Per recipe	59	1.5	467
Per ½ cup (83 gm) serving	12	0.3	93
Using Coolwhip			
Per recipe	143	3.1	399
Per ½ cup (83 gm) serving	29	0.6	80

Any Season Fruit Bowl

20 oz can chunk pineapple
11 oz can mandarin oranges
17 oz can dark sweet cherries

1¼ cups (150 gm) unpeeled
   apples, cut in pieces

Mix drained, canned fruits and apple pieces in a large bowl and serve.

Yield: 6 cups (1019 gm).

	Phenylalanine (mg)	Protein (gm)	Calories
Per recipe	115	4.4	1227
Per ½ cup (85 gm) serving	10	0.4	102

Golden Coins

A popular dish that makes vegetable eating easy for the whole family.

4 cups (540 gm) sliced fresh
carrots or a 20 oz bag frozen
sliced carrots
1 cup (140 gm) thinly sliced or
chopped onion
1 cup (110 gm) thinly sliced or
chopped green pepper
½ cup (125 gm) condensed
Campbell's Tomato Soup

½ cup granulated sugar
¼ cup vegetable oil
⅓ cup vinegar
½ teaspoon prepared (wet)
mustard
½ teaspoon Worcestershire
sauce
½ teaspoon salt
½ teaspoon pepper

Prepare vegetables, using a food processor for greatest convenience in preparing fresh carrots. Cook carrots until barely tender, or if using frozen carrots just allow to thaw completely. In a large bowl combine carrots, onion, and green pepper. In a small bowl mix together the soup, sugar, oil, vinegar, mustard, Worcestershire sauce, salt, and pepper. Pour over the vegetables and toss to coat completely with dressing. Cover and refrigerate for at least 1 hour, or preferably overnight, to marinate.

Yield: 5 cups (890 gm, without excess dressing).

Storage Tip
Keeps well, refrigerated, for up to 2 weeks.

	Phenylalanine (mg)	Protein (gm)	Calories
Per recipe	339	10.2	1564
Per ½ cup (45 gm) serving	34	1.0	156

Master Mix Pancakes

The easy way to make pancakes. This is an outstanding recipe, always ready for a satisfying breakfast. The batter also makes crispy, golden onion rings.

Pancake Master Mix

⅔ cup (83 gm) Wel-Plan Baking Mix
⅔ cup (83 gm) wheat starch
1⅓ cups (128 gm) sifted Softasilk cake flour (do not use regular flour)

4 teaspoons baking powder
1 teaspoon salt
3 tablespoons sugar
½ cup (56 gm) powdered Cremora or Coffee-Mate coffee creamer

Mix all ingredients together in a plastic container with airtight lid. Label with instructions for making pancakes. Store at room temperature indefinitely. Makes thirteen 4½-inch pancakes (420 gm dry mix).

To Make Pancakes

3½ tablespoons (32 gm) *Pancake Master Mix*
¼ teaspoon cinnamon (optional)

1 teaspoon vegetable oil
2½ to 3 tablespoons water

Mix all ingredients in a small bowl or measuring cup, using 2½ or 3 tablespoons water, depending on thickness of pancakes desired. Pour batter onto hot greased griddle. Cook on first side until bubbles appear and edges are slightly set, a minute or so; turn and brown other side.

Yield: one 4½-inch pancake.

	Phenylalanine (mg)	Protein (gm)	Calories
Per recipe *Pancake Master Mix*	536	11.6	1360
Per pancake	41	0.9	105

Variations

Low Master Mix Pancakes

Use 1 cup (110 gm) Wel-Plan Baking Mix, ⅔ cup (83 gm) wheat starch and only 1 cup (92 gm) sifted cake flour in the *Master Mix Pancakes* recipe. Prepare pancakes as for original recipe.

Yield: one 4½-inch pancake.

	Phenylalanine (mg)	Protein (gm)	Calories
Per recipe *Master Mix Pancakes*	398	8.7	1338
Per pancake	31	0.7	103

Onion Rings

1 recipe pancake batter (using 3½ tablespoons *Pancake Master Mix*)	eight ¼-inch onion rings, from a medium onion (100 gm) vegetable oil for frying

Dip onion rings in pancake batter. Fry until golden in oil heated to 375°. Remove to a paper towel to drain. Serve immediately.

Yield: 8 onion rings.

	Phenylalanine (mg)	Protein (gm)	Calories
Per recipe	70	2.0	363
Per onion ring	9	0.3	45

Mushroom Soup and Rice

An excellent family dish.

1 can condensed Campbell's
Cream of Mushroom Soup
1 soup can instant white rice
(1⅓ cups, 114 gm)
1 soup can water

1½ cups (201 gm) frozen carrot
slices
1½ cups (180 gm) frozen green
beans

Mix soup with water in a 2-quart casserole. Add rice and frozen vegetables, stirring until well mixed. Bake, covered, at 350° for 35 to 40 minutes or until rice and vegetables are done and most liquid is absorbed, or microwave on High for 12 to 14 minutes.

Yield: 4 cups (965 gm).

Note
To "extend" diet portion, remove ¼ cup serving of cassrole and add 2 to 4 tablespoons cooked Aproten Ditalini and a tablespoon or so of extra water to moisten. Reheat in microwave oven. Nutrient values for phenylalanine and protein will remain the same.

Family Portion
When casserole is baked, remove diet portion, then mix in 1 to 2 cups of cooked chicken pieces to remaining casserole and if desired, several tablespoons of grated Parmesan cheese. Microwave for an extra 1 to 2 minutes to heat through.

	Phenylalanine (mg)	Protein (gm)	Calories
Per diet recipe	935	21.4	828
Per ¼ cup (60 gm) serving	58	1.3	52

Quickie Tomato Mushroom Casserole

½ cup (55 gm) uncooked Aproten Ditalini, Wel-Plan Macaroni, or regular elbow macaroni
½ cup (115 gm) stewed tomatoes

⅓ cup (76 gm) condensed Campbell's Cream of Mushroom Soup (¼ can)
2 black olives, chopped (optional)
salt to taste

Cook, rinse, and drain pasta according to package directions. Meanwhile, chop stewed tomatoes into smaller pieces (do not drain). Mix tomatoes with undiluted mushroom soup in a small saucepan; add pasta and chopped olives and heat through. Season to taste.

Yield: 1½ cups (330 gm).

	Phenylalanine (mg)	Protein (gm)	Calories
Using low protein pasta			
Per recipe	121	3.2	285
Per ½ cup (110 gm) serving	40	1.1	95
Using regular pasta			
Per recipe	455	10.1	211
Per ½ cup (110 gm) serving	151	3.4	70

Goulash

½ cup (55 gm) uncooked
   Aproten Ditalini or Wel-Plan
   Macaroni
¾ cup (180 gm) cream-style
   corn

¾ cup tomato sauce or
   spaghetti sauce
   (without cheese or meat)
salt and pepper to taste

Cook, rinse, and drain pasta according to package directions. Mix pasta, corn, tomato or spaghetti sauce, and seasonings in a saucepan and heat, stirring occasionally until heated through.

Yield: 2¼ cups (550 gm).

Family Portion
Prepare any multiple of the recipe to suit family needs, using regular elbow macaroni. Add approximately ½ lb cooked ground beef per recipe.

	Phenylalanine (mg)	Protein (gm)	Calories
Per diet recipe	228	6.0	381
Per ¼ cup (61 gm) serving	25	0.7	42

No-Tuna Casserole

Great when the rest of the family is having "tuna casserole."

½ cup (55 gm) uncooked
   Aproten Ditalini or Wel-Plan
   Macaroni
3 tablespoons (66 gm)
   condensed Campbell's
   Cream of Mushroom Soup
1½ tablespoons water

1 tablespoon (9 gm)
   chopped onion
5 black olives, chopped
2 teaspoons (8 gm) frozen peas
2 tablespoons (13 gm) sliced
   celery

Cook, rinse, and drain pasta according to package directions. Mix soup with water; mix with pasta and remaining ingredients and place in a small, lightly greased casserole. Bake, covered, about 15 minutes at 350°, or microwave on High for 1 to 2 minutes.

Yield: 1¾ cups (244 gm).

	Phenylalanine (mg)	Protein (gm)	Calories
Per recipe	108	2.7	282
Per ¼ cup (35 gm) serving	15	0.4	40

Busy Day Casserole

⅓ cup (36 gm) uncooked
  Aproten Ditalini, Wel-Plan
  Macaroni, or regular elbow
  macaroni
1 tablespoon (8 gm) Durkee or
  Schilling Mushroom Gravy
  Mix, Brown Gravy Mix, or
  Onion Gravy Mix

⅓ cup water
⅓ cup (42 gm) canned Vege-All
  (remove lima beans)
salt to taste

Cook, rinse, and drain pasta according to package directions. Meanwhile, combine gravy mix with water in a small saucepan; bring to a boil over medium heat. Mix pasta and Vege-All in with gravy; heat through. Season to taste.

Yield: 1 cup (180 gm).

	Phenylalanine (mg)	Protein (gm)	Calories
Using low protein pasta			
Per recipe	90	2.0	173
Per ½ cup (90 gm) serving	45	1.0	86
Using regular pasta			
Per recipe	309	6.5	124
Per ½ cup (90 gm) serving	155	3.3	62

Mom's PKU Casserole

A larger quantity can be made to serve the whole family.

¼ cup (30 gm) cut frozen, fresh, or canned green beans
⅓ cup (45 gm) thinly sliced carrots
¼ cup (43 gm) diced potatoes

salt and pepper to taste
¼ teaspoon basil
2 tablespoons (28 gm) condensed Campbell's Cream of Mushroom Soup

Divide vegetables equally between 2 individual casseroles. Sprinkle salt, pepper, and basil over vegetables. Top each casserole with 1 tablespoon of undiluted soup. Cover and bake at 350° for 30 minutes, or microwave on High for 3 minutes or until vegetables are tender.

Yield: ¾ cup (130 gm).

	Phenylalanine (mg)	Protein (gm)	Calories
Per recipe	98	2.6	88
Per casserole (6 tablespoons, 65 gm)	49	1.3	44

Glorified Stew

1 can condensed Campbell's
   Vegetable Soup
⅔ cup (152 gm) condensed
   Campbell's Cream of
   Mushroom Soup (½ can)

1⅓ cups (227 gm) sliced
   potatoes
1 cup (135 gm) sliced carrots
½ teaspoon salt

In a bowl, mix undiluted soups together; mix in potatoes, carrots, and salt. Put in a 1- to 1½-quart casserole or baking dish, or individual casseroles; cover. Bake at 350° for 25 to 30 minutes, or microwave on High for 5 minutes or until vegetables are tender.

Yield: 3⅓ cups (800 gm).

Family Portion
Remove diet portion to an individual casserole. Add ¾ to 1 cup (½ lb) cooked ground beef to remainder of stew for a hearty main dish.

	Phenylalanine (mg)	Protein (gm)	Calories
Per diet recipe	681	17.8	580
Per ¼ cup (57 gm) serving	49	1.3	41

Quick Asparagus Casserole

14 oz can asparagus, drained
   or 1½ cups (270 gm) cooked
   frozen or fresh asparagus
⅔ cup (152 gm) condensed
   Campbell's Cream of
   Mushroom Soup (½ can)

¼ cup (16 gm) French's French
   Fried Onions

Mix asparagus with soup. Put into a 1-quart casserole or baking dish. Top with french fried onions. Bake at 350° for 20 minutes, or microwave on High for 3 to 4 minutes.

Yield: 2 cups (410 gm).

	Phenylalanine (mg)	Protein (gm)	Calories
Per recipe	378	12.2	276
Per ¼ cup (51 gm) serving	47	1.5	35

Quick Green Bean Casserole

For each serving desired:

1 tablespoon (14 gm) condensed
Campbell's Cream of
Mushroom Soup
1½ teaspoons water
¼ cup (30 gm) canned or
cooked, frozen, cut
green beans

1 tablespoon (4 gm) French's
French Fried Onions

Mix soup with water in a small casserole. Add green beans. Sprinkle french fried onions on top. Microwave on High for 45 seconds, or bake at 350° for 5 to 10 minutes or until heated through.

Yield: ¼ cup (45 gm).

	Phenylalanine (mg)	Protein (gm)	Calories
Per ¼ cup (45 gm) serving	42	1.2	49

Barbeque Beans

4 to 6 slices bacon cut in half
(remove for diet portion)
½ cup (70 gm) chopped onion
¾ cup catsup

¼ cup packed brown sugar
1½ tablespoons vinegar
⅓ cup liquid from beans
two 14½ oz cans cut green beans

In a skillet, fry bacon until done but not crisp. Remove bacon to paper toweling to drain. In 1 tablespoon bacon fat fry onions until tender, 1 to 2 minutes. In a measuring cup, mix together catsup, brown sugar, vinegar, and bean liquid. Mix onions, catsup mixture, and beans together in a 1½-quart casserole. Lay bacon on top. Microwave on High, covered, for 5 to 6 minutes; or bake at 325° for 45 minutes. For diet portion, remove bacon pieces. For family portion, serve beans with a bacon slice on top of each serving.

Yield: 3 cups (684 gm).

	Phenylalanine (mg)	Protein (gm)	Calories
Per diet recipe	296	10.1	665
Per ¼ cup (57 gm) serving	25	0.8	55

Quick Pizza Crust

1 cup (110 gm) Wel-Plan
   Baking Mix
½ teaspoon baking powder
dash of salt

1 tablespoon vegetable oil
¼ cup plus 2 teaspoons water
   with 1 scant drop yellow
   food coloring

Preheat oven to 425°. Stir together Baking Mix, baking powder, and salt in a medium bowl. Mix oil with water in a measuring cup. Gradually add liquid to dry ingredients, mixing thoroughly. Dough should be the consistency of soft biscuit dough; add a small amount of extra water or Baking Mix if necessary. Knead dough in your hands briefly, then pat into the bottom of a greased 9-inch pie pan. Spread with sauce and toppings of your choice (see pages 270–72). Bake for 12 to 18 minutes. (Do not overbake or the crust will become dry and tough.)

Yield: 1 pizza crust.

	Phenylalanine (mg)	Protein (gm)	Calories
Per pizza crust (not including sauce and topping)	4	0.3	503

Cracker Bars

Very similar to toffee candy, but with almost no effort.

20 Wel-Plan crackers	¾ cup (135 gm) Nestlé
1 cup margarine or butter	semisweet chocolate
1 cup packed brown sugar	chips

Preheat oven to 350°. Place crackers side by side on a lightly greased standard size cookie sheet. In a saucepan boil margarine and sugar for 5 minutes, stirring occasionally. Pour syrup over crackers, spreading evenly. Bake crackers for 5 minutes or until bubbly. Remove from oven and sprinkle with chocolate chips; return to oven for a minute or so to soften chips. Remove from oven and spread chocolate over bars. When cool cut each cracker square in half, making 40 bars.

Yield: 40 bars.

Note

You can easily make ½ of the recipe, placing 10 crackers on the cookie sheet (the sheet will only be ½ full, with 2 instead of 4 crackers in one of the rows).

	Phenylalanine (mg)	Protein (gm)	Calories
Per recipe	380	8.0	3536
Per bar	10	0.2	88

Creamy Lemon Pudding or Pie Filling

A tangy dessert with a thick and creamy consistency.

1 pkg (4 serving size) lemon
    Jell-O Instant Pudding and
    Pie Filling mix
¾ cup liquid Rich's Richwhip
    Topping

½ cup water
¼ cup bottled or fresh
    lemon juice

Mix all ingredients together in a medium bowl and beat on low speed with an electric mixer for 1 to 2 minutes, until smooth and creamy.

Yield: 1⅔ cups (420 gm).

	Phenylalanine (mg)	Protein (gm)	Calories
Per recipe	trace	trace	503
Per ½ cup (126 gm) serving	trace	trace	151

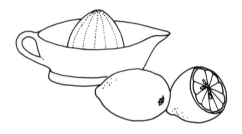

Instant Strawberry Ice Cream

Wonderful fresh strawberry flavor in a soft-serve type ice cream made in your food processor.

20 oz bag loose-frozen
   whole strawberries
   (6 cups, 600 gm)

¼ cup granulated sugar
8 oz carton liquid Rich's
   Richwhip Topping

    Pour strawberries into work bowl of a food processor with the steel blade in (a blender will not work satisfactorily); pulse on and off several times to break strawberries into fairly fine pieces. Add sugar and pulse several additional times. With food processor running, gradually pour Richwhip Topping through feed tube. Process until smooth (up to 45 seconds), scraping bowl once or twice as needed. Serve immediately. You may freeze leftovers; break into chunks and reprocess until smooth and creamy before serving.

Yield: 4½ cups.

Note
    Do not substitute strawberries packed in sugar syrup, or another non-dairy creamer.

	Phenylalanine (mg)	Protein (gm)	Calories
Per recipe	67	3.6	1159
Per ½ cup serving	7	0.4	129

310

Quick Banana Ice Cream

¼ cup orange juice
6-inch banana (80 gm),
   not overly ripe
12 large marshmallows
2 teaspoons granulated sugar
3 to 5 drops yellow food
   coloring

4 oz container Coolwhip
   (1¾ cups) or ½ cup liquid
   Rich's Richwhip Topping,
   whipped

In a covered blender at high speed, blend all ingredients except whipped topping about 1 to 2 minutes or until smooth. Do not use a fully ripe banana or the ice cream will have a dark color.

Fold banana mixture into whipped topping; pour into an 8- or 9-inch metal baking pan and freeze until firm. When frozen, repack into a covered plastic freezer container.

Yield: 2 cups.

	Phenylalanine (mg)	Protein (gm)	Calories
Using Richwhip			
Per recipe	73	2.4	721
Per ½ cup serving	18	0.6	180
Using Coolwhip			
Per recipe	157	4.0	653
Per ½ cup serving	39	1.0	163

Mock Angel Food

Tastes remarkably like Angel Food cake.

½-inch slice *Best White Bread*
¼ cup liquid Rich's Richwhip
  Topping

4 teaspoons vanilla protein-free
  frosting

Preheat oven to 400°. Cut crust from bread, then slice lengthwise and crosswise to form 4 squares. Put Richwhip Topping in a small dish; dip each square of bread, as you would for French toast. Allow each bread square to soak for about ½ minute, then turn over and soak again (you will only use about 2 tablespoons of the Richwhip Topping). Remove bread squares to a lightly greased or nonstick cookie sheet or pan. Bake for 3 to 4 minutes on each side. Allow to cool several minutes, then frost with a little phenylalanine-free frosting. Serve.

Yield: 1 serving.

Note
Pillsbury vanilla Ready-to-Spread Frosting Supreme is "free" and convenient to use.

	Phenylalanine (mg)	Protein (gm)	Calories
Per serving	11	0.2	353

Applesauce Dessert

1 cup (240 gm) applesauce
(chunky style is good)
2 teaspoons lemon juice
½ teaspoon cinnamon

1 cup (68 gm) Coolwhip or
whipped Rich's Richwhip
Topping

Stir lemon juice and cinnamon into applesauce until thoroughly mixed. Gently fold in Coolwhip. Chill. Pile into dessert glasses to serve.

Yield: 2 cups (318 gm).

	Phenylalanine (mg)	Protein (gm)	Calories
Using Richwhip			
Per recipe	12	0.4	377
Per ½ cup (80 gm) serving	3	0.1	94
Using Coolwhip			
Per recipe	63	1.4	336
Per ½ cup (80 gm) serving	16	0.4	84

Quick Apple Dessert

4 cups (480 gm) sliced tart
apples
⅓ cup granulated sugar
½ teaspoon cinnamon
¼ cup water

⅓ cup packed brown sugar
⅓ cup margarine or butter
⅔ cup (57 gm) Nabisco graham
cracker crumbs

Preheat oven to 350°. Put apples into a 9-inch pie or cake pan. Mix cinnamon with sugar. Sprinkle over apples. Pour water over top. Mix brown sugar, margarine, and cracker crumbs together in a small bowl; sprinkle mixture over apples. Bake for 30 minutes, or microwave on High for 8 minutes or until apples are tender.

Yield: 3⅓ cups (666 gm).

	Phenylalanine (mg)	Protein (gm)	Calories
Per recipe	219	4.8	1617
Per ¼ cup (50 gm) serving	16	0.4	121

Quick and Low Apple Dessert

1 cup (120 gm) sliced tart
apples
1½ tablespoons granulated
sugar
dash of cinnamon
1 tablespoon water
1½ tablespoons packed brown
sugar

1½ tablespoons margarine
or butter
2½ tablespoons (22 gm)
*Cinnamon Graham
Cracker* crumbs

Preheat oven to 350°. Put apples into a small baking pan or individual casserole. Continue with directions for *Quick Apple Dessert* (page 313). Bake for 20 minutes, or microwave on High for 3 to 4 minutes or until apples are tender.

Yield: ¾ cup (170 gm).

	Phenylalanine (mg)	Protein (gm)	Calories
Per recipe	22	0.6	454
Per ¼ cup (56 gm) serving	9	0.2	172

Amaretto Apples

5 cups (600 gm) tart apple
cubes (½-inch)
3 tablespoons margarine or
butter

¼ cup granulated sugar
¼ cup (40 gm) raisins
¼ cup amaretto liqueur
(almond-flavored)

Peel and cube apples. Melt margarine in a 2-quart baking dish. Add apples, sprinkle with sugar, and microwave on High, uncovered, for 3 minutes. Stir in raisins and liqueur and microwave on High for 3 to 5 minutes, until liquid reduces to a glaze and apples are tender.

Yield: 3 cups (680 gm).

Note

You can substitute ¼ cup water plus 1 teaspoon almond extract for amaretto liqueur. Add extra tablespoon sugar.

	Phenylalanine (mg)	Protein (gm)	Calories
Per recipe	74	3.0	1110
Per ½ cup (113 gm) serving	12	0.5	185

Honey-Glazed Apple Slices

Like apple crisp without the "crisp" and less sweet.

3 large cooking apples, peeled
2 tablespoons margarine or
  butter
2 tablespoons honey

1 teaspoon cornstarch
1 tablespoon orange liqueur
  or water
¼ teaspoon cinnamon

Quarter and core peeled apples (about 5 cups, 325 gm). Cut each quarter into 3 thick slices. Place apple slices in a 2-quart casserole; add margarine, cut in pieces. Microwave on High, uncovered, for 2 to 3 minutes, stirring once after 1 minute. Combine honey, cornstarch, water or liqueur, and cinnamon; pour over apples, stirring lightly to mix. Microwave on High, uncovered, 4 to 5 minutes or until apples are glazed and tender, stirring 2 or 3 times during cooking. Serve warm or cold.

Yield: 2 cups (490 gm).

	Phenylalanine (mg)	Protein (gm)	Calories
Per recipe	28	1.0	543
Per ½ cup (123 gm) serving	7	0.2	136

Maple Baked Bananas

6-inch banana
1 teaspoon margarine or butter
1 tablespoon maple or maple-
   flavored syrup

dash of cinnamon

Peel banana, cut in half, and slice each piece in half lengthwise. In a small dish, microwave margarine on High 30 to 45 seconds, until melted. Stir in maple syrup and cinnamon to taste. Place banana slices in dish, turning once to coat with syrup mixture. Microwave on High for 30 seconds. Turn bananas over and microwave on High for 30 seconds more. Serve warm.

Yield: 2 servings.

	Phenylalanine (mg)	Protein (gm)	Calories
Per recipe	45	1.2	204
Per serving	22	0.6	102

Strawberry Fool

A delightfully simple summer dessert for the whole family.

¾ cup (135 gm) mashed fresh
   strawberries
1½ tablespoons granulated
   sugar

8 oz container Coolwhip
   (3½ cups) or 8 oz carton
   liquid Rich's Richwhip
   Topping, whipped

Mix sugar into mashed strawberries and let stand 30 minutes. Fold strawberries into whipped topping. Garnish each serving with a whole fresh strawberry.

Yield: 3¾ cups.

	Phenylalanine (mg)	Protein (gm)	Calories
Using Richwhip			
Per recipe	11	0.8	754
Per ½ cup serving	2	0.1	101
Using Coolwhip			
Per recipe	179	4.0	618
Per ½ cup serving	24	0.5	82

Easy Crumb Topping

Use as a topping for any fruit crisp, for a fruit pie instead of a top crust, or to add crunch to a dessert of canned fruit pie filling.

4 Aproten Rusks, crushed fine
  (½ cup)
1½ tablespoons packed brown
  sugar

¼ teaspoon cinnamon or
  to taste
2 tablespoons melted
  margarine or butter

Mix sugar and cinnamon with rusk crumbs in a small bowl. Add melted margarine and mix well.

Yield: ½ cup.

	Phenylalanine (mg)	Protein (gm)	Calories
Per recipe	10	0.3	345
Per 1 tablespoon	1	trace	43

Cooking with Kids

This section includes a selection of recipes which require few ingredients, use simple preparation techniques, and are attractive and child appealing. They are designed for young children (as young as age 5 or 6) to prepare with adult help and supervision, or for older children to prepare by themselves. Readiness for help in recipe preparation or independent kitchen activities will depend on the individual child. You will need to use your judgment about when your own child is ready and what level of activity is appropriate.

For any child, food-related activities in the kitchen can be fun and rewarding. For children on a restricted diet, these activities have additional benefits. With young children, preparing special diet items offers you and your child a time to be together, and allows many opportunities to talk easily about diet. Your child will also learn what ingredients are used in special baking, and will develop measuring or weighing skills and an appreciation for accuracy. These experiences can foster pride in special diet foods, encourage the child to try the different foods that he or she has helped prepare, and facilitate their acceptance.

Do encourage *all* family members to taste what the child has made!

General Tips for Kids in the Kitchen

Even if your child is not interested in helping in the kitchen, try to make special cookies, cakes, and baked goods when he or she is around so there is the fun of tasting dough, licking beaters, etc.—something enjoyed by children of *all* ages.

Let your young child participate in simple activities like stirring batter, helping to knead bread dough, cutting out and decorating cookies, washing vegetables and fruits, or pulling apart lettuce for a salad.

Help your young child make a recipe by premeasuring or weighing ingredients into small dishes, then let him or her stir them together.

Let your young child be a "gopher" for recipe ingredients.

Try marking measuring cups and spoons with colored stick-on dots, then put the same color dots next to measurements on a recipe to help the child decide quickly which measuring utensil goes with which ingredient.

Let your child help choose what recipes he or she wants you to make by going through the cookbook.

Thumb-index your *Low Protein Food List* by category so your older child can look up phenylalanine values for foods being prepared for a meal.

Teach your older child to use a gram scale if you use one regularly.

Before you do your weekly grocery shopping, let your older child help plan menus. Let the child choose what he or she especially likes, including salad, vegetable/main dish, and dessert. Plan not only what the child on-diet would eat, but what the rest of the family would eat that is the same or similar. Planning with your child gives you the opportunity to talk about the "phe" or protein content of foods and gives him or her the satisfaction of making a decision.

Let your child help weigh or measure out portions of food that he or she will eat, whether or not the child has been involved in preparation.

Let your child help pack his or her own lunch for school, and help count "phes" or protein.

Let your child participate in cooking for others in the family, or in packing their lunches. Having experiences with high protein foods, other than eating them, will help defuse the mystery over these foods by letting the child "explore" forbidden foods (seeing texture of eggs being broken, etc.) and allowing him or her to enjoy serving these foods to others. By seeing what foods go into recipes for the rest of the family (e.g., eggs in cookies) your child will better understand why regular homemade cookies are not allowed or infrequently allowed. Preparing these foods together gives you an opportunity to talk about them and why they are not on the diet.

Easy Food Preparation Ideas for Kids

Let your child:
- Make sandwiches, choosing the filling from several choices offered, and using low protein bread or crackers (see page 523 for sandwich ideas).

- Create his or her own vegetable soup, using G. Washington's Seasoning and Broth, cut-up vegetables, and low protein pasta (see page 134 for guidelines in creating such a soup).
- Make his or her own salads with lettuce, assorted vegetables, and a "free" dressing.
- "Invent" desserts with Coolwhip or Richwhip Topping and either fresh or frozen fruit (whole or mashed), adding colored candy sprinkles or a cherry for a decorative touch.
- Use a handmixer to make low protein instant pudding (see page 399).
- Make Kool-Aid for the whole family.
- Help with formula preparation beginning at a very young age. As early as age 2 or 3 a child will enjoy pushing buttons on the blender, or getting the can of formula for you. Later, he or she can help measure or weigh formula powder, putting it into the blender. Routine involvement with formula preparation from a young age will prepare the child for mixing the formula independently at a relatively young age, and may foster positive acceptance of formula drinking.

Wicked Witches Brew

For your Halloween party. By leaving out the make-believe "toads," this is also a nice drink for winter holiday time!

32 oz (1 quart) apple cider	5 whole cloves
½ cup lemon juice	2 cinnamon sticks
1 teaspoon nutmeg	toads (make-believe)

1. Combine cider, lemon juice, nutmeg, cloves, cinnamon sticks, and make-believe toads in a medium saucepan.
2. Bring cider to a boil over low heat and simmer 10 minutes.
3. Cool cider slightly and serve, leaving the cloves, cinnamon sticks, and imaginary toads in the bottom of the pan. You can also serve the cider cold.

Makes 4½ cups (36 oz).

	Phenylalanine (mg)	Protein (gm)	Calories
Per recipe	24	1.2	509
Per ½ cup (4 oz) serving	3	0.1	57

(20 oz = 1 exchange)

Red Hot Soup

1 can condensed Campbell's
   Tomato Soup
¼ cup apple juice

1 cup water
a dash of cloves
a dash of cinnamon

1. Combine all ingredients in a saucepan or microwave-safe dish.
2. Mix, then heat on stove for several minutes or in microwave oven on High for 2 to 3 minutes, or until as hot as you like.
3. Serve.

Makes 2¼ cups (600 gm).

	Phenylalanine (mg)	Protein (gm)	Calories
Per recipe	109	3.1	244
Per ½ cup (133 gm) serving	24	0.7	54
	(1½ exchanges)		

Shawn's Pasta Soup Deluxe

A favorite recipe created by a young boy with PKU.

½ cup (45 gm) cauliflower,
broken into small flowerets
¼ cup (46 gm) Aproten Anellini
1 pkg G. Washington's Golden
Seasoning and Broth
1½ cups water
dash of salt

dash of garlic powder
dash of onion powder
1 teaspoon dried parsley flakes
(if you want)
1 teaspoon Betty Crocker
BacO's Bits (be sure
it is a *level* teaspoon)

1. Combine cauliflower pieces, uncooked pasta, broth powder, and water in a medium saucepan.
2. Cover pan and bring soup to a boil over high heat.
3. Turn heat down to low. Put cover back on the pan and let simmer 8 minutes.
4. Add salt and seasoning, and imitation bacon bits.
5. Serve.

Makes 1½ cups.

	Phenylalanine (mg)	Protein (gm)	Calories
Per recipe	79	1.9	189
Per ½ cup serving	26	0.6	63
	(2 exchanges)		

Snoopy Salad

1 lettuce leaf
1 canned pear half
1 canned prune
1 raisin

1 maraschino or candied
  cherry
2 canned mandarin orange
  segments

1. Wash a lettuce leaf and pat dry with a paper towel. Place on salad plate.
2. Using a fork, lift a nice big pear half, a prune, and 2 mandarin orange segments from their cans and 1 maraschino cherry from the jar and place on a paper towel to dry. Refrigerate remaining fruit for another time.
3. Place the pear half, cut side down, on the lettuce leaf. This will be Snoopy's head.
4. Cut the prune lengthwise in half with a scissors and take out the pit. Place one of the prune halves at the large end of pear half for the ear. Eat the other prune half!
5. Using a teaspoon, scoop out a tiny hole in the pear half for the eye. Place a raisin in the hole.
6. Cut the cherry in half with the scissors. Place one half at the top of the narrow end of the pear half for the nose. Eat the other half!
7. Use the mandarin orange segments for the collar.

Makes 1 salad.

	Phenylalanine (mg)	Protein (gm)	Calories
Per salad	15 (1 exchange)	0.6	72

Kids' Apple Salad

¼ cup (30 gm) cut-up,
   unpeeled apple
¼ cup (30 gm) shredded
   carrots

2 tablespoons (20 gm) raisins
2 tablespoons Miracle Whip
   Salad Dressing

1. Cut apple in small pieces.
2. Shred carrots using a grater.
3. In a small bowl combine apple pieces, grated carrots, and raisins.
4. Mix in Miracle Whip.
5. Put salad in refrigerator for 1 hour or more before serving.

Makes ⅔ cup (96 gm).

	Phenylalanine (mg)	Protein (gm)	Calories
Per recipe	31	1.1	231
Per ⅓ cup (48 gm) serving	15	0.6	115
	(1 exchange)		

Taco Salad

⅔ cup (35 gm) lettuce, torn
   in pieces
4 black olives, cut in pieces
   (optional)
¼ cup (60 gm) cut-up tomatoes
4 Doritos

2 to 4 tablespoons Kraft
   Catalina Salad Dressing
   (use as much as you want),
   or any favorite "free" salad
   dressing

Diet Portion
1. Tear lettuce into bite-sized pieces.
2. Cut up olives and tomatoes.
3. Put lettuce, olives, and tomatoes in a bowl.
4. Break each Dorito into several pieces. Mix into salad just before serving.
5. Top salad with salad dressing.

Makes 1½ cups (1 serving).

Family Portion
1. Make individual salads, like the *Diet Portion*, according to the number of people you want to serve.
2. Add shredded American or cheddar cheese on top, and sour cream or avocado pieces if desired. You could also add some cooked ground beef.

	Phenylalanine (mg)	Protein (gm)	Calories
Per 1½ cup diet serving	67	1.4	235
	(4½ exchanges)		

Variation

Low Taco Salad
Replace the Doritos with 4 low protein *Taco Chips* (page 110). Otherwise make the salad as in the original recipe.

Makes 1½ cups (1 serving).

	Phenylalanine (mg)	Protein (gm)	Calories
Per 1½ cup serving	43	1.2	220
	(3 exchanges)		

"Low Pro" Spaghettios®

½ cup (65 gm) uncooked   a little salt
   Aproten Anellini
3 tablespoons tomato sauce
   or spaghetti sauce
   (without meat or cheese)

1. Cook, rinse, and drain pasta according to directions on the package.
2. Mix pasta and tomato sauce or spaghetti sauce in a small sauce pan or microwave-safe dish
3. Add the amount of salt you like.
4. Heat on stove for a few minutes, or microwave on High for 1½ to 2 minutes, or until as hot as you like.
5. Serve.

Makes 1⅓ cups (320 gm).

	Phenylalanine (mg)	Protein (gm)	Calories
Per 1⅓ cup serving	30 (2 exchanges)	0.9	244

Trademark used with permission of Campbell Soup Company.

Kids' Vegetable Casserole

½ cup (55 gm) uncooked
    Aproten Ditalini or Wel-Plan
    Macaroni
⅔ cup (152 gm) condensed
    Campbell's Vegetarian
    Vegetable Soup (½ can)

¼ teaspoon salt

1. Cook, rinse, and drain pasta according to directions on the package.
2. In a saucepan or microwave-safe dish, mix undiluted soup, pasta, and salt.
3. Heat through on stove, or in microwave oven on High for 1½ to 2 minutes, or until as hot as you like.
4. Serve.

Makes 1½ cups (290 gm).

	Phenylalanine (mg)	Protein (gm)	Calories
Per recipe	163	3.5	333
Per ½ cup (97 gm) serving	54	1.2	111
	(3½ exchanges)		

Macaroni in a Mug

½ cup (55 gm) uncooked
  Aproten Ditalini or Wel-Plan
  Macaroni
¼ cup (56 gm) condensed
  Campbell's Old-Fashioned
  Vegetable Soup (take out
  the lima beans)

3 tablespoons tomato sauce
  or spaghetti sauce
  (without meat or cheese)

1. Cook, rinse, and drain pasta according to directions on the package.
2. Mix cooked pasta with undiluted soup and tomato sauce or spaghetti sauce in a small saucepan and heat for a few minutes; serve in a coffee mug or soup mug. Or put everything in a mug and microwave on High for 1½ minutes, or until as hot as you like.
3. Serve.

Makes 1 cup.

	Phenylalanine (mg)	Protein (gm)	Calories
Per 1 cup serving	78 (5½ exchanges)	2.3	251

Kids-Love-It Pizza

1 package Pillsbury Buttermilk Refrigerator Rolls (6 biscuits per package)

6 tablespoons tomato sauce or spaghetti sauce (without meat or cheese)

1. Preheat oven to 450°.
2. Lightly grease a cookie sheet or baking pan.
3. Remove biscuits from package.
4. With your hands, press each biscuit into a 3-inch circle on the cookie sheet or pan.
5. Spread 1 tablespoon sauce on each biscuit.
6. Sprinkle *Pizza Toppings* of your choice on one pizza. Have an adult help you figure how the pizza fits into your diet after you add toppings.
7. Let anyone else who wants a pizza put on his or her own toppings.

Makes 6 pizzas.

Pizza Toppings (choose one or more):

	Phenylalanine (mg)	Protein (gm)	Calories
chopped olives, 1 tablespoon	3	0.1	15
sliced mushrooms, 1 tablespoon	3	0.2	2
chopped onions, 1 tablespoon	3	0.1	3
chopped green peppers, 1 tablespoon	3	0.1	2

	Phenylalanine (mg)	Protein (gm)	Calories
Per recipe	467	10.0	329
Per pizza (not including toppings)	78 (5½ exchanges)	1.7	55

Jiffy Fudge

one-pound package (4 cups) of
  confectioner's sugar
⅓ cup Hershey's unsweetened
  cocoa (not instant)

¼ cup Rich's Coffee Rich
½ cup margarine or butter
2 teaspoons vanilla

1. Line an 8 × 8-inch baking pan with aluminum foil.
2. Put confectioner's sugar and cocoa through sifter, sifting into a 2-quart microwave-safe baking dish. Add the Coffee Rich and margarine. *Do not stir.*
3. Place baking dish in microwave oven; microwave on High for 2 to 2½ minutes, or until margarine is just melted.
4. Add vanilla, then stir with a wooden spoon until all the ingredients are well blended.
5. Scrape fudge from baking dish into the foil-lined pan; smooth the top with a knife or spatula. Place in freezer for ½ hour to set firm.
6. Cut into 36 pieces. Wrap individual pieces in plastic wrap and refrigerate or freeze.

Makes 36 pieces.

	Phenylalanine (mg)	Protein (gm)	Calories
Per recipe	409	8.7	2783
Per piece	11	0.2	77
	(1½ pieces are 1 exchange)		

331

Chocolate-Covered Cherries

10 oz jar maraschino cherries
    with stems (25 cherries)
½ cup (90 gm) Nestlé semisweet
    chocolate chips

1½ teaspoons vegetable
    shortening or vegetable oil

1. Put a sheet of waxed paper on top of a cookie sheet.
2. Remove cherries from the jar and place on a double layer of paper towels laid on the kitchen counter to dry. Pat with more paper towels to dry as much as possible.
3. Put chocolate chips in a small microwave-proof dish. Add shortening or oil.
4. Microwave chocolate chips on medium power for 3 minutes. Stir, then microwave for 2 more minutes.
5. Holding one cherry by the stem, dip it into the chocolate mixture to coat completely. Gently shake off excess chocolate, then place on the prepared cookie sheet.
6. Repeat step #5 with all of the remaining cherries. (You should have about 1 tablespoon of chocolate left after all the cherries have been dipped.)
7. Refrigerate cherries until chocolate is firm, then remove them to a covered container and store in the refrigerator.

Makes 25 cherries.

	Phenylalanine (mg)	Protein (gm)	Calories
Per recipe	189	4.4	695
Per cherry	8	0.2	28
	(½ exchange)		

Finger Gelatin

1 package Prono low protein
   gelled dessert mix (any
   flavor)

½ cup water
granulated sugar, if you want

1. In a small saucepan, mix Prono and water and bring to a boil over medium heat until dessert powder is dissolved. Or microwave on High in a microwave-safe dish for 1 minute or until it boils.
2. Pour mixture into a 7 × 4-inch loaf pan and let stand at room temperature until it is firm.
3. Cut into 12 pieces. Roll each piece in granulated sugar if desired.

Makes 12 pieces.

Storage Tip
Keeps well, covered, for up to a week or more. Refrigeration is not necessary.

	Phenylalanine (mg)	Protein (gm)	Calories
Per recipe	0	0	335
Per piece	0 ("free")	0	28

Prono Pops

1 cup boiling water
½ package (3 tablespoons)
    Prono low protein gelled
    dessert mix, any flavor

1 package Kool-Aid (of same or
    similar flavor as Prono)
¾ cup granulated sugar
1¾ cups cold water

1. Boil water in a saucepan, or put in a glass measuring cup and microwave on High for 2 to 2½ minutes.
2. Mix Prono powder, Kool-Aid powder, and sugar in a bowl.
3. Add boiling water to Prono and Kool-Aid. Stir until dissolved.
4. Add the cold water to the Kool-Aid mixture. Stir.
5. Pour mixture into 12 Tupperware Ice Tups molds, ¼ cup liquid in each one.
6. With adult help, place a plastic stick and top on each Ice Tup mold.
7. Freeze.

Makes 12 pops.

	Phenylalanine (mg)	Protein (gm)	Calories
Per recipe	9	0	633
Per pop	0 ("free")	0	53

Orange Juice Freeze

¾ cup (6 fl oz, ½ of 12 oz can) frozen orange juice concentrate, thawed

2 cups plus 2 tablespoons (17 fl oz) water

3 medium bananas (each 6 inches long; 342 gm)

8 oz can crushed pineapple in its own juice

1. In a large bowl, mix orange juice with the three cans of water.
2. Peel, then slice bananas using a table knife into the bowl of orange juice.
3. Open pineapple can and add pineapple and its juice to the orange juice mixture. Mix well.
4. Spoon mixture into twenty 3 oz Dixie cups or other small containers, trying to divide bananas as evenly as you can. Cover, or put uncovered small containers in a large plastic container. Freeze.
5. Eat as a breakfast fruit, a frozen salad, or as a snack, letting it get slightly slushy before eating.

Makes 20 Dixie cups.

	Phenylalanine (mg)	Protein (gm)	Calories
Per recipe	203	6.9	688
Per Dixie cup (¼ cup serving)	10	0.3	34
	(1 exchange)		

Banana Boats

1 medium banana   10 Nestlé semisweet chocolate chips
  (6 inches long)   8 mini marshmallows

1. Preheat oven to "broil" if you want to use a regular oven. (You can also use a microwave oven, which is easier.)
2. Peel banana. Cut in half so you have two 3-inch sections of banana.
3. Cut a V-shaped wedge lengthwise in each banana section. Remove the cut piece and eat, or save for something else.
4. Place the banana sections in a small baking pan or microwave-safe dish.
5. Fill the banana groove with a chocolate chip, then a marshmallow, and continue alternating until you have 4 marshmallows and 5 chocolate chips for each banana.
6. *For a regular oven,* cover pan with foil; put into oven on a rack 6 inches from broiler and broil for 5 minutes. Remove foil and broil, uncovered, for a few seconds until marshmallows are golden brown. *For a microwave oven,* microwave on High, uncovered, for 1½ minutes, or until marshmallows are puffy.
7. Eat while warm.

Makes 2 banana boats.

	Phenylalanine (mg)	Protein (gm)	Calories
Per recipe	66	1.7	181
Per banana boat	33	0.8	91
	(2½ exchanges)		

Blushing Baked Apple

1 medium-sized cooking apple (180 gm)
2 teaspoons brown sugar

2 teaspoons red cinnamon candies
1 teaspoon lemon juice

1. Preheat oven to 350° if you want to use a regular oven. (You can also use a microwave oven.)
2. Peel the top two-thirds of the apple with a potato peeler; then have an adult help core the apple to within ½ inch of the bottom. Place apple in a baking dish or microwave-safe dish.
3. Mix brown sugar with candies and lemon juice in a small dish; fill the apple cavity using a spoon.
4. Pour ½ cup water in the bottom of the pan.
5. *For a regular oven*, bake for 30 to 40 minutes or until apple is tender but still holds its shape. *For a microwave oven*, microwave on High for 5 to 6 minutes or until apple is tender.
6. Let apple cool slightly, then serve warm.

Makes 1 apple.

	Phenylalanine (mg)	Protein (gm)	Calories
Per apple	8 (½ exchange)	0.4	155

Grammys

1 regular graham cracker square or 1 low protein *Cinnamon Graham Cracker*

¼ teaspoon softened margarine or butter
¼ teaspoon granulated sugar
a little cinnamon

1. Using a table knife, spread the graham cracker with margarine.
2. Mix the sugar with a little cinnamon and sprinkle the mixture over the cracker.
3. *For a regular oven,* place cracker on a small pan and bake for 10 minutes at 275°. *For a microwave oven,* place cracker on paper towel or plate. Microwave on High for 30 to 45 seconds, until bubbly.
4. Let cool, then eat.

Makes 1 grammy.

	Phenylalanine (mg)	Protein (gm)	Calories
Using low protein graham cracker	trace ("free")	trace	53
Using regular graham cracker	21 (1½ exchanges)	0.4	42

Chocowich

2 slices *Best White Bread* or
   Best Homestyle Bread

1 tablespoon of your
   favorite jam
12 semisweet chocolate chips

1. Lightly toast the bread in a toaster or toaster oven.
2. Spread toast with jam.
3. Arrange chocolate chips on top of jam.
4. Top with second slice of toast.
5. Broil for 1 minute or until bread is golden brown.
6. Eat while hot.

Makes 1 sandwich.

	Phenylalanine (mg)	Protein (gm)	Calories
Per sandwich	32 (2 exchanges)	0.9	260

Mini S'more Snacks

1 regular graham cracker
  square or 1 low protein
  *Cinnamon Graham
  Cracker*
8 regular size Nestlé semisweet
  chocolate chips or
  ½ teaspoon Nestlé mini semisweet
  chocolate chips

1. Place cracker on paper towel or a plate. Top with chocolate chips, then marshmallows.
2. Put in microwave oven.
3. Microwave on High for 15 to 30 seconds, until marshmallows just start to puff.
4. Let cool slightly, then eat.

Makes 1 serving.

	Phenylalanine (mg)	Protein (gm)	Calories
Using low protein graham cracker	22 (½ exchange)	0.5	112
Using regular graham cracker	42 (3 exchanges)	0.9	101

Cookies

Cookies from the recipes in this section look and taste like regular cookies, though they will not generally brown as deeply (except the several recipes using an egg yolk). All have excellent flavor and texture and will be enjoyed by those on the diet as well as others.

The cookies in this section are not fragile, but sturdy, and travel and keep well. They are ideal for school lunches—or for anytime.

Special Tips

Most of the baked cookies and bars include vanilla Jell-O Instant Pudding and Pie Filling mix. Be sure to use the *instant* pudding mix (the cook-type mix will not work in these recipes). Be sure that you do *not* use pudding mix sweetened with aspartame.

The recipes using pudding mix are all adaptations of a basic recipe, using more or less water and with only slight alterations in other ingredients to make cookies of different shapes and textures. Many different variations of the recipes are obtained by adding chips, by using a different flavor pudding mix, etc.

The cookies using pudding mix are essentially "disaster proof." Even if the Baking Mix/wheat starch or water measurements are not exact, you will never have cookies that "spread all over the pan" as was the tendency in the past for many cookies containing wheat starch. The various recipes using pudding mix are all equally successful; they are also adaptable, and you may be interested in creating your own variations of the basic recipes.

There are three recipes which call for an egg yolk (*Crackly Molasses Cookies, Chocolate Chip Cookies,* and *Toffee Bars*). In order to separate the white from the yolk, the egg should be cold, not at room temperature. Separate the yolk as carefully as you can; a small amount of white will cling to it. Be sure to use a medium-sized egg (average weight 41 gm, including shell), not large or extralarge. Because of the great amount of phenylalanine/protein in the egg, if you use an egg larger than medium, the cookies will contain significantly more phenylalanine and protein than indicated for the recipe.

Preparing cookie dough in a food processor is a great convenience. Add ingredients in order listed in the recipe, using the steel blade to process briefly. If you are adding chocolate chips, be sure you do not overprocess or they will melt; do process until they *barely* begin to melt for a nice brown cookie that looks just like a "regular" one.

It is often difficult to make the exact number of cookies called for in recipes other than those for bar cookies. Especially for cookies that are relatively "high," it is convenient to weigh the dough on a gram scale. Then divide the total weight by the number of cookies called for in the recipe and you will find the weight needed per cookie. Weigh the dough for several cookies, to guide you in determining size, or weigh the dough for each cookie if you are especially concerned about the accuracy of phenylalanine/protein. For example, *Peanut Butter Cookies* yields 680 gm of dough. To make the 40 cookies called for, use 17 gm of dough per cookie (680 ÷ 40 = 17).

Bake only one pan of cookies at a time for most consistent results.

Let a hot cookie sheet cool before putting on another batch of cookie dough, or use two or more cookie sheets and alternate so the sheet is always cool for a new batch of dough.

Place cookie sheet in the middle rack of the oven to bake.

Always bake cookies in a *preheated* oven.

Cool hot cookies on a wire rack.

There are many recipes for chocolate chip cookies to choose from, since they seem to be the most popular. All of the varieties are excellent; find your favorite.
- *Chocolate Chip Cookies*, with egg yolk
- from *Basic Cookies*
  Method 1 drop cookies (least "traditional" in appearance).
  Method 2 rolled, then flattened with a flat-bottomed glass.
- from *Basic Cut-Out Cookies*
- from *Freezer Cookies*

Store cooled cookies according to their crispness:
- Store *soft cookies* (for example *Basic Cookies* using fruit or vegetable purée) in an airtight container, with a small piece of bread or apple for maintaining moisture.
- Store *bar cookies* in a single layer, or layer with waxed paper or plastic wrap.
- Store *crisp cookies* in a container or tin with a loose-fitting lid to retain crispness.

To cut bar cookies into the number indicated by the recipe:

8 × 8-inch pan,
16 bars

8 × 8-inch pan,
20 bars

8 × 8- or 9 by 9-inch pan,
25 bars

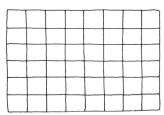

13 × 9 or 11 × 7-inch pan,
48 bars

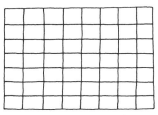

13 × 9 or 11 × 7-inch pan,
56 bars

All of the cookies freeze well in an airtight container for up to several months.

Freezing the *dough* works well and makes it easy to make fresh cookies with little effort. The dough for any cookie using pudding mix freezes exceptionally well. Freeze in small quantities to make a certain number of cookies (label the number); or just remove desired portion from the whole mass, as needed. The latter method relies on the accuracy of your memory as to the size cookie to make for a given phenylalanine/protein content, *or* first weighing your total mass of dough and then determining the weight of dough to use for each cookie. If the particular cookie variation contains almost no phenylalanine/protein, variability in the size of your cookie will not matter very much.

Two recipes containing peanut butter are included. Your child should have an explanation about why peanut butter is allowed in cookies but not on bread (*very* little in each cookie). You will want to use discretion in using these recipes—it may not be wise for some children.

Basic Cookies

A never-fail cookie with many variations that are all simply delicious.

½ cup vegetable shortening
⅓ cup softened margarine
  or butter
2 tablespoons granulated sugar
¼ cup packed brown sugar
1 pkg (4-serving size) vanilla
  Jell-O Instant Pudding and
  Pie Filling mix
1 teaspoon vanilla

⅓ cup plus 1 tablespoon water
  (*Method 1 only*)
3 tablespoons water (*Method 2*
  only)
2 cups (220 gm) Wel-Plan
  Baking Mix
1½ teaspoons baking powder
½ teaspoon salt

Preheat oven to 375°. In a medium mixing bowl, cream shortening and margarine with sugars. Add pudding mix and vanilla, mixing well. Gradually add water, mixing well. Stir together Baking Mix, baking powder, and salt; add to creamed mixture, mixing until thoroughly combined.

Method 1
Drop dough by teaspoonful onto an ungreased cookie sheet, 20 to 25 cookies per sheet. Slightly flatten each cookie with back of spoon, if you wish, as the cookies will not spread or flatten significantly during baking. Bake for 10 minutes. Let cookies cool slightly on baking sheet, then remove to wire cooling rack. Cookies will remain more soft than crisp.

Method 2
(This can be used for any of the variations which do not have added fruit or vegetable purée, to make a more traditional-appearing round, flat cookie).

Using your hands, shape dough into small walnut-sized balls, and place on an ungreased cookie sheet, 20 to 25 cookies per sheet. With a flat-bottomed glass or small dish dusted with Baking Mix, flatten balls to a ¼- to ⅜-inch thickness. For a crisp cookie, bake 12 minutes; for a softer cookie, bake 8 to 10 minutes.

Yield: 36 cookies.

Note
Wheat starch may be substituted for Baking Mix in this recipe with similar results.

Storage Tip
Baked cookies freeze well. Dough also freezes very well for up to 6 months in an airtight plastic container. To have a variety of cookies

available, prepare several batches using different variations; bake some now, freeze remainder of the dough for another time.

	Phenylalanine (mg)	Protein (gm)	Calories
Per recipe	48	1.5	2835
Per cookie	1	trace	79

Variations

Applesauce Raisin Cookies

Delete water and add ⅔ cup (160 gm) applesauce, ⅓ cup (53 gm) raisins, 1 teaspoon cinnamon, and ½ teaspoon nutmeg.

Yield: 36 cookies.

	Phenylalanine (mg)	Protein (gm)	Calories
Per recipe	91	3.5	3115
Per cookie	3	0.1	87

Applesauce Spice Cookies

Delete water and add ⅔ cup (160 gm) applesauce, 1 teaspoon cinnamon, and ½ teaspoon nutmeg.

Yield: 36 cookies.

	Phenylalanine (mg)	Protein (gm)	Calories
Per recipe	56	1.8	2956
Per cookie	2	0.1	82

Banana Chocolate Chip Cookies

Delete water and add ⅔ cup (154 gm) mashed ripe bananas and ¼ cup (45 gm) Nestlé mini semisweet chocolate chips.

Yield: 36 cookies.

	Phenylalanine (mg)	Protein (gm)	Calories
Per recipe	197	5.0	3217
Per cookie	5	0.1	89

Banana Spice Cookies

Delete water and add ⅔ cup (154 gm) mashed ripe bananas and 1 teaspoon cinnamon.

Yield: 36 cookies.

	Phenylalanine (mg)	Protein (gm)	Calories
Per recipe	106	3.1	2977
Per cookie	3	0.1	83

Butterscotch Cookies

Replace vanilla instant pudding with butterscotch instant pudding.

Yield: 36 cookies.

	Phenylalanine (mg)	Protein (gm)	Calories
Per recipe	48	1.5	2835
Per cookie	1	trace	79

Butterscotch Chip Cookies

Replace vanilla instant pudding with butterscotch instant pudding. Add ⅓ cup (56 gm) Nestlé butterscotch chips to dough.

Yield: 36 cookies.

	Phenylalanine (mg)	Protein (gm)	Calories
Per recipe	108	2.7	3142
Per cookie	3	0.1	87

Carrot Orange Cookies

Delete water and add ⅔ cup (67 gm) mashed, cooked, carrots and 1 teaspoon grated fresh orange rind.

Yield: 36 cookies.

	Phenylalanine (mg)	Protein (gm)	Calories
Per recipe	69	2.2	2864
Per cookie	2	0.1	80

Chocolate Chip Cookies

Add ¼ cup (45 gm) Nestlé mini semisweet chocolate chips to dough.

Yield: 36 cookies.

	Phenylalanine (mg)	Protein (gm)	Calories
Per recipe	139	3.4	3075
Per cookie	4	0.1	85

Chocolate Chip Cookies with Snap, Crackle, and Pop

Add ¼ cup (45 gm) Nestlé mini semisweet chocolate chips and ¾ cup (20 gm) Rice Krispies to dough.

Yield: 36 cookies.

	Phenylalanine (mg)	Protein (gm)	Calories
Per recipe	203	4.8	3155
Per cookie	6	0.1	88

Chocolate–Chocolate Chip Cookies

Add 1½ tablespoons Hershey's unsweetened cocoa (not instant) and ¼ cup (45 gm) Nestlé mini semisweet chocolate chips to dough.

Yield: 36 cookies.

	Phenylalanine (mg)	Protein (gm)	Calories
Per recipe	236	5.4	3107
Per cookie	7	0.1	86

Chocolate Fudge Cookies

Add 1½ tablespoons Hershey's unsweetened cocoa (not instant) to dough.

Yield: 36 cookies.

	Phenylalanine (mg)	Protein (gm)	Calories
Per recipe	145	3.5	2866
Per cookie	4	0.1	80

Coconut Cookies

Replace vanilla instant pudding with coconut cream instant pudding.

Yield: 36 cookies.

	Phenylalanine (mg)	Protein (gm)	Calories
Per recipe	48	1.5	2835
Per cookie	1	trace	79

Oatmeal Cookies

Add ¼ cup (24 gm) quick oatmeal to dough.

Yield: 36 cookies.

	Phenylalanine (mg)	Protein (gm)	Calories
Per recipe	286	6.0	2945
Per cookie	8	0.2	82

Oatmeal Chocolate Chip Cookies

Add ¼ cup (24 gm) quick oatmeal and ¼ cup (45 gm) Nestlé mini semisweet chocolate chips to dough.

Yield: 36 cookies.

	Phenylalanine (mg)	Protein (gm)	Calories
Per recipe	377	7.9	3185
Per cookie	10	0.2	88

Oatmeal Raisin Cookies

Add ¼ cup (24 gm) quick oatmeal and ⅓ cup (53 gm) raisins to dough.

Yield: 36 cookies.

	Phenylalanine (mg)	Protein (gm)	Calories
Per recipe	321	7.7	3103
Per cookie	9	0.2	86

Pumpkin Cookies

Delete water and add ⅔ cup (133 gm) canned pumpkin.

Yield: 36 cookies.

	Phenylalanine (mg)	Protein (gm)	Calories
Per recipe	95	3.0	2879
Per cookie	3	0.1	80

Pumpkin Chocolate Chip Cookies

Delete water and add ⅔ cup (133 gm) canned pumpkin and ¼ cup (45 gm) Nestlé mini semisweet chocolate chips.

Yield: 36 cookies.

	Phenylalanine (mg)	Protein (gm)	Calories
Per recipe	186	4.8	3120
Per cookie	5	0.1	87

Pumpkin Raisin Cookies

Delete water and add ⅔ cup (133 gm) canned pumpkin and ⅓ cup (53 gm) raisins.

Yield: 36 cookies.

	Phenylalanine (mg)	Protein (gm)	Calories
Per recipe	130	4.7	3038
Per cookie	4	0.1	84

Raisin Cookies

Add ½ cup (80 gm) raisins to dough.

Yield: 36 cookies.

	Phenylalanine (mg)	Protein (gm)	Calories
Per recipe	101	4.1	3074
Per cookie	3	0.1	85

Spritz Cookies

A traditional holiday cookie but attractive for any special occasion.

Prepare *Basic Cookies* dough using ⅓ cup plus 1 tablespoon water. Fill a cookie press and press out cookies using disc of your choice, onto an ungreased cookie sheet. Bake at 375° for 8 to 10 minutes. Sprinkle with colored candy sprinkles, colored sugar, or pipe on tinted *Decorator Frosting*, or decorate with candied cherries.

Yield: 40 cookies.

	Phenylalanine (mg)	Protein (gm)	Calories
Per recipe	48	1.5	2835
Per cookie	1	trace	71

Chocolate Chip Cookies on a Stick

These will be a big hit with all of the children for a school or home birthday party or special occasion. You can use the idea for any of the varieties of *Basic Cookies* (without added vegetable or fruit purée).

Basic Cookies dough, using only 3 tablespoons water and to which you have added 6 tablespoons (68 gm) Nestlé mini semisweet chocolate chips
18 Popsicle sticks (available at craft stores)
clear plastic wrap
¼ inch wide grosgrain gift ribbon, or yarn

Wrap prepared dough in plastic wrap and put in freezer for 1 hour or overnight. When ready to bake cookies, preheat oven to 375°. Divide dough into 18 equal pieces (approximately 35 gm each). Roll each into a ball with your hands. Place 8 or 9 balls on a cookie sheet sprayed with vegetable cooking spray or line with parchment baking paper. Push a Popsicle stick about ⅔ of the way into each ball (there should be almost as much dough on the top of the stick as under it). The free end of the Popsicle should remain parallel with the cookie sheet.

Bake cookies for 13 to 15 minutes. Remove to a cooling rack after a minute or so, being careful not to jar the sticks until cookies are completely cool. Repeat with remaining dough balls. When done, the cookies should have become flattened on the bottom and remain nicely rounded on top.

When cookies are completely cool, wrap them in an approximately 6-inch width of plastic wrap by placing a cookie on the diagonal of each piece of plastic wrap, then folding it around the cookie. Tie a piece of ribbon or yarn around each stick.

Yield: 18 cookies.

	Phenylalanine (mg)	Protein (gm)	Calories
Per recipe	185	4.4	3198
Per cookie	10	0.2	178

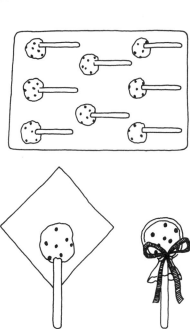

Basic Cut-Out Cookies

The dough is very easy to work with and makes a crisp, excellent, all-around cookie.

½ cup vegetable shortening
⅓ cup softened margarine or
   butter
2 tablespoons granulated sugar
¼ cup packed brown sugar
1 pkg (4-serving size) vanilla
   Jell-O Instant Pudding and
   Pie Filling mix

1 teaspoon vanilla
¼ cup water
2 cups (220 gm) Wel-Plan
   Baking Mix
½ teaspoon salt

In a medium mixing bowl, cream shortening and margarine with sugars. Add pudding mix and vanilla and mix well. Gradually add water, mixing well. Stir together Baking Mix and salt; add to creamed mixture, mixing until thoroughly combined. Dough will be quite stiff. Wrap in plastic wrap and refrigerate for several hours or put in freezer for 45 minutes.

Preheat oven to 375°. Roll dough out to about ⅛-inch thickness on surface dusted with Baking Mix, sprinkling top of dough with a small amount of Baking Mix (just enough to prevent rolling pin from sticking). Cut out using a 2-inch round cookie cutter, or any shape desired. Place on an ungreased cookie sheet 1 inch apart.

Bake for 6 to 8 minutes, depending on your preference for a softer or crisper cookie. After 5 minutes of baking, open oven; if cookies have "bubbled" slightly, quickly and gently flatten each one with a spatula, then return for remainder of baking time. Let cookies cool slightly on pan before removing to wire cooling rack. Frost or decorate as desired.

Yield: 75 two-inch cookies, more or less, depending on size of cutter.

Note
These make excellent sandwich-type cookies, using a round or simple-shaped cutter and filled with plain or tinted Decorator Frosting, Pinwheel Filling, or low protein frosting of your choice.

	Phenylalanine (mg)	Protein (gm)	Calories
Per recipe	48	1.5	2931
Per cookie	1	trace	39

Variations

Chocolate Chip Cookies

Add ¼ cup (45 gm) Nestlé mini semisweet chocolate chips to dough.
Roll dough ³⁄₁₆ inch thick. Cut out with 2-inch round cutter.

Yield: 48 two-inch cookies.

	Phenylalanine (mg)	Protein (gm)	Calories
Per recipe	139	3.4	3172
Per cookie	3	0.1	66

Fudge Circles

Add 2 tablespoons Hershey's unsweetened cocoa (not instant) along
with pudding mix and vanilla. For an Oreo-type sandwich cookie, cut
out using 2-inch or 3-inch round cutter (for 2-inch cutter, roll dough
⅛ inch thick; for 3-inch cutter, roll dough ³⁄₁₆ inch thick). Prick each
cookie with a fork before baking, if desired. Make sandwiches with
2 cookies and *Decorator Frosting* spread between, or use for an *Ice
Cream Sandwich.*

Yield: 75 two-inch cookies or 30 three-inch cookies.

	Phenylalanine (mg)	Protein (gm)	Calories
Per recipe	178	4.1	2973
Per 3-inch cookie	6	0.1	99
Per 2-inch cookie	2	0.1	40

Gingerbread Cookies

Delete water and add ¼ cup dark molasses. Add 1 to 1½ teaspoons cinnamon and ¾ to 1½ teaspoons ginger. Delete vanilla. Cut out with a 2½-inch gingerbread cutter.

Yield: 64 medium gingerbread cookies.

	Phenylalanine (mg)	Protein (gm)	Calories
Per recipe	48	1.5	3191
Per cookie	1	trace	50

Dutch Snowballs

Especially festive for Christmas, but a treat anytime.

Diet Portion

½ recipe *Basic Cut-Out*
    Cookies

20 Hershey's Chocolate Kisses
confectioner's sugar

Prepare *Basic Cut-Out Cookies* dough and chill it as directed. Preheat oven to 350°. Remove foil wrap from Kisses. Take small pieces of dough (15 gm) and form around the Kisses, rolling with your hands into smooth balls. Place on an ungreased cookie sheet (all 20 balls on one sheet). Bake for 12 minutes. Remove to wire cooking rack. While still slightly warm, roll in confectioner's sugar.

Yield: 20 cookies.

Family Portion

1 cup margarine or butter
¾ cup sugar
2 tablespoons sherry or orange
    liqueur
2⅓ cups sifted flour

1 cup finely chopped pecans or
    walnuts
50 Hershey's Chocolate Kisses
confectioner's sugar

Cream margarine, sugar, and sherry or liqueur in a mixing bowl. Add flour, then stir in nuts. Gather dough into a ball and wrap in plastic wrap; refrigerate at least 1 hour. Preheat oven to 350°. Continue as for *Diet Portion*. Test-bake one ball, adding a little more flour if cookie does not retain its round shape.

Yield: 50 cookies.

	Phenylalanine (mg)	Protein (gm)	Calories
Per diet recipe	388	9.5	3375
Per cookie	19	0.5	169

Rainbow Cookies

Charming multicolored cookies that kids will love. A nice holiday or everyday cookie that is sturdy for traveling in school lunches.

Basic Cut-Out Cookies dough, using only 3 tablespoons water
red, green, and yellow food coloring (or colors of your choice)

Divide dough into 3 approximately equal parts, putting each into a small bowl. Mix red, green, or yellow coloring into each piece of dough, using 6 to 8 drops of color for each, making a bright and perky pink, yellow, and green dough (or use cake decorating paste colors, which come in an array of shades). Wrap each piece of dough in plastic wrap and put in freezer for 1½ to 2 hours, until fairly firm.

Line a 7½ × 3¾-inch loaf pan with plastic wrap, allowing it to extend over the sides. With hands, pat a layer of green dough evenly in bottom of pan (do not add extra Baking Mix even if a little sticky or dough layers will not adhere together well). Press yellow dough into a rectangle approximately the same as the shape of the pan, using the plastic wrap it was covered with as a surface. Place yellow dough rectangle on top of green dough, pressing as needed to fit, smoothing top. Repeat this with pink layer. Cover pan with plastic wrap and freeze for 3 to 4 hours.

Preheat oven to 375°. Remove dough from pan, using plastic wrap extending from sides to lift out. With a sharp knife, cut dough in half lengthwise. Cut each strip into 20 pieces (about ⅜-inch thick)—each cookie will have 3 stripes of beautiful color. Place on ungreased cookie sheet, 16 to 20 cookies per sheet, and bake for 10 minutes.

Yield: 40 cookies.

Note

To make a smaller batch of cookies, make ½ the *Basic Cut-Out Cookies* recipe, using 1½ tablespoons water. Form dough into three 2-inch-wide by 7-inch-long strips with your hand, stacking them on plastic wrap. Wrap the dough in the plastic wrap, then in foil, and put in a plastic freezer bag to freeze.

	Phenylalanine (mg)	Protein (gm)	Calories
Per recipe	48	1.5	2835
Per cookie	1	trace	71

Variation

Neapolitan Cookies

Prepare as for *Rainbow Cookies* but leave one piece of dough plain, tint one pink, and add 2 teaspoons Hershey's unsweetened cocoa (not instant) to the third. Place chocolate layer on bottom, followed by plain, and pink.

Yield: 40 cookies.

	Phenylalanine (mg)	Protein (gm)	Calories
Per recipe	91	2.4	2849
Per cookie	2	0.1	71

Freezer Cookies

Make fresh-baked cookies that look like "store-bought" varieties in a few minutes using this technique.

Prepare *Basic Cut-Out Cookies* dough, using instant vanilla, butterscotch, or coconut cream pudding. Pack dough very firmly into 4 small, empty 6-oz juice cans with top end removed and bottom left intact (dough will fill 3½ cans). Cover each with plastic wrap and seal in a plastic bag or airtight container.

When you are ready to bake one or more cookies, take a can and open bottom with a can opener; push dough out the top, ¼ inch at a time (using the metal bottom to push dough). Slice off ¼-inch thick slices of dough for each cookie desired, using a sharp knife, placing on an ungreased cookie sheet. Rewrap leftover dough, leaving cut bottom of can in place. Bake cookies in preheated 375° oven for 12 to 15 minutes, depending on your preference for softer or crisper cookies.

Alternatively, you can roll dough into 1½-inch diameter cylinders, wrap in plastic wrap, and freeze, cutting off ¼-inch slices as desired.

Yield: 28 cookies.

	Phenylalanine (mg)	Protein (gm)	Calories
Per recipe	48	1.5	2835
Per cookie	2	0.1	101

Variations

Chocolate Chip Cookies

Use instant vanilla pudding. Add ¼ cup (45 gm) Nestlé mini semi-sweet chocolate chips to dough.

Yield: 28 cookies.

	Phenylalanine (mg)	Protein (gm)	Calories
Per recipe	139	3.4	3075
Per cookie	5	0.1	110

Chocolate–Chocolate Chip Cookies

Use instant vanilla pudding. Add 2 tablespoons Hershey's unsweetened cocoa (not instant) and ¼ cup (45 gm) Nestlé mini semisweet chocolate chips to dough.

Yield: 28 cookies.

	Phenylalanine (mg)	Protein (gm)	Calories
Per recipe	269	6.0	3117
Per cookie	10	0.2	111

Chocolate Fudge Cookies

Use instant vanilla pudding. Add 1½ tablespoons Hershey's unsweetened cocoa (not instant) to dough.

Yield: 28 cookies.

	Phenylalanine (mg)	Protein (gm)	Calories
Per recipe	145	3.5	2866
Per cookie	5	0.1	102

Oatmeal Cookies

Use instant vanilla pudding. Add ¼ cup (24 gm) quick oatmeal to dough.

Yield: 28 cookies.

	Phenylalanine (mg)	Protein (gm)	Calories
Per recipe	286	6.0	2945
Per cookie	10	0.2	105

Oatmeal Chocolate Chip Cookies

Use instant vanilla pudding. Add ¼ cup (24 gm) quick oatmeal and ¼ cup (45 gm) Nestlé mini semisweet chocolate chips to dough.

Yield: 28 cookies.

	Phenylalanine (mg)	Protein (gm)	Calories
Per recipe	377	7.9	3185
Per cookie	13	0.3	114

Note

Other possible variations using regular size chips, or raisins, will not work easily, as it is too difficult to cut the dough smoothly.

Chocolate Chip Cookies

These look and taste just like traditional chocolate chip cookies.

⅔ cup softened margarine or butter
½ cup granulated sugar
½ cup packed brown sugar
1 medium egg yolk (1 tablespoon, 15 gm)
1 teaspoon vanilla

⅓ cup (60 gm) Nestlé mini semisweet chocolate chips
2 cups plus 3 tablespoons (240 gm) wheat starch
½ teaspoon baking soda
½ teaspoon salt

Preheat oven to 375°. Cream margarine and sugars in medium mixing bowl. Add egg yolk and vanilla, mixing well. Add chocolate chips. Stir together wheat starch, baking soda, and salt; add to creamed ingredients and mix, first with a spoon, then with hands (as mixture will be quite dry) to form a clay-like dough. Drop by teaspoon onto an ungreased sheet, 16 cookies per sheet (cookies will spread during baking). Bake for 10 to 12 minutes. Let cool on pan slightly, then remove to cooling rack.

Yield: 54 cookies.

Note

It is wise to test-bake one cookie first. Add a little more wheat starch if it spreads too much; add a little water if it does not spread enough.

	Phenylalanine (mg)	Protein (gm)	Calories
Per recipe	336	7.0	3374
Per cookie	6	0.1	62

Variation

Crispy Raisin Cookies

Delete chocolate chips and add ½ cup (80 gm) raisins.

Yield: 54 cookies.

	Phenylalanine (mg)	Protein (gm)	Calories
Per recipe	268	7.1	3293
Per cookie	5	0.1	61

Crackly Molasses Cookies

Crisp round cookies with a crackly top, like traditional ginger cookies.

½ cup vegetable shortening
1 cup packed brown sugar
2 tablespoons molasses
1 medium egg yolk
   (1 tablespoon, 15 gm)

2 cups (220 gm) wheat starch
½ teaspoon baking soda
¼ teaspoon salt
1 teaspoon cinnamon
¼ teaspoon cloves

Preheat oven to 375°. In a medium mixing bowl, cream shortening and sugar. Add molasses and egg yolk, mixing well. Mix together wheat starch, baking soda, salt, cinnamon, and cloves; add to creamed ingredients and mix, first with a spoon, then with hands (as mixture will be quite dry) to form a clay-like dough. Form dough into small balls. Roll each ball in sugar. Place cookies on an ungreased cookie sheet, 16 to 20 cookies per sheet. Bake for 10 to 12 minutes. Let cool on pan slightly, then remove to cooling rack.

Yield: 48 cookies.

Note
It is wise to test-bake one cookie first. Add a little more wheat starch if it spreads too much; add a little water if it does not spread enough.

	Phenylalanine (mg)	Protein (gm)	Calories
Per recipe	142	3.0	2870
Per cookie	3	0.1	60

Variations

Both variations have approximately the same nutrient content as the original recipe.

Crackly Lemon or Orange Cookies

Delete molasses, cinnamon, and cloves. Add 1 tablespoon lemon or orange rind and 4 tablespoons lemon or orange juice.

Yield: 48 cookies.

Rocky Road Bars

Dense, chewy, and delicious.

½ cup (90 gm) Nestlé butterscotch chips
¼ cup margarine or butter
⅓ cup packed brown sugar
1 cup (110 gm) wheat starch
¼ teaspoon salt

1¼ teaspoons baking powder
1 cup (40 gm) mini
marshmallows
⅓ cup (60 gm) Nestlé semisweet chocolate chips

Preheat oven to 350°. Melt butterscotch chips and margarine in a medium saucepan over low heat (or microwave on High for 2 minutes in a 1½-quart baking dish). Remove from heat. Add sugar, wheat starch, salt, and baking powder and mix well (mixture will be dry). Mix in marshmallows and chocolate chips. Firmly pat mixture into a greased 8-inch square baking pan. Bake for 15 minutes. Loosen with a knife from sides of pan while still warm. Cut into bars when cool.

Yield: 20 bars.

	Phenylalanine (mg)	Protein (gm)	Calories
Per recipe	267	5.8	2075
Per bar	13	0.3	104

Toffee Bars

Thin rich bars that are always a favorite.

¾ cup softened margarine or
    butter
1 cup packed brown sugar
1 medium egg yolk
    (1 tablespoon, 15 gm)

1 teaspoon vanilla
2¼ cups (248 gm) wheat starch
⅔ cup (120 gm) Nestlé semi-
    sweet chocolate chips

Preheat oven to 350°. In a medium mixing bowl, cream margarine and sugar. Mix in egg yolk and vanilla. Mix in wheat starch, first using a spoon, then hands (as mixture will be dry) to make a soft clay-like dough. Press dough evenly into an ungreased 13 × 9-inch baking pan. Bake for 15 minutes. Remove from oven and sprinkle chocolate chips over top. Return to oven for about 1 minute, then remove and spread chocolate smoothly over top. Cut into bars while slightly warm.

Yield: 56 bars.

	Phenylalanine (mg)	Protein (gm)	Calories
Per recipe	341	7.2	3757
Per bar	6	0.1	67

Variation

Butterscotch Toffee Bars

Replace chocolate chips with ⅔ cup (120 gm) Nestlé butterscotch chips.

Yield: 56 bars.

	Phenylalanine (mg)	Protein (gm)	Calories
Per recipe	226	4.7	3774
Per bar	4	0.1	67

Party Fudge Bars

Great for school parties or holidays.

Fudge Mixture

1 cup granulated sugar
1½ tablespoons margarine or
    butter
⅓ cup Rich's Coffee Rich

5 large marshmallows
½ cup (90 gm) Nestlé semi-
    sweet chocolate chips

Rice Krispie Mixture

¼ cup margarine or butter
24 large marshmallows

5 cups (135 gm) Rice Krispies
    cereal

Prepare Fudge Mixture. Combine sugar, margarine, and Coffee Rich in a saucepan; bring to a boil over medium heat (or microwave on High for 1 minute in a 1½-quart baking dish). Stir in marshmallows and chips, heating until melted (or microwave on High for 45 to 60 seconds). Cover and set aside.

Prepare Rice Krispie Mixture. Melt margarine in a saucepan (or microwave on High for 30 seconds in a 2-quart baking dish). Add marshmallows and cook over low heat until marshmallows are melted, stirring frequently (or microwave on High 1½ to 2 minutes). Mix in cereal and stir until well coated.

Press ⅔ of *Rice Krispie Mixture* evenly into a lightly greased 13 × 9-inch pan, using greased hands. Pour *Fudge Mixture* over top, spreading evenly. Top with rest of *Rice Krispie Mixture* (some of fudge layer will show through). Sprinkle with colored candy sprinkles. Cut into bars when cool. Refrigerate to retain crispness.

Yield: 56 bars.

	Phenylalanine (mg)	Protein (gm)	Calories
Per recipe	826	18.8	3696
Per bar	15	0.3	66

Puffed Wheat 'N Rice Bars

½ cup margarine or butter
½ cup light Karo corn syrup or maple syrup
1 cup packed brown sugar
1 teaspoon vanilla

1 teaspoon cinnamon
2 cups (32 gm) Quaker Puffed Wheat cereal
6 cups (81 gm) Quaker Puffed Rice cereal

In a large saucepan, heat margarine, syrup, sugar, vanilla, and cinnamon. After mixture is full of bubbles, boil for 1½ minutes. Quickly stir in the cereals; press firmly into a greased 13 × 9-inch pan. Cut into bars when cool. Refrigerate to retain crispness.

Yield: 40 bars.

	Phenylalanine (mg)	Protein (gm)	Calories
Per recipe	419	9.4	2550
Per bar	10	0.2	64

Rice Krispie Marshmallow Treats

¼ cup margarine or butter
40 large marshmallows

5 cups (135 gm) Rice Krispies cereal

Melt margarine in a large saucepan (or microwave on High for 45 to 60 seconds in a 3-quart baking dish). Add marshmallows and cook over low heat, stirring frequently (or microwave on High for 2 to 3 minutes, stirring twice). Add cereal and stir until well coated. Using greased hands or a spatula, firmly press mixture evenly into a lightly greased 13 × 9-inch pan. Cut into bars when cool.

Yield: 48 bars.

	Phenylalanine (mg)	Protein (gm)	Calories
Per recipe	574	14.1	1841
Per bar	12	0.3	38

Crispy Date Bars

A nice holiday cookie for the whole family.

¼ cup margarine or butter
1 cup (150 gm) finely chopped
   dates
½ cup packed brown sugar
1 tablespoon water

1 teaspoon vanilla
3 cups (81 gm) Rice Krispies
   cereal
confectioner's sugar

In a medium saucepan, melt margarine over low heat. Add dates, sugar, and water. Continue cooking for 2 to 3 minutes, until dates are soft. Add vanilla and Rice Krispies, mixing well. Firmly press into a lightly greased 11 × 7-inch pan. Dust with confectioner's sugar sprinkled through a fine mesh strainer or sifter. Cut into bars when cool.

Yield: 48 bars.

	Phenylalanine (mg)	Protein (gm)	Calories
Per recipe	368	9.3	1557
Per bar	8	0.2	32

Brownies

Chocolaty-rich and delicious cake-type brownies.

½ cup vegetable shortening
¼ cup packed brown sugar
7 tablespoons (70 gm)
    vanilla Jell-O Instant
    Pudding and Pie Filling mix
3 tablespoons Hershey's
    unsweetened cocoa
    (not instant)

½ cup water
1 cup (110 gm) Wel-Plan
    Baking Mix
¾ teaspoon baking powder
¼ teaspoon salt

Preheat oven to 375°. In a medium mixing bowl, cream shortening with sugar. Add pudding mix and cocoa, mixing well. Gradually add water, mixing well. Stir together Baking Mix, baking powder, and salt; add to creamed mixture, mixing until thoroughly combined.

Spread batter into a greased 8- or 9-inch square baking pan, smoothing top with backside of a spoon. Bake 15 minutes. Cool on wire rack, then cut into bars. Nice frosted with *Chocolate Buttercream Frosting* or *Basic Buttercream Frosting*. For a festive occasion, use green-tinted frosting, plain or flavored with mint, and add colored candy sprinkles.

Yield: 16 bars.

Storage Tip

For freezing unfrosted cookies, place cut brownies on a cookie sheet and freeze, then place in a freezer bag or stack in a Tupperware or other plastic freezer container. This technique prevents any sticking together.

	Phenylalanine (mg)	Protein (gm)	Calories
Per recipe	203	4.4	1800
Per bar	13	0.3	113

Chocolate Chip Bars

Sure to be a favorite.

½ cup vegetable shortening
¼ cup packed brown sugar
5 tablespoons (50 gm)
    vanilla Jell-O Instant
    Pudding and Pie Filling mix
⅓ cup water

1 cup (110 gm) Wel-Plan
    Baking Mix
¾ teaspoon baking powder
¼ teaspoon salt
¼ cup (45 gm) Nestlé semi-
    sweet chocolate chips

Preheat oven to 375°. In a medium mixing bowl, cream shortening with sugar. Add pudding mix, mixing well. Gradually add water, mixing well. Stir together Baking Mix, baking powder, and salt; add to creamed mixture, mixing until thoroughly combined. Mix in chocolate chips. Spread batter into a greased 8- or 9-inch square baking pan, smoothing top with back of a spoon. Bake 25 minutes. Cool on wire rack, then cut into bars.

Yield: 16 bars.

Storage Tip

For freezing, place cut bars on a cookie sheet and freeze, then place in a freezer bag or stack in a Tupperware or other plastic freezer container. This technique prevents any sticking together.

	Phenylalanine (mg)	Protein (gm)	Calories
Per recipe	99	2.3	1978
Per bar	6	0.1	124

Variations

Butterscotch Brownies

Replace vanilla instant pudding with butterscotch instant pudding. Delete chocolate chips.

Yield: 16 bars.

	Phenylalanine (mg)	Protein (gm)	Calories
Per recipe	8	0.4	1737
Per bar	1	trace	109

Raisin Bars

Replace chocolate chips with ½ cup (80 gm) raisins.

Yield: 16 bars.

	Phenylalanine (mg)	Protein (gm)	Calories
Per recipe	62	3.0	1977
Per bar	4	0.2	124

Peanut Butter Cookies

These look and taste very much like regular peanut butter cookies despite the small amount of peanut butter (see the special tips on pages 342 and 344).

½ cup vegetable shortening
¼ cup softened margarine or butter
2 tablespoons (32 gm) creamy peanut butter (be sure measure is level)
2 tablespoons sugar
¼ cup packed brown sugar

1 pkg (4-serving size) vanilla Jell-O Instant Pudding and Pie Filling mix
¼ cup water
2 cups (220 gm) Wel-Plan Baking Mix
1½ teaspoons baking powder
¼ teaspoon salt

Preheat oven to 375°. In a medium mixing bowl, cream shortening, margarine, and peanut butter with sugars. Add pudding mix and mix well. Gradually add water, mixing well. Stir together Baking Mix, baking powder, and salt; add to creamed mixture, mixing until thoroughly combined.

With hands, roll small pieces of dough into walnut-sized balls. Place on ungreased cookie sheet, 15 per pan. Dip a fork in Baking Mix. Press fork tines into each dough ball, flattening. Bake for 10 to 12 minutes. Let cookies cool slightly on baking sheet, then remove to cooling rack.

Yield: 40 cookies.

	Phenylalanine (mg)	Protein (gm)	Calories
Per recipe	529	10.8	2986
Per cookie	13	0.3	75

Variation

Low Peanut Butter Cookies

Use only 1 tablespoon peanut butter and increase margarine to ⅓ cup. These have a slight peanut butter taste and still look like regular peanut butter cookies though they will not brown as much.

Yield: 40 cookies.

	Phenylalanine (mg)	Protein (gm)	Calories
Per recipe	292	5.6	3016
Per cookie	7	0.2	76

Peanut Butter Bars

See the special tip on page 344.

⅓ cup vegetable shortening
2 tablespoons (32 gm) creamy
   peanut butter (be sure
   measure is level)
¼ cup packed brown sugar
5 tablespoons (50 gm)
   vanilla Jell-O Instant
   Pudding and Pie Filling mix

⅓ cup water
1 cup (110 gm) Wel-Plan
   Baking Mix
¾ teaspoon baking powder
¼ teaspoon salt

Preheat oven to 375°. In a medium mixing bowl, cream shortening and peanut butter with brown sugar. Add pudding mix. Gradually add water. Stir together Baking Mix, baking powder, and salt; add to creamed mixture, mixing until thoroughly combined. Spread batter into a greased 8- or 9-inch square baking pan, smoothing top with back of a spoon. Bake 25 minutes. Cool on wire rack, then cut into bars.

Yield: 25 bars.

	Phenylalanine (mg)	Protein (gm)	Calories
Per recipe	496	9.8	1815
Per bar	20	0.4	73

Cakes

Cakes in this section all have excellent texture and flavor, even the recipes lowest in phenylalanine/protein. "Higher" recipes are also provided for diets with a higher phenylalanine or protein allowance, or for birthdays and other special occasions. However, even the cakes using wheat starch and/or Wel-Plan Baking Mix would be acceptable to most persons not on the diet—especially if they are unaware of the special ingredients used.

Special Tips

Cake flour is used in several recipes, where it was desirable for the best texture. For purchasing and measuring, see *Using the Recipes*.

In several of the recipes (*Quick-Mix Cake, Banana Cake,* and *Sunshine Cake*) a medium egg is called for. Be sure to use a medium-sized egg (average weight 41 gm, including shell), not large or extra-large. Because of the great amount of phenylalanine/protein in the egg, if you use an egg larger than medium, the cake will contain significantly more phenylalanine and protein than indicated for the recipe.

Be sure to use an electric mixer, when indicated, for cake with a light texture and cupcakes with a nicely rounded top. Blend for only the amount of time stated—overbeating may cause some cracking and underbeating will cause the cake to be heavy in texture.

If the recipe does not call for use of an electric mixer, beat batter by hand until smooth (30 to 45 seconds).

A microwave oven can be used for baking cupcakes quickly. Use about 2 tablespoons cake batter per cupcake. Microwave on High for 2 to 3 minutes. The cupcakes may be slightly less even in texture than when baked in a regular oven, but are nice and light. You may get more cupcakes than the recipe indicates when using the microwave method; recalculate nutrient content accordingly.

Use waxed paper, cut to size, on the bottom of the pan for a layer cake for easiest removal. Lay your pan on a piece of waxed paper, then trace an outline in pencil and cut out. Grease the sides and bottom of pan, then insert the waxed paper circle.

Place cupcakes or cake on a center rack in the oven to bake.

Don't open the oven until the minimum baking time stated in the recipe has passed or the cake or cupcakes may fall.

Always bake cake or cupcakes in a *preheated* oven. Put cake or cupcakes in the preheated oven immediately after preparing the batter for optimal rising and a light texture.

After baking, let layer cake cool 10 to 15 minutes in the pan on a wire cooling rack. Loosen around all sides with a knife and turn cake out onto a plate (cake will be "upside down"), then flip the cake back onto the wire rack or a plate.

Frost cake or cupcakes only after they are thoroughly cool. Brush off crumbs first (for a layer cake, freeze before frosting if cake seems crumbly).

Store cake or cupcakes in a cake keeper or covered airtight container at room temperature, or in the refrigerator for up to several days. The cakes also freeze well and can be quickly "freshened" in a microwave oven.

Most unfrosted cakes or cupcakes will become a little moist on top after 24 hours in the refrigerator. If they are not to be eaten right away, the moisture can be avoided by freezing the cakes right away, or by frosting the cakes when cooled.

Birthday Cake

Excellent texture and flavor. The whole family can enjoy this.

1 cup (110 gm) Wel-Plan
  Baking Mix
½ cup (55 gm) wheat starch
½ cup (48 gm) sifted Softasilk
  cake flour (do not use
  regular flour)
¾ cup granulated sugar

2 teaspoons baking powder
½ teaspoon salt
⅔ cup water
1 drop yellow food coloring
⅓ cup vegetable oil
½ teaspoon vanilla

Preheat oven to 350°. In a medium mixing bowl, stir together Baking Mix, wheat starch, cake flour, sugar, baking powder, and salt. Mix water, yellow coloring, vegetable oil, and vanilla together in a liquid measuring cup; add to dry ingredients, mixing on medium speed of an electric mixer for 1½ minutes. Scrape batter into a greased 8- or 9-inch pan or twelve 2½-inch diameter muffin cups greased or lined with cupcake liners. Bake 20 minutes for cupcakes or 30 to 35 minutes for cake (cake will not be brown on top when done).

Yield: 12 cupcakes or one 8- or 9-inch single layer cake.

Note
  Mixing with an electric mixer, as directed, is important for producing cake with a light texture.

Storage Tip
  The edge of the cake or cupcakes may become a little dry on standing. Store in an airtight container with a small piece of bread or apple to minimize drying.

	Phenylalanine (mg)	Protein (gm)	Calories
Per recipe	196	4.4	1982
Per cupcake or ¹⁄₁₂ cake	16	0.4	165

Variations

Both variations have approximately the same nutrient content as the original recipe.

Orange Cake

Add 1 teaspoon fresh orange rind with the dry ingredients. Replace the ⅔ cup water with ⅓ cup of fresh or canned orange juice and ⅓ cup water. Excellent frosted with *Orange Buttercream Frosting.*

Spice Cake

Add ¾ teaspoon cinnamon, ¼ teaspoon cloves, and ⅛ teaspoon nutmeg with the dry ingredients. Excellent frosted with *Simple Caramel Frosting.*

Tastes-Like-Devil's-Food Cake

An updated version of a favorite recipe from the first edition of *Low Protein Cookery*.

½ cup granulated sugar
¼ cup Miracle Whip Salad
   Dressing
2 tablespoons Hershey's
   unsweetened cocoa
   (not instant)
½ cup cold water

½ cup (55 gm) Wel-Plan
   Baking Mix
½ cup (55 gm) wheat starch
1 teaspoon baking soda
¼ teaspoon salt
½ teaspoon vanilla

Preheat oven to 350°. In a medium mixing bowl, combine sugar, Miracle Whip, cocoa, and a small amount of the water. When cocoa and salad dressing are well blended, add remaining water and mix. Stir together Baking Mix, wheat starch, baking soda, and salt. Add to chocolate mixture and blend untl smooth. Add vanilla and mix well. Pour batter into a greased 8-inch square or round cake pan or ten 2½-inch diameter muffin cups greased or lined with cupcake liners. Bake 20 minutes for cupcakes or 20 to 25 minutes for cake.

Yield: 10 cupcakes or one 8-inch single layer cake.

	Phenylalanine (mg)	Protein (gm)	Calories
Per recipe	150	3.1	1124
Per cupcake or ¹⁄₁₀ of cake	15	0.3	112

Variation

Chocolate Snack Cakes

These mimic Hostess Suzie-Qs.

Pour batter into a greased 8-inch square pan. Bake as directed. When cool, cut cake in half, then make 10 rectangular bars by cutting 4 equally placed slices in the opposite direction; remove from pan. Split each bar by cutting in half horizontally, using a serrated knife. Fill each bar with *Pinwheel Filling,* making a "sandwich." Wrap each "sandwich" individually in plastic wrap.

Yield: 5 snack cakes.

	Phenylalanine (mg)	Protein (gm)	Calories
Per snack cake	30	0.7	366

Chocolate Pinwheels

One of the more addictive recipes in this book for those with a sweet tooth, they mimic Hostess Chocolate Ho Hos. Easy, attractive, and child-appealing, these make wonderful school treats or snacks and are especially nice for parties. No one would ever guess they are "low protein."

½ recipe *Tastes-Like-Devil's-*   1 recipe *Pinwheel Filling*
 Food Cake

Preheat oven to 350°. Prepare cake batter as directed for *Tastes-Like-Devil's-Food Cake.* Using a 10¾ (or 11) × 7-inch baking pan (use *only* this size pan, or see *Note*) cut a piece of waxed paper 12 to 13 inches long and place in baking pan, pushing paper into edges and corners to make a smooth bottom and allowing paper to protrude on all four sides; grease waxed paper lightly or spray with vegetable cooking spray (such as "Pam").

Pour cake batter into prepared pan and spread as evenly as possible, making a layer that is quite thin. Bake for 12 to 13 minutes. After removing pan from oven, immediately lift out cake, using protruding waxed paper sides; transfer to a counter top, waxed paper side down. Let cool 20 to 30 minutes.

While cake is cooling, prepare *Pinwheel Filling.* When cake is cool, spread filling evenly on cake, keeping frosting crumb-free by piling it thickly on several places and carefully spreading with a knife or spatula.

With long side facing you, begin rolling cake, as for a jelly roll or cinnamon rolls, at first using wax paper to help you start the roll, then pulling off waxed paper as you continue rolling, keeping the roll quite tight. If you get a little cracking as you roll, don't worry, as the roll will be held together by the filling. Cut into 10 slices. When they are completely cool, wrap individual slices in plastic wrap, or place in an airtight container in a single layer.

Yield: 10 pinwheels.

Note

If you do not have an 11 × 7-inch baking pan, you may prepare one whole recipe of *Tastes-Like-Devil's-Food Cake* batter and use a 15 × 11-inch jelly roll pan or cookie sheet with sides. One sheet of waxed paper will just cover the bottom and enough of the sides. After baking do not remove cake from pan. Let cool. Using a double recipe of filling, carefully spread on cooled cake, then cut cake in half, forming two 11 × 7-inch rectangles. Roll each half as per original recipe, starting with the outside and rolling to the center.

Even if you are using an 11 × 7-inch pan, you may still want to make a whole recipe of cake batter. Use ¾ cup batter for pinwheels and ¾ cup batter to make 6 cupcakes; or bake one pan of pinwheels, then another, using ¾ cup batter for each.

Storage Tip

These keep well for up to a week in the refrigerator and also freeze exceptionally well (they can be eaten directly from the freezer as they will not become hard-frozen).

	Phenylalanine (mg)	Protein (gm)	Calories
Per recipe	75	1.7	1267
Per pinwheel (including filling)	7	0.2	127

Vanilla Pinwheels

These taste similar to Hostess Twinkies, but come in a different shape. Kids love them and they travel and keep well.

⅓ cup (36 gm) Wel-Plan
  Baking Mix
3 tablespoons (21 gm) wheat
  starch
2 tablespoons (18 gm) Softasilk
  cake flour (do not use
  regular flour)
¼ cup granulated sugar

¾ teaspoon baking powder
⅛ teaspoon salt
⅓ cup water
1 drop yellow food coloring
2 tablespoons vegetable oil
¼ teaspoon vanilla
1 recipe *Pinwheel Filling*

Preheat oven to 350°. In a medium mixing bowl, stir together Baking Mix, wheat starch, cake flour, sugar, baking powder, and salt. Mix water, yellow coloring, vegetable oil, and vanilla together in a liquid measuring cup; add to dry ingredients, mixing for 1 minute.

Follow directions for *Chocolate Pinwheels* for preparing baking pan, baking (cake will not be browned on top when done), cooling, filling, rolling, cutting, and storing. Do not overbake the cake, as it will become too dry to roll well.

Yield: 10 pinwheels.

Note
Filling or cake batter could be flavored or tinted with food coloring as desired. Colored candy sprinkles pressed into the filling after slicing the cake also add a decorative touch.

Storage Tip
These keep well for up to a week in the refrigerator and also freeze exceptionally well (they can be eaten directly from the freezer as they will not become hard-frozen).

	Phenylalanine (mg)	Protein (gm)	Calories
Per recipe	73	1.8	1410
Per pinwheel (including filling)	7	0.2	141

Pinwheel Filling

1 cup unsifted confectioner's sugar

2 tablespoons white vegetable shortening (such as Crisco)

1 tablespoon plus ½ teaspoon water

½ teaspoon vanilla

dash of salt

Place all ingredients in a mixing bowl. Mix with an electric mixer until well combined, about 20 to 30 seconds.

Yield: filling for 10 *Chocolate* or *Vanilla Pinwheels.*

	Phenylalanine (mg)	Protein (gm)	Calories
Per recipe	0	0.0	708
Per pinwheel	0	0.0	71

Ice Cream Cone Cupcakes

A very cute idea for a birthday party. Everyone would enjoy them. Other cake batters in this section could also be used.

1 recipe *Tastes-Like-Devil's-Food Cake*

9 Nabisco Comet Cups (small waffle-type ice cream cones)

low protein frosting of your choice

Preheat oven to 350°. Prepare cake batter. Fill each comet cup with about ¼ cup batter, using a ¼-cup measure to scoop out batter. Place filled cups upright on an ungreased baking pan and bake for 30 minutes, or until cake is rounded on top and springs back when tapped lightly with a finger. Cool on a wire rack, then frost with your favorite low protein frosting. Decorate, if desired, with candy corn, jelly beans, Lifesavers, candy sprinkles, or any "free" candy.

Yield: 9 cupcake cones.

Note
The cones are best eaten the same day that they are made, since the cone will not retain its crispness. For using this idea with other cake recipes, one comet cone equals 15 mg phenylalanine, 0.3 gm protein, 18 calories; add to these the appropriate cake calculations.

	Phenylalanine (mg)	Protein (gm)	Calories
Per recipe	312	6.5	1274
Per cupcake cone (not including frosting)	35	0.7	142

Applesauce Cake

An excellent "low" birthday cake or cupcakes. Unfrosted cupcakes also make excellent breakfast muffins.

¼ cup softened margarine
    or butter
¼ cup packed brown sugar
¼ cup granulated sugar
½ cup (120 gm) applesauce
½ cup water
¾ cup (83 gm) Wel-Plan Baking
    Mix

¾ cup (83 gm) wheat starch
2 teaspoons baking powder
½ teaspoon baking soda
¼ teaspoon salt
½ teaspoon cinnamon

Preheat oven to 350°. In a medium mixing bowl, cream margarine and sugars until well blended. Mix in applesauce and water. Stir together Baking Mix, wheat starch, baking powder, baking soda, salt, and cinnamon; blend into creamed mixture, mixing on medium speed of an electric mixer for 1½ minutes. Pour batter into a greased 8- or 9-inch round or square baking pan or twelve 2½-inch diameter muffin cups greased or lined with cupcake liners. Bake 18 to 20 minutes for cupcakes or 25 to 30 minutes for cake.

Yield: 12 cupcakes or one 8- or 9-inch single layer cake.

Note
Mixing with an electric mixer, as directed, is important for producing cake with a light texture.

	Phenylalanine (mg)	Protein (gm)	Calories
Per recipe	41	1.2	1526
Per cupcake or ¹⁄₁₂ of cake	3	0.1	127

Variations

Applesauce Raisin Cake

Add ½ cup (80 gm) raisins to cake batter.

Yield: 12 cupcakes or one 8- or 9-inch single layer cake.

	Phenylalanine (mg)	Protein (gm)	Calories
Per recipe	95	3.8	1766
Per cupcake or ¹⁄₁₂ of cake	8	0.3	147

Banana Cake

Replace the applesauce with ½ cup (115 gm) mashed ripe banana. Prepare and bake as indicated. Excellent frosted with *Banana Butter- cream Frosting,* or leave plain and serve as a muffin.

Yield: 12 cupcakes or one 8- or 9-inch single layer cake.

	Phenylalanine (mg)	Protein (gm)	Calories
Per recipe	78	2.1	1541
Per cupcake or ¹⁄₁₂ of cake	7	0.2	128

Carrot Cake

An excellent low protein version of an all-time favorite cake.

¼ cup vegetable oil
¼ cup packed brown sugar
¼ cup granulated sugar
¾ cup (89 gm) shredded or
  grated carrots
½ cup (140 gm) crushed
  pineapple, undrained
¾ cup (83 gm) Wel-Plan Baking
  Mix

¾ cup (83 gm) wheat starch
2 teaspoons baking powder
½ teaspoon baking soda
¼ teaspoon salt
1½ teaspoons cinnamon
¼ cup water

Preheat oven to 350°. In a medium mixing bowl, blend oil with sugars, using an electric mixer on low speed. Mix in shredded carrots and crushed pineapple with juice. Stir together Baking Mix, wheat starch, baking powder, baking soda, salt, and cinnamon. Add water and dry ingredients to bowl and mix on medium speed for 1½ minutes. Pour batter into a greased 8- or 9-inch round or square baking pan or twelve 2½-inch diameter muffin cups greased or lined with cupcake liners. Bake 25 to 30 minutes for cake or 18 to 20 minutes for cupcakes.

Yield: 12 cupcakes or one 8- or 9-inch single layer cake.

Note
Mixing with an electric mixer, as directed, is important for producing cake with a light texture.

	Phenylalanine (mg)	Protein (gm)	Calories
Per recipe	53	1.9	1622
Per cupcake or ¹⁄₁₂ of cake	4	0.2	135

Chocolate and Cherry Christmas Cakes

These extra-moist and rich cakes will remind you of a steamed pudding dessert. Both diet and family portions can be made out of one can of pie filling.

1 cup (110 gm) Wel-Plan
   Baking Mix
⅓ cup granulated sugar
½ teaspoon baking soda
2 teaspoons cinnamon
⅛ teaspoon salt
3 tablespoons water
¼ cup vegetable oil

1 teaspoon vanilla
½ of a 21 oz can Comstock or
   Wilderness Cherry Pie
   Filling
¼ cup (45 gm) Nestlé semisweet chocolate chips
confectioner's sugar

Preheat oven to 350°. In a large mixing bowl stir together Baking Mix, sugar, baking soda, cinnamon, and salt. Combine water, oil, and vanilla in a liquid measuring cup; add to dry mixture and mix well. Stir in cherry pie filling and chocolate chips (batter will turn pinkish but after baking will not retain this color). Spoon batter into eight 2½-inch greased muffin cups (the cakes will stick to paper liners). Bake for 45 minutes. Remove from pan; cool. Sift confectioner's sugar on top of each cupcake or decorate with red and green candied cherries.

Yield: 8 cupcakes.

Family Portion
For the rest of the family, cupcakes can be made using the diet recipe but replacing Baking Mix with regular flour and replacing the water with 1 egg; also, add ½ cup chopped walnuts to batter if desired.

Storage Tip
The cakes keep well, refrigerated, for several weeks. They also freeze well in an airtight container.

	Phenylalanine (mg)	Protein (gm)	Calories
Per diet recipe	137	3.6	1688
Per cupcake	17	0.5	211

Quick-Mix Cake

For those with a higher tolerance for phenylalanine/protein or for a special occasion. Either version 1 or version 2 makes a delicious cake.

1. 1 box Duncan Hines Moist Deluxe Cake Mix (Banana, Butterscotch, Tropical Fruit, Raspberry, Orange, Lemon, or French Vanilla flavor)
   1⅓ cups plus 1 tablespoon water
   ½ cup applesauce
   1 medium egg (box will call for 3 eggs)

2. 1 box Pillsbury Moist Supreme Cake Mix (Funfetti, French Vanilla, White, or Yellow flavor)
   1⅓ cups water
   ½ cup applesauce
   1 medium egg (box will call for 2 eggs)

Preheat oven to 350°. Prepare cake mix as directed, substituting applesauce for the oil. Pour batter into 30 greased 2½-inch muffin cups, two 8- or 9-inch round or square baking pans, or a 13 × 9-inch baking pan. For layer cakes, it is advisable to line the bottom of the pan with waxed paper for easier removal. Bake cupcakes for 20 to 25 minutes, an 8- or 9-inch cake for 25 to 35 minutes, or a 13 × 9-inch cake for 30 to 35 minutes.

Yield: 30 cupcakes, or two 8- or 9-inch cake layers, or one 13 × 9-inch cake.

Note

Duncan Hines cake mix produces the best one-egg cake, but Pillsbury cake mix is also good (just slightly more fragile). Both cakes will be somewhat more fragile than usual but when thoroughly cooled can be easily frosted with a fairly soft frosting. The substitution of applesauce for oil reduces the fragility of the cake, especially for the Duncan Hines mix. Betty Crocker cake mix produces a one-egg cake that is too fragile and is not recommended.

The phenylalanine content given for these recipes is an estimate based on the "rounded" protein content provided on the box. Precise analysis of the mixes is not available. Because the phe content is high, it is advisable to use these recipes only if you are working with a substantial amount of dietary phenylalanine.

	Phenylalanine (mg)	Protein (gm)	Calories
Duncan Hines or Pillsbury			
Per recipe	1218	24.0	2418
Per cupcake or $^1/_{30}$ sheet cake	41	0.8	81
Per $^1/_{16}$ of 2-layer cake	76	1.5	162

Banana Cake

Excellent for the whole family.

1 cup (96 gm) sifted Softasilk
    cake flour (do not use
    regular flour)
⅔ cup granulated sugar
1¼ teaspoons baking powder
¼ teaspoon baking soda
¼ teaspoon salt

¼ cup vegetable shortening
½ cup (116 gm) mashed ripe
    banana
1 medium egg
2 tablespoons water
½ teaspoon vanilla

Preheat oven to 350°. In a mixing bowl, stir together cake flour, sugar, baking powder, baking soda, and salt. Add remaining ingredients and blend with an electric mixer on medium speed for 2 minutes. Pour batter into a greased 8- or 9-inch round or square baking pan. Bake for 25 to 30 minutes. Remove to cooling rack. When cake is cool, frost with low protein frosting of your choice, or dust with confectioner's sugar.

Yield: One 8- or 9-inch single layer cake.

	Phenylalanine (mg)	Protein (gm)	Calories
Per recipe	717	14.7	1480
Per ¹⁄₁₆ cake	45	0.9	93

Sunshine Cake

For a birthday or special occasion.

1¼ cups (120 gm) sifted
  Softasilk cake flour (do not
  use regular flour)
⅔ cup granulated sugar
2 teaspoons baking powder
¼ teaspoon salt
¼ cup vegetable oil

¼ cup Rich's Coffee Rich
¼ cup water
1 medium egg
½ teaspoon vanilla
2 to 3 drops yellow food
  coloring

Preheat oven to 350°. In a mixing bowl, mix together cake flour, sugar, baking powder, and salt. Add remaining ingredients and blend with an electric mixer on medium speed for 2 minutes. Pour batter into a greased 8- or 9-inch round or square baking pan. Bake for 25 to 30 minutes. Remove to cooking rack. When cake is cool, frost with low protein frosting of your choice.

Yield: One 8- or 9-inch single layer cake.

	Phenylalanine (mg)	Protein (gm)	Calories
Per recipe	778	15.7	1537
Per ¹⁄₁₆ of cake	49	1.0	96

Variations

Both variations have approximately the same nutrient content as the original recipe.

Orange Cake

Replace the ¼ cup water with ¼ cup orange juice. Add 1 teaspoon grated fresh orange rind.

Yield: one 8- or 9-inch single layer cake.

Spice Cake

Add 1 teaspoon cinnamon, ½ teaspoon nutmeg, ¼ teaspoon cloves along with dry ingredients.

Yield: one 8- or 9-inch single layer cake.

Shortcake

Like the traditional shortcake biscuit.

⅔ cup (73 gm) Wel-Plan Baking
   Mix
2 teaspoons baking powder
¼ teaspoon salt
1 tablespoon granulated sugar

3 tablespoons vegetable
   shortening
2 tablespoons Rich's Coffee
   Rich or water

Preheat oven to 400°. In a small mixing bowl, stir together Baking Mix with baking powder, salt, and sugar. Cut in shortening with a fork, 2 knives, or a pastry blender until like coarse meal. Add Coffee Rich or water and stir with a fork until dough is evenly moistened. Divide dough into 3 equal parts. On a lightly greased baking sheet press dough out with hands into three 2½- or 3-inch diameter rounds, about ½-inch thick. Bake for 15 minutes, until light golden brown. Serve warm or cold, split in half or kept whole, topped with sliced or mashed fruit or fruit pie filling and whipped non-dairy topping.

Yield: 3 shortcakes.

Note
   Use a yellow shortening such as Fluffo or Butter-Flavored Crisco for a nice color, or add a scant drop of yellow food coloring to Coffee Rich or water.

	Phenylalanine (mg)	Protein (gm)	Calories
Per recipe	8	0.3	705
Per shortcake	3	0.1	235

Donuts

Diet Portion

1½ cups plus 1 tablespoon
   (172 gm) Wel-Plan Baking
   Mix
1¼ teaspoons baking powder
¼ teaspoon salt
½ teaspoon cinnamon
¼ cup granulated sugar

¼ cup Rich's Coffee Rich
¼ cup water
1½ tablespoons vegetable oil
¼ teaspoon vanilla
drop of yellow food coloring
vegetable oil for frying

In a medium mixing bowl, stir together Baking Mix, baking powder, salt, cinnamon, and sugar. Combine Coffee Rich, water, oil, vanilla, and yellow coloring in a liquid measuring cup; stir into dry ingredients, mixing until smooth. Sprinkle a small amount of Baking Mix on the dough to prevent sticking, then gather dough in your hands and form into a ball. Pat or roll dough to a thickness of about ⅜ inch on a surface dusted with Baking Mix. Cut with a 2½-inch donut cutter (greased to prevent dough from sticking). Reroll dough as necessary to get 6 donuts and 6 holes.

In a pan or deep fryer with a minimum of 1 inch of oil, fry donuts several at a time, for 1 minute on each side in hot oil, using a candy thermometer to check temperature for most predictable results (375°).

Yield: 6 donuts and 6 donut holes.

Note

Donuts may crack slightly on one side, like "homestyle" donuts. They will look and taste very similar to the *Family Portion* but will be golden brown rather than deeper brown and will not get quite as large.

Good rolled in confectioner's sugar while warm, or frosted with low protein frosting of your choice.

As long as you are going to the trouble of making donuts, why not make some for the whole family?

2 cups flour	½ cup milk
1 teaspoon baking powder	1 slightly beaten egg
½ teaspoon salt	3 tablespoons vegetable oil
½ teaspoon cinnamon	½ teaspoon vanilla
½ cup granulated sugar	vegetable oil for frying

Prepare batter, cut out, and fry as for *Diet Portion*. These will brown more quickly than the diet donuts. Makes 12 donuts plus 12 donut holes.

Storage Tip

Both diet and family donuts keep well for several days in an airtight container. They also freeze well. Putting them in a microwave oven for a few seconds will make them taste "fresh-baked."

	Phenylalanine (mg)	Protein (gm)	Calories
Per diet recipe	18	0.7	1054
Per donut	3	0.1	151
Per donut hole	1	trace	44

Basic Buttercream Frosting

¼ cup softened margarine or
   butter
3 cups sifted confectioner's
   sugar

¼ cup Rich's Coffee Rich
1 teaspoon vanilla (or other
   flavoring such as almond,
   orange, maple, or mint)

In a medium mixing bowl, cream margarine and ½ cup of the confectioner's sugar. Add a small amount of Coffee Rich and blend well. Continue adding sugar, then Coffee Rich, beating well after each addition. Mix in flavoring. Frosts 12 cupcakes (2 tablespoons per cupcake) or one 8- or 9-inch single layer cake.

Yield: 1½ cups.

	Phenylalanine (mg)	Protein (gm)	Calories
Per recipe	35	1.3	2833
Per 2 tablespoons or ¹⁄₁₂ of recipe	3	0.1	236

Variations

Banana Buttercream Frosting

Replace the Coffee Rich with ¼ cup (58 gm) mashed ripe banana. Add ½ teaspoon lemon juice.

Yield: 1½ cups.

	Phenylalanine (mg)	Protein (gm)	Calories
Per recipe	45	1.7	2800
Per 2 tablespoons or ¹⁄₁₂ of recipe	4	0.1	233

Chocolate Buttercream Frosting

Add 3 tablespoons Hershey's unsweetened cocoa (not instant), blending well.

Yield: 1½ cups.

	Phenylalanine (mg)	Protein (gm)	Calories
Per recipe	230	5.2	2896
Per 2 tablespoons or ½₂ of recipe	19	0.4	241

Orange Buttercream Frosting

Replace the Coffee Rich with ¼ cup orange juice. Add 1½ teaspoons fresh grated orange rind.

Yield: 1½ cups.

	Phenylalanine (mg)	Protein (gm)	Calories
Per recipe	31	1.5	2775
Per 2 tablespoons or ½₂ of recipe	3	0.1	231

Strawberry Buttercream Frosting

Replace the Coffee Rich with ¼ cup (65 gm) mashed frozen or fresh strawberries (with juice).

Yield: 1½ cups.

	Phenylalanine (mg)	Protein (gm)	Calories
Per recipe	29	1.5	2766
Per 2 tablespoons or ½₂ of recipe	2	0.1	231

Decorator Frosting

An excellent "free" recipe that keeps well in the refrigerator in a tightly covered container and also freezes well.

1 lb (4 cups) sifted
   confectioner's sugar
½ cup vegetable shortening
¼ cup cold water

½ teaspoon flavoring of your
   choice (vanilla, almond,
   orange, maple, etc.)
dash of salt

Place all ingredients in a mixing bowl. Mix with an electric mixer just until well combined, 20 to 30 seconds. Frosts 16 cupcakes (2 tablespoons per cupcake) or one 8- or 9-inch double layer cake.

Yield: 2 cups.

	Phenylalanine (mg)	Protein (gm)	Calories
Per recipe	0	0.0	2731
Per 2 tablespoons or ¹⁄₁₆ of recipe	0	0.0	171

Simple Caramel Frosting

1 cup packed brown sugar
½ cup Rich's Coffee Rich
2 cups sifted confectioner's
   sugar

½ teaspoon vanilla

Mix sugar and Coffee Rich in a small saucepan and bring just to a bubbling boil. Remove from heat and stir in confectioner's sugar and vanilla. Let cool. Add 2 to 3 tablespoons additional Coffee Rich or water, or enough to make a smooth spreading consistency. Frosts 12 cupcakes (2 tablespoons per cupcake) or one 8- or 9-inch single layer cake.

Yield: 1½ cups.

	Phenylalanine (mg)	Protein (gm)	Calories
Per recipe	22	0.5	1780
Per 2 tablespoons or ¹⁄₁₂ of recipe	2	trace	148

Puddings

Special Tips

For convenience, it is possible to make low protein pudding from Jell-O Pudding and Pie Filling mix by replacing milk with non-dairy creamer. However, thickening will be affected by this substitution and the instructions below should be followed. Instant pudding is the most successful and has the best flavor, but cook-type pudding can also be made. Use vanilla, lemon, butterscotch, banana cream, or coconut cream pudding mix (chocolate varieties are high in protein).

Instant Pudding Varieties

1 pkg (4-serving size) Jell-O
    Instant Pudding and Pie
    Filling mix
¼ cup liquid Rich's Richwhip
    Topping (do not substitute
    Rich's Coffee Rich, as it will
    not thicken)

¾ cup water

Add Richwhip and water to pudding mix in a bowl. Beat with an electric mixer, hand beater, or wire whip until thickened. Chill.

Yield: 1¾ cups.

	Phenylalanine (mg)	Protein (gm)	Calories
Per recipe	8	0.2	520
Per ½ cup serving	2	0.1	149

Cook-type Pudding Varieties

Method 1 (preferred method)

1 pkg (4-serving size) Jell-O
    Pudding and Pie Filling mix
2 teaspoons cornstarch

⅓ cup liquid Rich's Richwhip
    Topping
1 cup plus 2 tablespoons water

Mix cornstarch with dry pudding mix. Add Richwhip and water. Cook in a saucepan over medium heat until bubbly and thickened (or microwave in a 1-quart casserole on High for 1½ minutes, stir well, then microwave on High for another 45 seconds).

Yield: 1½ cups.

	Phenylalanine (mg)	Protein (gm)	Calories
Per recipe	0	0.0	597
Per ½ cup serving	0	0.0	199

Method 2

Use ⅔ cup Rich's Coffee Rich and ¾ cup water in place of liquid ingredients in Method 1.

Yield: 1½ cups.

	Phenylalanine (mg)	Protein (gm)	Calories
Per recipe	29	0.5	614
Per ½ cup serving	10	0.2	205

Orange Tapioca Pudding

A favorite among cookbook taste-testers.

4 cups water
1 pkg (4-serving size) cook-type
vanilla Jell-O Pudding and
Pie Filling mix
1 pkg (4-serving size) tapioca
Jello-O Pudding and Pie
Filling mix

1 pkg (4-serving size) orange
Jell-O or Prono low protein
gelled dessert mix
2 cups (137 gm) Coolwhip or
whipped Rich's Richwhip
Topping

Put water in large saucepan; mix in pudding mixes and Jell-O or Prono. Bring to a boil over medium heat, stirring. Chill for 1 to 2 hours. Mix in whipped topping. Chill.

Yield: 6 cups (1230 gm).

	Phenylalanine (mg)	Protein (gm)	Calories
Using Prono and Richwhip			
Per recipe	0	0	1382
Per ½ cup (102 gm) serving	0	0	115
Using Prono and Coolwhip			
Per recipe	103	2.0	1299
Per ½ cup (102 gm) serving	9	0.2	108
Using Jell-O and Richwhip			
Per recipe	148	7.2	1391
Per ½ cup (102 gm) serving	12	0.6	116
Using Jell-O and Coolwhip			
Per recipe	251	9.2	1308
Per ½ cup (102 gm) serving	21	0.8	109

Strawberrioca

10 oz pkg frozen strawberries
2 tablespoons quick-cooking
tapioca

¼ cup granulated sugar
2 teaspoons lemon juice

Thaw and drain strawberries, reserving juice. Add water to the juice to make 1½ cups. In a medium saucepan, mix the strawberry juice with the tapioca and sugar. Let stand for 5 minutes; then bring to a boil, stirring occasionally. Remove from heat. Stir in strawberries and lemon juice. Chill.

Yield: 2¼ cups (542 gm).

	Phenylalanine (mg)	Protein (gm)	Calories
Per recipe	22	1.5	462
Per ½ cup (120 gm) serving	5	0.3	103

Peach Tapioca

16 oz can sliced peaches,
drained
2 tablespoons quick-cooking
tapioca

2 tablespoons granulated sugar
1 tablespoon lemon juice
1 drop yellow food coloring

Drain peaches, reserving juice. Cut peaches into bite-sized pieces. Add water to peach juice to make 1 cup. Combine tapioca, peach juice, and sugar in a medium saucepan and let stand 5 minutes. Cook, stirring frequently, until tapioca is thickened and clear. Add lemon juice, peaches, and food coloring. Chill.

Yield: 2¼ cups (530 gm).

	Phenylalanine (mg)	Protein (gm)	Calories
Per recipe	41	1.3	190
Per ½ cup (118 gm) serving	9	0.3	42

Pumpkin Pudding

A nice alternative to pumpkin pie.

12 large marshmallows
2 teaspoons lemon juice
½ cup (100 gm) canned
  pumpkin
2½ tablespoons packed brown
  sugar

¼ teaspoon each cinnamon,
  nutmeg, and ginger
4 oz container Coolwhip (1¾
  cups), or ½ cup liquid
  Rich's Richwhip Topping,
  whipped

In a double boiler, heat marshmallows and lemon juice until marshmallows are melted (about 10 to 12 minutes), stirring several times. Add pumpkin, sugar, and spices and cook for 5 minutes, stirring several times during cooking. Chill mixture about 20 minutes. Fold in whipped topping. Chill.

Yield: 2 cups (317 gm).

	Phenylalanine (mg)	Protein (gm)	Calories
Using Richwhip			
Per recipe	70	2.3	761
Per ½ cup (79 gm) serving	18	0.6	190
Using Coolwhip			
Per recipe	154	3.9	693
Per ½ cup (79 gm) serving	39	1.0	173

Grape Pudding

¾ cup (6 fl. oz, ½ of 12 oz can)
  frozen grape juice
  concentrate, thawed
1½ cups (12 fl oz) water

3 tablespoons cornstarch
⅓ cup granulated sugar (or less
  if desired)

Mix all ingredients together in a medium saucepan. Cook over medium heat, stirring slowly until mixture thickens and becomes clear. Chill.

Yield: 2½ cups (635 gm).

	Phenylalanine (mg)	Protein (gm)	Calories
Per recipe	60	2.8	676
Per ½ cup (127 gm) serving	12	0.6	135

Miracle Strawberry Pudding

10 oz pkg frozen strawberries, thawed

1 pkg (4-serving size) cook-type vanilla Jell-O Pudding and Pie Filling mix

2 tablespoons granulated sugar

2 teaspoons lemon juice

1 tablespoon margarine or butter

Drain strawberries, reserving juice. Add cold water to juice to make 1½ cups. In a saucepan, combine pudding mix, sugar, lemon juice, and measured liquid; mix well. Cook and stir over medium heat until mixture comes to a full boil. Add margarine and mix until melted. Remove from heat and add strawberries. Chill.

Yield: 2¼ cups (562 gm).

	Phenylalanine (mg)	Protein (gm)	Calories
Per recipe	28	1.6	787
Per ½ cup (125 gm) serving	6	0.4	175

Variation

Frozen Strawberry Pudding Cups

After pudding has chilled, fold in 1 cup (68 gm) Coolwhip. Pour into 6 individual paper baking cups. Freeze firm.

Yield: 3 cups (630 gm).

	Phenylalanine (mg)	Protein (gm)	Calories
Per recipe	79	2.6	940
Per ½ cup (105 gm) serving	13	0.4	157

Miracle Cherry Pudding

1 pkg (4-serving size) cook-type
   vanilla Jell-O Pudding and
   Pie Filling mix
¼ cup granulated sugar
¼ teaspoon salt
½ cup water

2 teaspoons lemon juice
16 oz can pitted red sour
   cherries
1 tablespoon margarine or
   butter
3 drops red food coloring

Combine pudding mix, sugar, salt, water, and lemon juice in a medium saucepan. Blend until smooth. Add undrained cherries. Cook and stir over medium heat until mixture comes to a full boil. Remove from heat. Add margarine and red food coloring. Chill.

Yield: 2¾ cups (685 gm).

	Phenylalanine (mg)	Protein (gm)	Calories
Per recipe	47	2.1	852
Per ½ cup (125 gm) serving	9	0.4	155

Variation

Frozen Cherry Pudding Cups

After pudding has chilled, fold in 1 cup (68 gm) Coolwhip. Pour into 6 individual paper baking cups. Freeze firm.

Yield: 3½ cups (753 gm).

	Phenylalanine (mg)	Protein (gm)	Calories
Per recipe	98	3.0	1005
Per ½ cup (108 gm) serving	14	0.4	144

Golden Pudding

1½ cups orange juice

1 pkg (4-serving size) lemon
Jell-O Instant Pudding and
Pie Filling mix

In a mixing bowl, combine orange juice and pudding mix. Beat by hand according to pudding package directions. Chill.

Yield: 1⅔ cups (445 gm).

	Phenylalanine (mg)	Protein (gm)	Calories
Per recipe	45	2.2	528
Per ½ cup (134 gm) serving	14	0.7	160

Variation

Frozen Golden Pudding Cups

After pudding has chilled, fold in ¾ cup (51 gm) Coolwhip. Pour into 6 individual paper baking cups. Freeze firm.

Yield: 2¼ cups (496 gm).

	Phenylalanine (mg)	Protein (gm)	Calories
Per recipe	83	3.0	643
Per ½ cup (110 gm) serving	25	0.9	195

Lemon Pudding

1 pkg (4-serving size) lemon
   cook-type Jell-O Pudding
   and Pie Filling mix

½ cup granulated sugar
2¼ cups water

Mix pudding mix, sugar, and water in a saucepan. Cook and stir over medium heat until mixture comes to a full boil. Cool, stirring occasionally. Chill.

Yield: 2½ cups (660 gm).

	Phenylalanine (mg)	Protein (gm)	Calories
Per recipe	0	0.0	746
Per ½ cup (132 gm) serving	0	0.0	149

Variation

Frozen Lemon Pudding Cups

After pudding has chilled, fold in 1¼ cups (86 gm) Coolwhip. Pour into 6 individual paper baking cups. Freeze firm.

Yield: 3½ cups (746 gm).

	Phenylalanine (mg)	Protein (gm)	Calories
Per recipe	65	1.2	940
Per ½ cup (107 gm) serving	9	0.2	134

Brownie Pudding

Like a brownie on top with a rich pudding underneath. Diet recipe is as delicious as the family recipe and was a favorite among taste-testers.

Diet Portion

⅓ cup plus 1 tablespoon (41 gm) Wel-Plan Baking Mix
¼ cup granulated sugar
¾ teaspoon baking powder
pinch of salt
2 teaspoons Hershey's unsweetened cocoa (not instant)

2 tablespoons Rich's Coffee Rich or water
1 tablespoon water
2 teaspoons vegetable oil
¼ teaspoon vanilla

Topping

⅓ cup packed brown sugar
2 teaspoons Hershey's unsweetened cocoa (not instant)

⅓ cup boiling water

Preheat oven to 350°. In a medium bowl, stir together Baking Mix, sugar, baking powder, salt, and cocoa. Add Coffee Rich, water, vegetable oil, and vanilla; mix well. Spread mixture into a small greased baking dish, such as a Corning Ware individual casserole (approximately 2 cup capacity, 5 × 5 inches). Blend brown sugar and additional cocoa in a small bowl. Sprinkle over top of batter in a thick layer. Slowly pour hot water over all. Bake for 25 to 30 minutes. Serve warm or cold.

Yield: 1 cup (275 gm).

Family Portion

1 cup flour
¾ cup granulated sugar
2 teaspoons baking powder
¼ teaspoon salt
2 tablespoons Hershey's
    unsweetened cocoa (not
    instant)

½ cup milk
2 tablespoons vegetable oil
1 teaspoon vanilla

Topping

1 cup packed brown sugar
2 tablespoons Hershey's
    unsweetened cocoa (not
    instant)

1 cup boiling water

Prepare as for *Diet Portion*, using an 8- or 9-inch round or square baking pan. Bake at 350° for 45 minutes.

	Phenylalanine (mg)	Protein (gm)	Calories
Per diet recipe	93	1.9	769
Per ¼ cup (68 gm) serving	23	0.5	192

Holiday Steamed Pudding

A traditional, rich, holiday pudding that can be made well in advance. The diet recipe is as delicious as the family recipe; prepare them side by side.

Diet Portion

⅓ cup packed brown sugar
⅓ cup margarine or butter
⅓ cup (40 gm) grated carrots
⅓ cup (56 gm) grated potatoes
⅓ cup (53 gm) raisins
½ cup (55 gm) Wel-Plan Baking
   Mix

¼ teaspoon salt
¼ teaspoon baking soda
¼ teaspoon cinnamon
⅛ teaspoon nutmeg
dash of cloves

Cream brown sugar and margarine in a medium bowl. Mix in grated carrots, potatoes, and raisins. In a measuring cup, combine Baking Mix, salt, baking soda, and spices; stir into other mixture until evenly mixed and moist. Pack into a greased wide-mouthed 1-pint canning jar. Secure lid on jar. Boil in covered pot of water (water should be at least ½ way up sides of jar) for 3 hours. Serve pudding warm, with 1 tablespoon *Sauce* per serving.

Yield: 1½ cups (303 gm).

Sauce

½ cup packed brown sugar
2 tablespoons margarine
¼ cup cold water
1 tablespoon cornstarch

¼ teaspoon salt
½ to 1 teaspoon maple, rum, or
   vanilla flavoring

Combine all ingredients in a small saucepan. Bring to a boil, stirring until thickened, about 2 minutes. Makes ⅔ cup.

Family Portion

1 cup packed brown sugar	½ teaspoon salt
1 cup margarine or butter	1 teaspoon baking soda
1 cup grated carrots	1 teaspoon cinnamon
1 cup grated potatoes	½ teaspoon nutmeg
1 cup raisins	⅛ teaspoon cloves
1⅓ cups flour	

Prepare as for *Diet Portion*, packing pudding mixture into three greased wide-mouthed 1-pint canning jars. Steam as for *Diet Portion*. Serve warm, with *Sauce*.

Storage Tip
Pudding will keep in unopened jar in refrigerator for 3 months or in freezer for at least 6 months.

	Phenylalanine (mg)	Protein (gm)	Calories
Per diet recipe	133	4.1	1229
Per ¼ cup (51 gm) serving	22	0.7	205
Per ¼ cup (51 gm) serving plus 1 tablespoon sauce	24	0.7	313

Pies and Pastry

If you are not in the habit of making pies very often, when you do want to make a pie, preparing a filling that will suit the entire family is certainly desirable. So for convenience, most of the recipes in this section are designed to make both a small diet pie (using a low protein crust) and a regular-sized pie (using regular pie crust—either home made or commercially prepared) for the rest of the family, both using the same filling.

Nutrient values for the pies generally do not include values for the crust, because there are several low protein crust recipes from which to choose, and because many of the pie fillings could be served as a dessert without crust (for example, the "dream" pie recipes make excellent, light pudding-type desserts). Be sure to add in the appropriate nutrient values for crust (a minimal addition of phenylalanine/protein if you use the basic low protein pastry recipes in this section).

Favorite Pie Crust got its name from the enthusiastic response of taste-testers and recipe-testers. The dough is easy to work with and the overall quality of the baked pastry is excellent. Nevertheless, the dough is a little more fragile than regular pie crust dough and it may be somewhat difficult to make a normal-sized pie without some cracking or tearing. It works beautifully for small pies or tarts, as directed in the recipes, and also for making turnovers (using all Wel-Plan Baking Mix, rather than the mixture of Baking Mix and wheatstarch which the recipe calls for, makes an exceptionally sturdy crust). The *Basic Pie Crust* recipe also works well, but will not brown as much as *Favorite Pie Crust*.

Apple Pie

1 cup granulated sugar
1½ tablespoons cornstarch
½ teaspoon cinnamon
¼ teaspoon nutmeg
⅛ teaspoon salt

7½ cups (900 gm) peeled,
  thinly sliced, tart apples
regular dough for 2-crust pie
  and your choice of low
  protein pie crust dough

Preheat oven to 425°. Mix sugar with cornstarch, cinnamon, nutmeg, and salt. Slice apples into a large bowl, sprinkling sugar-spice mixture over them as you slice them. Let fruit mixture stand for 15 to 30 minutes. Meanwhile, prepare regular pie dough and low protein pie dough for 2-crust pies.

Diet Portion
Roll out low protein dough to a 6- to 7-inch circle and place in a 4-inch pie pan. Cut dough even with edge of pan. Fill with 1¼ cups (250 gm) apple mixture. Roll out top crust to a 6- to 7-inch circle. Cut top vents. Place on top of pie. Trim to ½ inch beyond lower crust dough. Fold overhanging dough under bottom dough. Crimp edges or press with a fork. Bake for 30 to 40 minutes or until apples are tender.

Family Portion
Use remaining apple mixture to fill an 8- or 9-inch regular pie crust. Bake for 45 to 50 minutes or until apples are tender.

Yield: 7½ cups filling.

	Phenylalanine (mg)	Protein (gm)	Calories
Per recipe filling	45	2.0	1355
Per ½ of 4-inch pie (not including crust)	4	0.2	113

Blueberry Pie

4 cups (640 gm) fresh
  blueberries
2 teaspoons lemon juice
1 cup granulated sugar
1½ tablespoons tapioca
1 teaspoon cinnamon

¼ teaspoon nutmeg
⅛ teaspoon salt
regular dough for 2-crust pie
  and your choice of low
  protein pie crust dough

Preheat oven to 425°. Wash and drain blueberries; place in a bowl. Mix in lemon juice. Mix together sugar, tapioca, cinnamon, nutmeg, and salt; mix with blueberries. Let fruit mixture stand for 15 to 30 minutes. Meanwhile, prepare regular pie dough and low protein pie dough for 2-crust pies.

Diet Portion
Roll out low protein dough to a 6- to 7-inch circle and place in a 4-inch pie pan. Cut dough even with edge of pan. Fill with ¾ cup (140 gm) of blueberry mixture. Roll out top crust to a 6- to 7-inch circle. Cut out top vents. Place on top of pie. Trim to ½ inch beyond lower crust dough. Fold overhanging dough under bottom dough. Crimp edges or press with a fork. Bake for 20 to 30 minutes.

Family Portion
Use remaining blueberry mixture to fill an 8- or 9-inch regular pie crust. Bake for 30 to 45 minutes.

Yield: 4 cups filling.

	Phenylalanine (mg)	Protein (gm)	Calories
Per recipe filling	154	4.3	1142
Per ½ of 4-inch pie (not including crust)	15	0.4	108

Cherry Pie

Two 1 lb cans sour red
cherries, drained, or 3½
cups (580 gm) fresh sour
cherries
½ cup juice from cherries
1½ cups granulated sugar
2½ tablespoons tapioca

¼ teaspoon almond extract
(optional)
5 to 7 drops red food coloring
regular dough for 2-crust pie
and your choice of low
protein pie crust dough

Preheat oven to 425°. Mix all ingredients in a mixing bowl; let stand 30 minutes. Meanwhile, prepare regular pie dough and low protein pie dough for 2-crust pies.

Diet Portion

Roll out low protein dough to a 6- to 7-inch circle and place in a 4-inch pie pan. Cut dough even with edge of pan. Fill with ¾ cup (200 gm) cherry mixture. Roll out top crust to a 6- to 7-inch circle, cutting top vents; or cut dough in ½-inch strips for a lattice-top pie. Place dough on top of pie, completing as for a regular 2-crust pie or lattice-top pie. Crimp edges or press with a fork. Bake for 20 to 30 minutes.

Family Portion

Use remaining cherry mixture to fill an 8- or 9-inch regular pie crust, using either a full top crust or lattice top crust. Bake for 30 to 35 minutes.

Yield: 4¼ cups filling.

	Phenylalanine (mg)	Protein (gm)	Calories
Per recipe filling	154	7.0	1584
Per ½ of 4-inch pie (not including crust)	13	0.6	138

Fresh Peach Pie

6 cups (950 gm) sliced fresh
  peaches
2 to 3 tablespoons tapioca
1 cup granulated sugar
½ teaspoon cinnamon

¼ teaspoon salt
regular dough for 2-crust pie
  and your choice of low
  protein pie crust dough

Preheat oven to 425°. Slice peaches into a large bowl. Mix tapioca, sugar, cinnamon, and salt together; mix into peaches (use 3 table-spoons tapioca for very juicy peaches). Let fruit mixture stand for 15 to 30 minutes. Meanwhile, prepare regular pie dough and low protein pie dough for 2-crust pies.

Diet Portion

Roll out low protein dough to a 6- to 7-inch circle and place in a 4-inch pie pan. Cut dough even with edge of pan. Fill with ¾ cup (225 gm) peach mixture. Roll out top crust to a 6- to 7-inch circle, cutting top vents; or cut dough in ½-inch strips for a lattice-top pie. Place dough on top of pie, completing as for a regular 2-crust pie or lattice-top pie. Crimp edges or press with a fork. Bake for 20 to 30 minutes.

Family Portion

Use remaining peach mixture to fill an 8- or 9-inch regular pie crust, using either a full top crust or lattice top crust. Bake for 30 to 35 minutes.

Yield: 6 cups filling.

	Phenylalanine (mg)	Protein (gm)	Calories
Per recipe filling	207	6.7	1188
Per ½ of 4-inch pie (not including crust)	13	0.4	74

Pumpkin Pie

Amazingly like "regular" pumpkin pie. Also good as a pudding.

¼ cup (50 gm) canned
  pumpkin
1½ teaspoons cornstarch
2 tablespoons packed brown
  sugar
⅓ cup Rich's Coffee Rich
2 tablespoons (18 gm) cook-
  type vanilla Jell-O Pudding
  and Pie Filling mix

½ teaspoon pumpkin pie
  spice (or combination of
  cinnamon, nutmeg, and
  ginger)
4-inch unbaked pie shell,
  using low protein pie crust
  dough of your choice

Preheat oven to 425°. Mix all ingredients in a bowl. Pour into unbaked pie shell. Bake for 30 minutes.

Yield: ⅔ cup (180 gm) filling.

	Phenylalanine (mg)	Protein (gm)	Calories
Per recipe	32	0.8	301
Per ½ of 4-inch pie (not including crust)	16	0.4	151

Strawberry Dream Pie

Also excellent as a pudding, as are any of the "Dream Pie" fillings in this section.

1 pkg (4-serving size) cook-type vanilla Jell-O Pudding and Pie Filling mix

1 pkg (4-serving size) strawberry Jell-O or Prono low protein gelled dessert mix

2 cups water

1 teaspoon lemon juice (optional)

4 oz container Coolwhip (1¾ cups) or ½ cup liquid Rich's Richwhip Topping, whipped

1 cup (105 gm) sliced fresh strawberries

Graham Cracker Crust or low protein crust of your choice

Combine pudding mix, Jell-O or Prono, water, and lemon juice in a saucepan. Cook and stir over medium heat until mixture comes to a boil. If using Jell-O, pour into a bowl and chill about an hour or until thickened (to speed chilling, place bowl of pudding mixture into a larger bowl of ice and water; stir until thickened). If using low protein gelled dessert mix, let sit at room temperature for 1 hour. Blend in whipped topping and strawberries. Pour into a 9-inch graham cracker crust. Chill until set, 1 to 2 hours. Cut pie in 8 pieces for a ½-cup serving of filling.

Family Portion plus Diet Portion

Use ½ cup filling for a baked 4-inch low protein pie crust or *Low Protein Graham Cracker Crust*, using remainder of filling for regular crust for the rest of the family.

Yield: 4 cups (845 gm) filling.

Note

Filling made with Prono will not set firmly; it is best used as a pudding or put in a 4-inch pie pan.

	Phenylalanine (mg)	Protein (gm)	Calories
Using Prono and Richwhip			
Per recipe filling	9	0.6	992
Per ½ cup (⅛ pie, not including crust)	1	0.1	124
Using Prono and Coolwhip			
Per recipe filling	99	2.2	924
Per ½ cup (⅛ pie, not including crust)	12	0.3	116
Using Jell-O and Richwhip			
Per recipe filling	157	7.8	992
Per ½ cup (⅛ pie, not including crust)	20	1.0	124
Using Jell-O and Coolwhip			
Per recipe filling	241	9.4	924
Per ½ cup (⅛ pie, not including crust)	30	1.2	115

Blueberry Dream Pie

1 pkg (4-serving size) cook-type vanilla Jell-O Pudding and Pie Filling mix

1 pkg (4-serving size) blackberry or blueberry Jell-O

2 cups water

1 teaspoon lemon juice (optional)

4 oz container Coolwhip (1¾ cups) or ½ cup liquid Rich's Richwhip Topping, whipped

1 cup (160 gm) fresh, frozen, or canned and drained blueberries

Graham Cracker Crust or low protein crust of your choice

Prepare as for *Strawberry Dream Pie.*

Yield: 4 cups (900 gm) filling.

	Phenylalanine (mg)	Protein (gm)	Calories
Using Jell-O and Richwhip			
Per recipe filling	166	7.7	1001
Per ½ cup (⅛ pie, not including crust)	21	1.0	125
Using Jell-O and Coolwhip			
Per recipe filling	250	9.3	933
Per ½ cup (⅛ pie, not including crust)	31	1.2	117

Peach Dream Pie

1 pkg (4-serving size) cook-type vanilla Jell-O Pudding and Pie Filling mix

1 pkg (4-serving size) peach Jell-O or orange Prono low protein gelled dessert mix

2 cups water

1 teaspoon lemon juice (optional)

4 oz container Coolwhip (1¾ cups) or ½ cup liquid Rich's Richwhip Topping, whipped

1 cup (160 gm) diced fresh or canned peaches

Graham Cracker Crust or low protein crust of your choice

Prepare as for *Strawberry Dream Pie.*

Yield: 4 cups (900 gm) filling.

Note

Filling made with Prono will not set firmly; it is best used as a pudding or in a 4-inch pie pan.

	Phenylalanine (mg)	Protein (gm)	Calories
Using Prono and Richwhip			
Per recipe filling	35	1.1	1029
Per ½ cup (⅛ pie, not including crust)	4	0.1	129
Using Prono and Coolwhip			
Per recipe filling	119	2.7	961
Per ½ cup (⅛ pie, not including crust)	15	0.3	120
Using Jell-O and Richwhip			
Per recipe filling	183	8.3	1029
Per ½ cup (⅛ pie, not including crust)	23	1.0	129
Using Jell-O and Coolwhip			
Per recipe filling	267	9.9	961
Per ½ cup (⅛ pie, not including crust)	33	1.2	120

Grasshopper Pie

1 pkg (4-serving size) cook-type vanilla Jell-O Pudding and Pie Filling mix

1 pkg (4-serving size) lime Jell-O or Prono low protein gelled dessert mix

1¾ cups water

2 tablespoons creme de menthe or 2 teaspoons mint flavoring plus 1 tablespoon water

4 oz container Coolwhip (1¾ cups) or ½ cup liquid Rich's Richwhip Topping, whipped

Chocolate Cookie Crust or *Graham Cracker Crust*

Combine pudding mix, Jell-O or Prono, and water in a saucepan. Cook and stir over medium heat until mixture comes to a boil. Add creme de menthe, or mint flavoring and extra water. If using Jell-O, pour mixture into a bowl and chill about an hour or until thickened (to speed chilling, place bowl of pudding mixture into a larger bowl of ice and water; stir until thickened). If using low protein gelled dessert mix, let sit at room temperature for 1 hour. Blend in whipped topping. Pour into a 9-inch pie shell. Chill until set, 1 to 2 hours. Cut pie into 10 pieces for a ⅓-cup serving of filling.

Family Portion plus Diet Portion

Use ½ cup filling for a 4-inch *Low Chocolate Cookie Crust* or *Low Graham Cracker Crust*, using the remainder of filling for regular crust for the rest of the family.

Yield: 3⅓ cups (740 gm) filling.

Note

Filling made with Prono will not set firmly; it is best used as a pudding or in a 4-inch pie pan.

	Phenylalanine (mg)	Protein (gm)	Calories
Using Prono and Richwhip			
Per recipe filling	0	0.0	960
Per ⅓ cup (¹⁄₁₀ pie, not including crust)	0	0.0	96
Using Prono and Coolwhip			
Per recipe filling	84	1.6	892
Per ⅓ cup (¹⁄₁₀ pie, not including crust)	8	0.2	89
Using Jell-O and Richwhip			
Per recipe filling	148	7.2	960
Per ⅓ cup (¹⁄₁₀ pie, not including crust)	15	0.7	96
Using Jell-O and Coolwhip			
Per recipe filling	232	8.8	892
Per ⅓ cup (¹⁄₁₀ pie, not including crust)	23	0.9	89

Chocolate-Filled Turnovers

Attractive and delicious lunchbox treats or snacks.

½ cup granulated sugar
¼ cup cornstarch
1 tablespoon Hershey's
  unsweetened cocoa (not
  instant)

½ cup Rich's Coffee Rich
2 tablespoons margarine or
  butter
½ teaspoon vanilla
1 recipe *Favorite Pie Crust*

In a small saucepan, combine sugar, cornstarch, and cocoa. Stir in Coffee Rich and margarine. Cook over medium heat, stirring until bubbly. Cook 1 minute longer, continuing to stir. Mix in vanilla. Refrigerate.

Prepare pie crust dough while filling is cooling. On a surface dusted with Baking Mix, roll dough to ⅛-inch thickness. Cut ten 4-inch circles, rerolling dough scraps as necessary. Place about 1 tablespoon filling on ½ of each circle, leaving a ½-inch margin around edge of the dough. Wet edge of one half of dough circle with a little water, using your fingers. Fold over and press edges together with fingertips, then press again with tines of a fork. Trim uneven dough edges with a knife. Prick turnovers with a fork several times.

Transfer filled pastries to an ungreased baking sheet. Sprinkle with a little sugar. Bake in preheated 400° oven for 20 minutes.

Yield: 10 turnovers.

Note

For *Favorite Pie Crust* use 2 cups (220 gm) Wel-Plan Baking Mix and no wheat starch for an exceptionally sturdy crust. The pies could be easily transported for lunch.

To conveniently make 4-inch circles, use the wide part of a canning funnel to cut out pie dough.

Storage Tip

These keep well at room temperature or refrigerated, for up to 5 days. They also freeze well for up to several months in an airtight container.

	Phenylalanine (mg)	Protein (gm)	Calories
Per recipe	114	2.5	3087
Per turnover	11	0.3	309

Fruit-Filled Turnovers

1 cup (295 gm) Comstock or
Wilderness pie filling (apple,
apricot, blueberry, cherry,
peach, pineapple, or
strawberry)

1 recipe *Favorite Pie Crust*

If using apple filling, add a little cinnamon and nutmeg to taste. Prepare pie crust dough and roll out as directed for *Chocolate-Filled Turnovers*, placing about 1½ tablespoons filling on each dough circle. Bake as directed for *Chocolate-Filled Turnovers*.

Yield: 10 turnovers.

Note
   See Note for *Chocolate-Filled Turnovers*.

	Phenylalanine (mg)	Protein (gm)	Calories
Per recipe	55	2.0	2473
Per turnover	6	0.2	247

Favorite Pie Crust

1 cup (110 gm) Wel-Plan
  Baking Mix
1 cup (110 gm) wheat starch
1 tablespoon granulated sugar
½ teaspoon salt

¼ teaspoon baking powder
⅔ cup yellow shortening (Fluffo
  or Butter-Flavored Crisco)
3½ tablespoons cold water
2 teaspoons vinegar

Combine Baking Mix, wheat starch, sugar, salt, and baking powder in a mixing bowl. Cut in shortening with a pastry blender, fork, or 2 knives until mixture resembles coarse bread crumbs. Combine water and vinegar in a separate dish; dribble over dry ingredients, blending in with a fork until all of dough clings together. Form dough into a smooth ball.

Roll dough out to ⅛-inch thickness on a surface dusted with Baking Mix, in the size of circle directed in individual recipes. A pastry cloth or wooden surface works best. Bake in preheated 425° oven for 10 minutes or bake as directed in individual recipes.

Yield:
  Enough dough for one of the following:
  15 pot pies (using about 25 gm each).
  12 small turnovers (using about 30 gm each).
  6 large turnovers (using about 60 gm each).
  six 4-inch diameter pies (using about 60 gm each).

Note
  One drop of yellow food coloring can be added to the water if you do not have yellow shortening. Use all Wel-Plan Baking Mix for an exceptionally sturdy crust if you do not feel adept at working with pie dough, or to prepare a crust that travels well. The recipe as given makes a crust which is very similar to regular crust in tenderness.

Storage Tip

The dough freezes well in an airtight container. Baked crusts may also be frozen for up to several months but may become a little fragile.

	Phenylalanine (mg)	Protein (gm)	Calories
Per recipe	15	0.6	2165
Per pot pie or small turnover	1	0.1	180
Per 4-inch pie or large turnover	3	0.1	361

Basic Pie Crust

¾ cup (83 gm) Wel-Plan Baking
   Mix
¾ cup (83 gm) wheat starch
⅓ cup plus 1 tablespoon yellow
   shortening (Fluffo or Butter-
   Flavored Crisco)

½ teaspoon salt
¼ cup cold water

Combine Baking Mix, wheat starch, and salt in a mixing bowl. Cut in shortening with a pastry blender, fork, or 2 knives until mixture resembles coarse bread crumbs. Dribble water over dry ingredients, blending in with a fork until all of dough clings together. Form dough into a smooth ball.

Roll dough out to ⅛-inch thickness on a surface dusted with Baking Mix, in the size of circle directed in individual recipe. A pastry cloth or wooden surface works best. Bake in preheated 425° for 10 minutes or bake as directed in individual recipes.

Yield:
   Enough dough for one of the following:
   12 pot pies (using about 25 gm each).
   10 small turnovers (using about 30 gm each).
   5 large turnovers (using about 60 gm each).
   five 4-inch diameter pies (using about 60 gm each).

Note
   This pastry will brown a little, but not as much as *Favorite Pie Crust.* One drop of yellow food coloring can be added to the water if you do not have yellow shortening.

Storage Tip
   The dough freezes well. Baked crusts may also be frozen for up to several months but may become a little fragile.

	Phenylalanine (mg)	Protein (gm)	Calories
Per recipe	12	0.5	1388
Per pot pie or small turnover	1	trace	139
Per 4-inch pie or large turnover	2	0.1	278

Graham Cracker Crust

1 cup (86 gm) graham cracker
   crumbs (from 13 squares)
¼ cup granulated sugar

¼ cup melted margarine or
   butter

Crush graham crackers with a rolling pin. In a bowl, mix graham cracker crumbs with sugar and melted margarine. Pat crumb mixture into a 9-inch pie pan. Refrigerate at least 1 hour before filling.

Yield: one 9-inch pie crust (1½ cups crumbs, 194 gm).

	Phenylalanine (mg)	Protein (gm)	Calories
Per recipe	271	5.2	990
Per ⅒ pie (19 gm)	27	0.5	97
Per ⅛ pie (24 gm)	33	0.6	122

Low Graham Cracker Crust

Save all of your "trimmings" from *Cinnamon Graham Crackers* for this delicious crust which is nearly indistinguishable from the regular version.

⅓ cup plus 1 tablespoon (55
   gm) *Cinnamon Graham
   Cracker* crumbs

1 tablespoon granulated sugar
1½ tablespoons melted
   margarine or butter

Finely crush graham crackers with a rolling pin. Mix sugar into crumbs in a small bowl. Add melted margarine and mix well. Press crumb mixture into a 4-inch pie pan. Refrigerate at least 1 hour before filling.

Yield: one 4-inch pie crust.

	Phenylalanine (mg)	Protein (gm)	Calories
Per recipe	14	0.3	481
Per ½ of 4-inch pie crust	7	0.1	241

Chocolate Cookie Crust

1 cup (110 gm) Nabisco
    Famous Chocolate Wafers,
    crushed (from 16 cookies)

2 tablespoons granulated sugar
¼ cup melted margarine or
    butter

Crush cookies with a rolling pin. In a bowl, mix together cookie crumbs and sugar. Mix in melted margarine. Pat crumb mixture into a 9-inch pie pan. Refrigerate at least 1 hour before filling.

Yield: one 9-inch pie crust (1½ cups crumbs, 194 gm).

	Phenylalanine (mg)	Protein (gm)	Calories
Per recipe	390	7.8	992
Per ¹⁄₁₀ pie crust (19 gm)	38	0.8	97
Per ⅛ pie crust (24 gm)	48	1.0	122

Low Chocolate Cookie Crust

½ cup (55 gm) crushed *Fudge
    Circles*
2 teaspoons granulated sugar

1½ tablespoons melted
    margarine or butter

Finely crush cookies with a rolling pin. Mix sugar with crumbs in a small bowl. Add melted margarine and mix well (mixture will be quite moist but will become firm on chilling). Press firmly into a 4-inch pie pan. Refrigerate at least 1 hour before filling.

Yield: one 4-inch pie crust.

	Phenylalanine (mg)	Protein (gm)	Calories
Per recipe	20	0.8	455
Per ¼ of 4-inch pie crust	5	0.2	114

Candy

Special Tips

A number of the recipes in this section contain the white or butterscotch "bark" (candy coating) that is used to make almond bark candy. There are brands of this product that contain protein and brands that do not. Protein-free brands were used in the recipes in this section. If you use brands that are not protein-free, be sure to add the extra phenylalanine to the recipe totals.

Because the brands of almond bark are known to change their ingredients periodically, and a product that was once protein-free may become no longer protein-free, it is important always to check the ingredient list on the product label. If the product contains whey or milk solids it is not protein-free. (Please see the introductory section of the Low Protein Food List, pp. 14–15, if you are not familiar with unusual ingredients that may be listed on the almond bark label; on these pages there is a list of less-familiar ingredients that do or do not contain protein and phenylalanine.)

Also, please check the Diet-Related Information section of the National PKU News Web site (www.pkunews.org) for additions and changes to the Low Protein Food List for PKU. These lists will include information on known almond bark brands and their phenylalanine content. This will never be an all inclusive list, however, and you may discover other suitable brands. The almond bark product is usually only available from mid to late October until the end of the holiday season, but keeps for up to a year or more at room temperature. Ener-G Foods carries one brand of the almond bark, which can be mail-ordered at any time of the year (please see contact information, page 32).

Marshmallow Treats

1½ lb protein-free premix for almond bark (see page 432)
3 to 4 drops green food coloring

4 cups (157 gm) mini marshmallows
candy sprinkles, jimmies, or colored sugar (optional)

Melt bark according to package directions. Mix in food coloring. Remove from heat and let cool several minutes. Add marshmallows (marshmallows will melt slightly if bark is too hot, but this makes for an interesting effect too). Quickly drop by teaspoon onto waxed paper. Cool.

Yield: 50 pieces.

	Phenylalanine (mg)	Protein (gm)	Calories
Per recipe	60	2.2	4155
Per piece	1	trace	83

Marshmallow Rice Krispie Candy

1½ lbs protein-free premix for butterscotch bark (see page 432)
2 cups (54 gm) Rice Krispies cereal

2 cups (78 gm) mini marshmallows

Melt bark according to package directions. Remove from heat and let cool several minutes. Add cereal and marshmallows (marshmallows will melt slightly if bark is too hot, but this makes for an interesting effect too). Quickly drop by teaspoon onto waxed paper. Cool.

Yield: 50 pieces.

	Phenylalanine (mg)	Protein (gm)	Calories
Per recipe	204	5.0	4116
Per piece	4	0.1	82

Peppermint Bark

20 Brach's Starlight Mints,
   crushed (½ cup) or ½ cup
   crushed peppermint candy
   canes

1 lb protein-free premix for
   almond bark (see page 432)
2 drops red food coloring

Crush mints or candy canes (an easy way to do this is to place them in a heavy plastic bag, then pound with a rolling pin until finely crushed). Melt bark according to package directions. Mix in food coloring and crushed mints. Quickly pour mixture onto an ungreased standard-sized cookie sheet, spreading thinly over the entire surface. Let cool, then break into pieces of desired size.

Yield: about 50 pieces.

	Phenylalanine (mg)	Protein (gm)	Calories
Per recipe	0	0	2415
Per piece	0	0	48

Candy Pretzels

½ lb protein-free premix for almond bark (see page 432) or 1 cup vanilla Pillsbury Ready-To-Spread Frosting Supreme

Candy sprinkles, jimmies, or colored sugar
55 mini 3-ring pretzels (1 inch diameter) (70 gm)

Melt bark according to package directions. If using frosting, melt in top of a double boiler. Remove from heat but keep over hot water. Dip pretzels, one at a time, into melted bark or frosting using a pair of tongs to hold them; shake gently to remove excess coating. Place each dipped pretzel on waxed paper, then immediately sprinkle with candy or sugar for a decorative effect. Let cool.

Yield: 55 pretzels.

Storage Tip
Store in airtight container. If vanilla frosting is used, coating may crack slightly on standing. These freeze well if premix for almond bark is used.

	Phenylalanine (mg)	Protein (gm)	Calories
Per recipe	315	6.5	1484
Per pretzel	6	0.1	27

Chocolate Bon-Bons

Mimic the appearance and flavor of commercial filled chocolates with surprisingly little effort. Nice for Christmas, or make into egg shapes for Easter.

½ cup softened margarine or
    butter
1 lb. (4 cups) sifted con-
    fectioner's sugar
1 tablespoon water
1½ teaspoons vanilla, orange,
    almond, or desired flavoring

½ cup (90 gm) Nestlé semi-
    sweet chocolate chips
¾ lb protein-free premix for
    almond bark (see page 432)
candy sprinkles, jimmies,
    colored sugar, or *Decorator*
    Frosting

In a medium bowl, cream margarine. Gradually add sugar, then water and flavoring as mixture becomes dry. Mix well. Refrigerate dough (or place in freezer for approximately 1 hour) until firm enough to handle. Shape into 45 small balls, using your hands to roll them, and place on a cookie sheet. If necessary, refrigerate again for several hours (or put in freezer for approximately 1 hour), until firm.

Melt premix for almond bark according to package directions. Add chocolate chips and stir until melted and well mixed. Using a spoon, dip balls one by one into hot chocolate mixture; set on waxed paper placed on a cookie sheet (you will inevitably have some drips around each bon-bon which can easily be broken off later). Immediately sprinkle with candy sprinkles or sugar for a decorative effect, or decorate with frosting when cool. Store in an airtight container. The candy keeps well at room temperature for several weeks, or can be refrigerated or frozen for a longer time.

Yield: 45 bon-bons.

Note

You will not use all of the chocolate mixture. Calculations are based on using all but 3 tablespoons (60 gm), which is too little to comfortably dip additional bon-bons.

	Phenylalanine (mg)	Protein (gm)	Calories
Per recipe	229	5.2	4886
Per bon-bon	5	0.1	109

Variation

Pastel Bon-Bons

Especially good with an orange- or lemon-flavored center (for additional flavor, add several teaspoons of grated fresh orange or lemon rind).

Omit chocolate chips. Color melted premix for almond bark with small amounts of powdered food colors (available from cake decorating supply stores. *Do not use liquid or paste colors*, as the candy coating will immediately thicken). Leaving the coating white and making a colored center is also nice. Prepare and coat as for *Chocolate Bon-Bons.*

Yield: 45 bon-bons.

	Phenylalanine (mg)	Protein (gm)	Calories
Per recipe	24	1.5	4405
Per bon-bon	trace	trace	98

Vanilla Butterballs

½ cup softened margarine or
  butter
1 tablespoon vanilla
2 cups sifted confectioner's
  sugar

2 to 3 drops food coloring
  (optional)
candy sprinkles, jimmies, or
  colored sugar (optional)

In a small mixing bowl, thoroughly cream margarine. Add vanilla and confectioner's sugar, beating until smooth. Color with food coloring if desired. By teaspoon, drop onto waxed paper placed in a baking pan or on a cookie sheet; or pipe into rosette shapes using a pastry bag with a large star tip for an easy and very attractive special treat. Sprinkle with colored candy sprinkles, jimmies, or colored sugar if desired. Freeze for at least several hours, then remove candy to a plastic container with tight-fitting cover, separating layers with waxed paper. Refreeze. Best served directly from the freezer.

Yield: 32 butterballs.

	Phenylalanine (mg)	Protein (gm)	Calories
Per recipe	47	1.2	1749
Per butterball	1	trace	55

Variation

Chocolate Butterballs

Add 2 teaspoons Hershey's unsweetened cocoa (not instant) along with confectioner's sugar.

Yield: 32 butterballs.

	Phenylalanine (mg)	Protein (gm)	Calories
Per recipe	90	2.1	1763
Per butterball	3	0.1	55

438

Million Dollar Candy Bars

Delicious, generous-sized candy bars with little protein, mimicking commercial "100 Grand Bars."

1 recipe *Caramels*
1 lb protein-free premix for
  almond bark (see page 432)
½ cup (90 gm) semisweet
  chocolate chips

⅔ cup (18 gm) Rice Krispies
  cereal

Prepare *Caramels*, pouring candy mixture into a well-greased 11 × 7-inch pan. Cool as directed, then cut into 35 pieces (6 cuts lengthwise, 4 cuts crosswise to make 35 rectangles). Melt bark according to package directions. Add chocolate chips and stir until melted. Mix in Rice Krispies.

Using a toothpick or spoon, dip caramel pieces in warm coating. Place on a cookie sheet lined with waxed paper and let harden. If any coating mixture remains after all caramel pieces are dipped, dribble remaining coating over already dipped pieces. When hardened, wrap candy bars individually in plastic wrap.

Yield: 35 candy bars.

	Phenylalanine (mg)	Protein (gm)	Calories
Per recipe	150	3.2	5898
Per candy bar	4	0.1	169

Caramels

½ cup margarine or butter
1⅓ cups packed brown sugar
½ cup light Karo corn syrup

¾ cup plus 2 tablespoons
   Rich's Richwhip Topping
½ teaspoon vanilla

Melt margarine in a large saucepan. Add sugar, syrup, and Rich-whip Topping. Bring mixture to a boil over moderate heat. Reduce heat slightly, allowing mixture to continue a steady boil. Cook, stirring occasionally, until candy thermometer fastened to the side of the pan registers precisely 245°, about 15 to 25 minutes. Stir in vanilla. Pour mixture into a well-greased 11 × 7- or 8 × 8-inch pan; let cool at room temperature, then refrigerate one hour or more. Cut into small squares. Wrap each piece in plastic wrap.

Yield: 49 caramels.

	Phenylalanine (mg)	Protein (gm)	Calories
Per recipe	47	1.0	2912
Per caramel	1	trace	59

Easy Fudge

2 pkg (4-serving size) cook-type
   Jell-O Pudding and Pie
   Filling mix (vanilla,
   butterscotch, coconut
   cream, or banana cream
   flavor)

¼ cup margarine or butter
½ cup water
1 lb (4 cups) sifted
   confectioner's sugar

Combine pudding mix, margarine, and water in a saucepan; bring to a boil over medium heat, stirring constantly. Remove from heat. Quickly mix in confectioner's sugar until well blended. Pour into a greased 8-inch square pan. Chill, then cut into pieces. Store, covered, in refrigerator. Fudge will remain somewhat soft.

Yield: 36 pieces.

Note
For variation, flavor vanilla fudge with ¼ teaspoon almond, orange, or peppermint extract and tint with food coloring if desired.

	Phenylalanine (mg)	Protein (gm)	Calories
Per recipe	24	0.9	2497
Per piece	1	trace	69

440

Chocolate Fudge

The all-time favorite fudge recipe from a marshmallow creme jar, adapted without sacrificing any of its delicious flavor.

1½ cups granulated sugar
6 tablespoons margarine or
   butter
⅓ cup Rich's Coffee Rich

1 cup (180 gm) Nestlé semisweet chocolate chips
   (6 oz bag)
1 cup (100 gm) Kraft Marshmallow Creme (½ of 7 oz jar)
1½ teaspoons vanilla

Combine sugar, margarine, and Coffee Rich in a large saucepan. Bring to a full boil over medium heat, stirring constantly. Boil until a candy thermometer fastened to the side of the pan registers 232° (soft ball stage), approximately 3 to 5 minutes. Remove from heat; mix in chocolate chips and marshmallow creme until melted. Add vanilla. Pour into a greased 8-inch square pan. Chill at least 2 hours before cutting.

Yield: 49 pieces.

	Phenylalanine (mg)	Protein (gm)	Calories
Per recipe	464	10.1	3179
Per piece	9	0.2	65

Two-Flavor Fudge

A favorite holiday treat from the first edition of *Low Protein Cookery.*

2 cups packed brown sugar
1 cup granulated sugar
1 cup liquid Rich's Richwhip
    Topping or Rich's Coffee
    Rich
½ cup margarine or butter

2 cups (78 gm) mini
    marshmallows
6 oz pkg Nestlé butterscotch
    chips
6 oz pkg Nestlé semisweet
    chocolate chips
1 teaspoon vanilla

Combine brown sugar, granulated sugar, non-dairy creamer, and margarine in a saucepan. Bring to a slow boil over low heat, stirring frequently; let boil vigorously for 15 minutes, stirring occasionally. Remove from heat. Add marshmallows, butterscotch chips, and chocolate chips; stir until melted and mixture is smooth. Blend in vanilla. Pour into a greased 8- or 9-inch square pan. Chill until firm. Cut into 64 pieces.

Yield: 64 pieces.

	Phenylalanine (mg)	Protein (gm)	Calories
Using Richwhip			
Per recipe	602	12.8	5147
Per piece	9	0.2	80
Using Coffee Rich			
Per recipe	770	16.0	5011
Per piece	12	0.3	78

Caramel Fudge

¾ cup margarine or butter
2 cups packed brown sugar
¼ cup Rich's Coffee Rich

1 teaspoon vanilla
3 cups sifted confectioner's sugar

In a large saucepan, melt margarine with brown sugar. Bring to a boil over medium heat, stirring constantly. Boil 2 minutes, continuing to stir constantly. Add Rich's Coffee Rich and continue cooking and stirring just until mixture comes to a boil; remove from heat. Cool to lukewarm, at room temperature. Mix in vanilla. Gradually add the confectioner's sugar, beating vigorously until the mixture is a thick, fudge-like consistency, about 2 minutes. Spread into a greased 8- or 9-inch square pan. Chill at least 2 hours before cutting. Keep refrigerated in an airtight container.

Yield: 49 pieces.

	Phenylalanine (mg)	Protein (gm)	Calories
Per recipe	82	2.3	4075
Per piece	2	trace	83

Variation

Caramel Snowballs

Prepare *Caramel Fudge* as directed. After it has chilled, cut it into 64 pieces. Take each piece in your hand and roll it into a ball. Put 1½ cups (120 gm) shredded coconut into a bowl or onto a plate. Roll balls in coconut. Keep refrigerated in an airtight container.

Yield: 64 balls.

	Phenylalanine (mg)	Protein (gm)	Calories
Per recipe	59	5.8	4685
Per ball	4	0.1	73

No-Peanuts Brittle

1 cup granulated sugar
½ cup light Karo corn syrup
½ cup water
⅛ teaspoon salt

1 teaspoon vanilla
½ teaspoon margarine or
  butter
1 teaspoon baking soda

Mix sugar, syrup, water, and salt together in a medium saucepan. Cook over medium heat until a candy thermometer fastened to the side of the pan registers 300° (hard crack stage), stirring occasionally, about 20 minutes. Mix in vanilla and margarine, then baking soda (mixture will become light and foamy after soda is added). Quickly pour onto a greased cookie sheet and spread thinly. Cool, then break into small pieces of desired size.

For Microwave Oven
Omit water. In a 1½-quart casserole, mix sugar, corn syrup, and salt. Microwave on High for 4 minutes. Add vanilla and margarine. Stir, then microwave on High for 2 minutes. Add baking soda and stir gently until light and foamy. Spread in pan as above.

Yield: about 35 pieces.

	Phenylalanine (mg)	Protein (gm)	Calories
Per recipe	0	0.0	1292
Per piece	0	0.0	37

Variation

Coconut Brittle

Add ½ cup (40 gm) shredded coconut just before pouring candy mixture onto cookie sheet.

Yield: about 35 pieces (342 gm).

	Phenylalanine (mg)	Protein (gm)	Calories
Per recipe	59	1.2	1495
Per piece (10 gm)	2	trace	43

Never-Fail Toffee

1 cup margarine or butter
1 cup granulated sugar
½ teaspoon salt
1 tablespoon water

1 teaspoon vanilla
½ cup (90 gm) Nestlé semisweet chocolate chips

Combine margarine, sugar, salt, water, and vanilla in a large sauce-pan. Bring to a boil over medium heat, stirring constantly. Continue boiling over medium heat, stirring constantly until candy thermome-ter attached to side of pan registers 300° (hard crack stage), 7 to 10 minutes. As you approach the end-point, the mixture should darken in color (continue cooking for a short time if it does not).

Quickly pour mixture into a greased 8- or 9-inch square pan. Let cool for a few minutes (it will harden quickly). Sprinkle chocolate chips over top of very warm toffee; when they are slightly melted, be-gin spreading them to cover toffee completely. When toffee is com-pletely cool and chocolate has hardened, break into bite-sized pieces. (Since pieces will be irregular, to get an accurate count of phenyl-alanine/protein, weigh pieces on a gram scale. Each 24 gm is 1 ex-change. For convenience, package in small labeled plastic bags after weighing.)

Yield: about 50 pieces (410 gm).

	Phenylalanine (mg)	Protein (gm)	Calories
Per recipe	276	5.7	2879
Per piece (8 gm)	6	0.1	58

Orange Balls

Melt-in-your-mouth confections.

2 cups (182 gm) crushed
  graham crackers
½ cup sifted confectioner's
  sugar
¼ cup melted margarine or
  butter

¼ cup undiluted frozen orange
  juice concentrate, thawed
confectioner's sugar

In a bowl, mix sugar with graham cracker crumbs. Blend in melted margarine and orange juice. Refrigerate mixture for 2 hours or more. Form into small walnut-sized balls; roll them in confectioner's sugar. Store in covered container in refrigerator. These are best after standing for 24 hours.

Yield: 24 balls.

	Phenylalanine (mg)	Protein (gm)	Calories
Per recipe	678	15.0	1533
Per ball	28	0.6	64

Low Orange Balls

These use your leftover trimmings from *Cinnamon Graham Crackers*.

2 cups (220 gm) crushed
  *Cinnamon Graham
  Crackers*
½ cup sifted confectioner's
  sugar

¼ cup melted margarine or
  butter
¼ cup undiluted frozen orange
  juice concentrate, thawed
confectioner's sugar

Follow directions for *Orange Balls*.

Yield: 24 balls.

	Phenylalanine (mg)	Protein (gm)	Calories
Per recipe	73	2.5	1865
Per ball	3	0.1	78

446

Cinnamon Munch

⅓ cup granulated sugar
1½ teaspoons cinnamon
¼ cup margarine or butter
4 cups (100 gm) Rice Chex
    cereal

2 cups (360 gm) Brach's Spice
Drops

Mix sugar and cinnamon together in a small bowl; set aside. Melt margarine in a large skillet over low heat. Add cereal. Stir gently until cereal is coated with margarine. Continue to heat and stir 5 minutes more. Sprinkle ½ the cinnamon-sugar mixture over the cereal; stir, then sprinkle with remaining cinnamon-sugar. Continue to heat and stir for 1 minute. Cool. Add spice drops and mix well.

Yield: 6 cups (552 gm).

Storage Tip
For convenience in calculating phenylalanine or protein, premeasure or weigh desired portions and put in labeled plastic bags.

	Phenylalanine (mg)	Protein (gm)	Calories
Per recipe	249	5.8	1419
Per ¼ cup (23 gm) serving	10	0.2	59

Rock 'N Roll Raisin Mix

A nutritious snack food for those allowed a more liberal amount of phenylalanine or protein.

½ cup margarine or butter
1 tablespoon Worcestershire
    sauce
½ teaspoon salt
1 teaspoon chili powder or
    several drops of tabasco
    sauce
2 cups (76 gm) pretzel sticks

2 cups (54 gm) Ralston Corn
    Chex cereal
2 cups (50 gm) Ralston Rice
    Chex cereal
1½ cups (240 gm) raisins

In a large saucepan, melt margarine with Worcestershire sauce, salt, and chili powder or tabasco sauce. Add pretzels and cereals. Mix gently but thoroughly. Spread out on a cookie sheet and bake at 250° for 45 minutes, stirring several times during baking. Add raisins and bake for 15 minutes more. Cool. Store in an airtight container.

Yield: 8 cups (520 gm).

Storage Tip
For convenience in calculating phenylalanine or protein, premeasure or weigh desired portions and put in labeled plastic bags.

	Phenylalanine (mg)	Protein (gm)	Calories
Per recipe	884	22.6	2254
Per ¼ cup (16 gm) serving	28	0.7	70

Caramel Popcorn

Delicious served warm. Great for a party.

½ cup margarine or butter
½ cup packed brown sugar
1 cup (39 gm) mini
    marshmallows or 7 large
    marshmallows cut in pieces

12 cups (75 gm) popped
    popcorn (about 6 table-
    spoons kernels before
    popping)

In a medium saucepan, combine margarine, brown sugar, and marshmallows and stir over medium heat until mixture comes to a boil. Pour over popcorn and mix well. Serve immediately.

Yield: 12 cups (300 gm).

	Phenylalanine (mg)	Protein (gm)	Calories
Per recipe	543	11.0	1596
Per ½ cup (13 gm)	23	0.5	67

Popcorn Balls

8 cups (50 gm) popped popcorn
    (approximately 4 to 5 table-
    spoons kernels before
    popping)
⅔ cup granulated sugar

½ cup water
2½ tablespoons light Karo corn
    syrup
⅛ teaspoon salt
½ teaspoon vinegar

Pop the corn, then keep covered in a pan set in a warm oven. Bring remaining ingredients to a boil in a medium saucepan, stirring occasionally. Cook, without stirring, until a candy thermometer fastened to the side of the pan registers 250° (firm ball stage) or a small amount of the mixture forms a firm ball when dropped in cold water. Remove from heat and quickly pour over warm popcorn; mix well. Working quickly, using greased hands, form into 20 small balls. Store in an airtight container or wrap individually in plastic wrap.

Yield: 20 popcorn balls.

	Phenylalanine (mg)	Protein (gm)	Calories
Per recipe	320	6.4	818
Per ball (10 gm)	16	0.3	41

Caramel Corn

Rivals the best commercial caramel corn anywhere, at a fraction of the cost.

1 cup packed brown sugar
¼ cup dark Karo corn syrup
½ cup margarine or butter
¼ teaspoon salt
¼ teaspoon baking soda

12 cups (75 gm) popped popcorn (about 6 tablespoons kernels before popping)

In a medium saucepan, mix together brown sugar, syrup, margarine, and salt. Bring to a boil over medium heat, stirring occasionally. Continue boiling slowly for 5 minutes, stirring constantly; remove from heat. Add baking soda and mix well. Quickly pour mixture over popped corn. Spread caramel corn on a large baking dish (15 × 11 inches or 13 × 9 inches). Bake at 225° for 1 hour, stirring several times. Remove from oven and let cool, stirring once as caramel corn begins to cool. Store in airtight container. The caramel corn also freezes well.

For convenience in calculating phenylalanine or protein, premeasure or weigh desired portions and put in labeled plastic bags.

For Microwave Oven

Combine brown sugar, syrup, margarine, and salt in a 1-quart glass measuring cup. Microwave, uncovered, on High for 2½ to 3 minutes, or until mixture boils, stirring once. Boil mixture on High for 2½ minutes without stirring. Place popped corn in a large bowl. Pour hot syrup over, mixing to coat.

Take approximately half of the caramel corn and spread in a 13 × 9- or 10 × 10-inch microwave-proof dish. Microwave uncovered on High for 3 minutes, stirring several times. Caramel corn will be very sticky at this point, but will quickly become crisp on cooling. Remove caramel corn to a bowl to cool. Repeat process with remaining popped corn. Stir a few times while caramel corn is cooling.

Yield: 12 cups (350 gm).

	Phenylalanine (mg)	Protein (gm)	Calories
Per recipe	528	10.4	1284
Per ½ cup (15 gm) serving	22	0.4	54

Frozen Desserts

The ice cream and sherbet recipes in this section are made by either of two processes:

1. "Still-frozen," where the mixture is frozen in a freezer and typically (but not always) stirred once or twice during the freezing process to break up ice crystals and make the finished product smoother.

2. "Churned" in an ice cream freezer.

Special Tips for Making Ice Cream and Sherbet

Still-Frozen Technique

The ice cream and sherbets made by the "still-frozen" technique have a very good flavor. However, the texture will be somewhat different from that of commercially-made ice cream and sherbet in being coarser and not having the same melting characteristics as the recipes using an ice cream freezer. The whipped topping used in these recipes minimizes the problem of coarseness to a significant extent.

A food processor is a handy tool for making still-frozen ice cream. Prepare ice cream mixture as directed in work bowl of processor using metal blade; leave metal blade in and cover bowl. Freeze mixture until soft-frozen. Remove from freezer and pulse several times. Return to freezer and repeat process one or more times for greatest smoothness. Scrape mixture into a plastic freezer container and freeze firm.

Churned Technique

The recipes designated for preparation in an ice cream freezer were designed specifically for the churning mechanism and are not suitable for the still-freezing technique.

The low protein ice cream and sherbet that are made in an ice cream freezer are wonderful. The flavor and texture are superb and rival most commercially made products. They are in fact superior to some store-bought ice creams and sherbets, in the opinion of discriminating cookbook taste-testers. If the members of your family enjoy eating ice cream, they are sure to find these recipes delicious, and it would be very worthwhile to invest in an ice cream freezer and regularly make your own ice cream—for the whole family. When using an electric freezer or a freezer like the Donvier (see below), you will find it surprisingly simple and quick.

All of the "churned" ice cream recipes in this section were tested with a Waring brand "Ice Cream Parlor" electric freezer. This particular machine is no longer made. There are now many other electric freezers that make it even easier to make your own ice cream. The new style of ice cream freezer uses an inner cylinder that is frozen in your own refrigerator freezer, and requires no salt or ice, as the Waring machine required. Brands of electric ice cream freezers such as Krups and Simac are available for about $60 through department stores, kitchen specialty stores, and kitchen mail-order catalogs. Most of the newer machines hold only 1 quart (4 cups) of ice cream. Some of the recipes in this section are designed to make 1½ quarts (6 cups; the capacity of the old Waring brand), so you will need to cut the recipe in half in order not to exceed the machine's smaller capacity.

There also are several brands of ice cream makers that are not electric, but require just several hand cranks every few minutes until the ice cream is fairly stiff (20–30 minutes). A Donvier "Chillfast Ice Cream Maker" is one such model. It works well for making low protein ice cream. Like the electric machines described above, it requires no salt or ice and uses a pre-frozen inner cylinder. It is fun and easy for children to help with making ice cream in this kind of ice cream freezer. Either a 1-pint or 1-quart capacity size is available in many department stores and kitchen specialty stores. The 1-quart size will hold ½ of the churned ice cream recipes in this section. Be sure to beat the liquid ice cream mixture with an electric mixer for several minutes until it is light and frothy before pouring it into the inner cylinder for freezing; otherwise the ice cream will not attain the volume indicated in the recipe and will not be as light in texture, since hand cranking does not incorporate air as an electric machine does.

Vanilla Ice Cream (Churned)

There are few things more appealing and delicious on a warm day than a scoop of smooth, creamy, homemade ice cream. You'll be delighted with this one and its many variations.

2 cups Rich's Coffee Rich
two 8 oz cartons liquid Rich's
  Richwhip Topping
¾ cup granulated sugar

2 to 3 teaspoons vanilla
⅛ teaspoon salt
4 drops yellow food coloring

Mix all ingredients in can of a 2-quart ice cream freezer. Stir briefly, until sugar dissolves. Freeze according to ice cream freezer manufacturer's instructions. Transfer ice cream to a plastic freezer container and freeze firm.

Yield: 6 cups.

Note

If you want a lower protein ice cream, replace the Rich's Coffee Rich with 1 cup Rich's Richwhip Topping diluted with 1 cup water. Subtract the 90 mg phenylalanine and 1.8 gm protein per recipe for vanilla and all flavor variations (this will make the vanilla flavor "free"). The ice cream will remain softer and will be less like regular ice cream than the original recipe, but it is still good.

Sugar may be reduced to ½ or ¼ cup, if desired.

	Phenylalanine (mg)	Protein (gm)	Calories
Per recipe	88	1.4	2547
Per ½ cup serving	7	0.1	212

Variations

Banana Orange Ice Cream

Omit vanilla. Add ¾ cup (173 gm) mashed bananas, ¼ cup orange juice, and ¼ cup granulated sugar along with other ingredients.

Yield: 7 cups.

	Phenylalanine (mg)	Protein (gm)	Calories
Per recipe	161	3.5	2927
Per ½ cup serving	11	0.3	209

Chocolate Ice Cream

Add ½ cup (152 gm) Hershey's chocolate syrup along with other ingredients.

Yield: 6½ cups.

	Phenylalanine (mg)	Protein (gm)	Calories
Per recipe	255	5.4	2963
Per ½ cup serving	20	0.4	228

Chocolate Chip or *Mint Chocolate Chip Ice Cream*

Add ½ cup (90 gm) Nestlé mini semisweet chocolate chips after churning is complete. For *Mint Chocolate Chip,* replace vanilla with 2 teaspoons mint flavoring and add 3 to 6 drops green food coloring along with other ingredients.

Yield: 6½ cups.

	Phenylalanine (mg)	Protein (gm)	Calories
Per recipe	270	5.1	3028
Per ½ cup serving	21	0.4	233

Chocolate-Chocolate Chip Ice Cream

Add ½ cup (152 gm) Hershey's chocolate syrup along with other ingredients. Add ½ cup (90 gm) Nestlé mini semisweet chocolate chips after churning is complete.

Yield: 7 cups.

	Phenylalanine (mg)	Protein (gm)	Calories
Per recipe	437	9.1	3444
Per ½ cup serving	31	0.7	246

Fresh Peach Ice Cream

Omit vanilla. Add 1 cup (250 gm) mashed fresh or frozen peaches, sweetened with ⅓ cup granulated sugar, along with other ingredients. Add 4 drops of red and 3 drops of yellow food coloring if desired.

Yield: 7 cups.

	Phenylalanine (mg)	Protein (gm)	Calories
Per recipe	142	3.1	2913
Per ½ cup serving	10	0.2	208

Peppermint Ice Cream

Add ½ cup crushed peppermint candy and 3 drops of red food coloring if desired, along with other ingredients. An easy way to crush candy is to place it in a heavy plastic bag, then pound it with a rolling pin until finely crushed.

Yield: 6½ cups.

	Phenylalanine (mg)	Protein (gm)	Calories
Per recipe	88	1.4	2933
Per ½ cup serving	7	0.1	226

Pineapple Ice Cream

Omit vanilla. Add 1 cup (280 gm) drained, crushed pineapple along with other ingredients.

Yield: 7 cups.

	Phenylalanine (mg)	Protein (gm)	Calories
Per recipe	116	2.5	2715
Per ½ cup serving	8	0.2	194

Raspberry Ice Cream

Omit vanilla. Add 1 cup raspberry purée with seeds strained out (from 1 pint raspberries), sweetened with ½ cup granulated sugar, along with other ingredients.

Yield: 7 cups.

	Phenylalanine (mg)	Protein (gm)	Calories
Per recipe	175	3.6	3056
Per ½ cup serving	12	0.3	218

Strawberry Ice Cream

Omit vanilla. Add a 10 oz package frozen strawberries, thawed, drained, and mashed (or 1 cup fresh mashed strawberries sweetened with ⅓ cup granulated sugar) along with other ingredients. Add 2 to 3 drops red food coloring if desired.

Yield: 7 cups.

	Phenylalanine (mg)	Protein (gm)	Calories
Per recipe	110	2.9	2816
Per ½ cup serving	8	0.2	201

Vanilla Custard Ice Cream (Churned)

This makes a richer ice cream than plain *Vanilla Ice Cream (Churned)* and its variations, with additional "body."

1 pkg (4-serving size) cook-type vanilla Jell-O Pudding and Pie Filling mix
⅓ cup granulated sugar
2 cups Rich's Coffee Rich

two 8 oz cartons liquid Rich's Richwhip Topping
1 teaspoon vanilla
1 to 2 drops yellow food coloring

Heat pudding mix, sugar, and Coffee Rich in a medium saucepan until boiling; boil gently several minutes (or microwave on High for 3 minutes in a 1½-quart baking dish; stir, then microwave on High for 3 to 4 minutes, until just slightly thickened). Cover and chill thoroughly, several hours or overnight.

Pour chilled custard into can of a 2-quart ice cream freezer; mix in liquid Richwhip and vanilla. Freeze according to ice cream freezer manufacturer's instructions. Transfer ice cream to plastic freezer container and freeze firm.

Any of the variations given for *Vanilla Ice Cream (Churned)* can be made with this recipe; nutrient content will be the same for phenylalanine and protein.

Yield: 6 cups.

	Phenylalanine (mg)	Protein (gm)	Calories
Per recipe	88	1.4	2547
Per ½ cup serving	7	0.1	212

Ice Cream Sandwiches

12 *Fudge Circles*, 3-inch
   diameter
3 cups Peach, Peppermint,
   Pineapple, Raspberry,
   Strawberry, or Vanilla Ice
   Cream from *Vanilla Ice
   Cream (Churned)* recipe

Prepare *Fudge Circles*, baking for only 5 minutes for a softer texture. Spread ice cream in an 11 × 7-inch baking pan. Freeze hard again. Quickly cut out 6 circles of ice cream with the same (or a slightly smaller) cookie cutter that you used to cut out *Fudge Circles.*

Using a spatula, place an ice cream circle on a cookie, topping with another cookie. Press firmly together. Repeat with remaining cookies and ice cream. Freeze, stacked in a covered container. Return ice cream "scraps" to your original ice cream container. Until the sandwiches have "aged" for 1 to 2 weeks the cookie part of the sandwich will be hard when eaten directly from the freezer; after that time it will be nice and soft, like a commercial ice cream sandwich, because of moisture from the ice cream. Frozen sandwiches will keep well for several months.

Yield: 6 ice cream sandwiches.

Making ice cream sandwiches requires a very cold freezer (0° or colder works optimally). This idea also works beautifully with any of the low protein sherbet recipes. Each sandwich uses about ¼ cup ice cream or sherbet; thus you can do your own calculating. You may also make mini ice cream or sherbet sandwiches, nice for small children, by using 2-inch diameter *Fudge Circles*. Each mini sandwich will use about 1½ tablespoons ice cream or sherbet.

	Phenylalanine (mg)	Protein (gm)	Calories
Per recipe	108	0.8	1792
Per ice cream sandwich	18	0.1	299

Vanilla Ice Milk (Churned)

If you are unable to obtain Rich's Richwhip Topping to make *Vanilla Ice Cream (Churned)*, try this recipe.

4 cups (1 quart) Rich's Coffee
   Rich
¾ cup granulated sugar

2 to 3 teaspoons vanilla
⅛ teaspoon salt
4 drops yellow food coloring

Mix all ingredients in can of a 2-quart ice cream freezer. Stir briefly, until sugar dissolves. Freeze according to ice cream freezer manufacturer's instructions. Transfer ice cream to a plastic freezer container and freeze firm.

Yield: 6 cups.

Note
For flavors, choose any of the *Vanilla Ice Cream (Churned)* variations, adding an extra 90 mg phenylalanine and 1.8 gm protein per recipe.

	Phenylalanine (mg)	Protein (gm)	Calories
Per recipe	176	2.7	1955
Per ½ cup serving	15	0.2	163

Vanilla Ice Cream (Still-Frozen)

1 cup water
⅓ cup granulated sugar
3 tablespoons light Karo corn syrup
½ cup Rich's Coffee Rich
8 oz container Coolwhip (3½ cups) or 8 oz carton liquid Rich's Richwhip Topping, whipped

2 teaspoons vanilla
2 to 3 drops yellow food coloring (optional)

In a small saucepan mix together water, sugar, and syrup; heat until sugar dissolves. Remove from heat and chill. Mix in Coffee Rich, then gradually add liquid mixture to whipped topping, mixing well. Add vanilla and food coloring. Pour into a metal baking pan and cover with foil. Freeze until soft-frozen, then stir to blend in sugar syrup which will have partially settled on the bottom. Pack into a plastic freezer container and freeze firm.

Yield: 4 cups.

	Phenylalanine (mg)	Protein (gm)	Calories
Using Richwhip			
Per recipe	22	0.3	1266
Per ½ cup serving	3	trace	158
Using Coolwhip			
Per recipe	190	3.6	1130
Per ½ cup serving	24	0.4	141

Variations

Chocolate Chip Ice Cream

Add ¼ cup (45 gm) Nestlé mini semisweet chocolate chips after ice cream is soft-frozen.

Yield: 4 cups.

	Phenylalanine (mg)	Protein (gm)	Calories
Using Richwhip			
Per recipe	113	2.2	1506
Per ½ cup serving	14	0.3	188
Using Coolwhip			
Per recipe	281	5.4	1370
Per ½ cup serving	35	0.7	171

Fresh Peach Ice Cream

Omit vanilla. Replace Coffee Rich with ½ cup (125 gm) mashed fresh peaches and 2 tablespoons sugar. Add 1 to 2 drops of yellow food coloring and 1 to 2 drops of red if desired.

Yield: 4 cups.

	Phenylalanine (mg)	Protein (gm)	Calories
Using Richwhip			
Per recipe	27	0.9	1244
Per ½ cup serving	3	0.1	155
Using Coolwhip			
Per recipe	195	4.1	1108
Per ½ cup serving	24	0.5	138

Peppermint Ice Cream

Add ⅓ cup crushed peppermint candy after ice cream is soft-frozen. Add 1 to 2 drops red food coloring if desired. An easy way to crush candy is to put it in a heavy plastic bag, then pound it with a rolling pin until finely crushed.

Yield: 4 cups.

	Phenylalanine (mg)	Protein (gm)	Calories
Using Richwhip			
Per recipe	22	0.3	1574
Per ½ cup serving	3	trace	197
Using Coolwhip			
Per recipe	190	3.6	1438
Per ½ cup serving	24	0.4	180

Pineapple Ice Cream

Replace Coffee Rich with ½ cup (140 gm) drained, crushed pineapple. Add 1 to 2 drops yellow food coloring if desired.

Yield: 4 cups.

	Phenylalanine (mg)	Protein (gm)	Calories
Using Richwhip			
Per recipe	36	0.9	1350
Per ½ cup serving	5	0.1	169
Using Coolwhip			
Per recipe	204	4.1	1214
Per ½ cup serving	26	0.5	152

Chocolate Ice Cream (Still-Frozen)

½ cup granulated sugar
3 tablespoons Hershey's
    unsweetened cocoa (not
    instant)
1¼ cups water
3 tablespoons light Karo corn
    syrup

8 oz container Coolwhip (3½
    cups) or 8 oz carton liquid
    Rich's Richwhip Topping,
    whipped

In a small saucepan, mix together sugar and cocoa. Add water and syrup; stir over medium heat until mixture comes to a boil. Remove from heat and chill. Gradually add cooled chocolate mixture to whipped topping, blending well. Pour into an 8-inch square or round metal baking pan and cover with foil. Freeze until soft-frozen, then stir to blend in chocolate mixture which will have partially settled on the bottom. Pack into a plastic freezer container and freeze firm.

Yield: 4½ cups.

	Phenylalanine (mg)	Protein (gm)	Calories
Using Richwhip			
Per recipe	195	3.9	1275
Per ½ cup serving	22	0.4	142
Using Coolwhip			
Per recipe	363	7.2	1139
Per ½ cup serving	40	0.8	127

Strawberry Ice Cream (Still-Frozen)

10 oz pkg frozen strawberries, thawed

8 oz container Coolwhip (3½ cups) or 8 oz carton liquid Rich's Richwhip Topping, whipped

¾ cup water

Mix undrained strawberries with whipped topping in a mixing bowl. Add water and mix well. Pack into a plastic freezer container and freeze firm.

Yield: 4½ cups.

	Phenylalanine (mg)	Protein (gm)	Calories
Using Richwhip			
Per recipe	22	1.5	909
Per ½ cup serving	2	0.2	101
Using Coolwhip			
Per recipe	190	4.7	773
Per ½ cup serving	21	0.5	86

Orange Sherbet (Churned)

A faithful replication of commercial sherbet in texture and appearance but unanimously declared superior in flavor by taste-testers.

1 cup Rich's Coffee Rich
¾ cup liquid Rich's Richwhip
  Topping
1½ cups water
¾ cup (6 fl oz, ½ of 12 oz can)
  frozen orange juice
  concentrate, thawed

½ cup granulated sugar
⅛ teaspoon salt
12 drops red food coloring
12 drops yellow food coloring

Pour Coffee Rich and Richwhip Topping directly into can of a 2-quart ice cream freezer. Mix in water, orange juice concentrate, sugar, salt, and food coloring (this amount of food coloring gives a beautiful orange color). Stir briefly, to dissolve sugar. Freeze according to ice cream freezer manufacturer's instructions. Transfer sherbet to a plastic freezer container and freeze firm.

Yield: 5½ cups.

Note

If you are unable to obtain Richwhip Topping, use a total of 1½ cups Rich's Coffee Rich and an extra ¼ cup water. Add an extra 22 mg phenylalanine and 0.5 gm protein per recipe for *Orange Sherbet, Grape Sherbet,* or *Lemonade Sherbet.*

	Phenylalanine (mg)	Protein (gm)	Calories
Per recipe	134	5.1	1546
Per ½ cup serving	12	0.5	141

Variations

Grape Sherbet

Follow directions for *Orange Sherbet,* replacing orange juice with ¾ cup (6 fl oz, ½ of 12 oz can) frozen grape juice concentrate and deleting food coloring.

Yield: 5½ cups.

	Phenylalanine (mg)	Protein (gm)	Calories
Per recipe	134	2.8	1440
Per ½ cup serving	12	0.4	153

Lemonade Sherbet

Follow directions for *Orange Sherbet,* replacing orange juice with ¾ cup (6 fl oz, ½ of 12 oz can) of frozen lemonade concentrate; delete red food coloring and use 3 to 6 drops yellow food coloring.

Yield: 5½ cups.

	Phenylalanine (mg)	Protein (gm)	Calories
Per recipe	52	0.7	1610
Per ½ cup serving	5	0.1	146

Orange Sherbet (Still-Frozen)

Real sherbet flavor, but more like ice cream in richness.

1 cup water
½ cup granulated sugar
¾ cup (6 fl oz, ½ of 12 oz can) frozen orange juice concentrate, thawed
8 oz container Coolwhip (3½ cups) or 8 oz carton liquid Rich's Richwhip Topping, whipped

6 drops red food coloring
3 drops yellow food coloring

In a small saucepan, boil water and sugar for 5 minutes (stirring is unnecessary). Cool to lukewarm or. cooler. In a mixing bowl, blend sugar syrup, orange juice concentrate, and whipped topping. Mix in coloring. Put into a plastic freezer container and freeze firm.

Yield: 4 cups.

	Phenylalanine (mg)	Protein (gm)	Calories
Using Richwhip			
Per recipe	90	4.4	1169
Per ½ cup serving	11	0.6	146
Using Coolwhip			
Per recipe	258	7.7	1033
Per ½ cup serving	32	1.0	129

Variations

Grape Sherbet

Replace orange juice with ¾ cup (6 fl oz, ½ of 12 oz can) of frozen grape juice concentrate. Delete food coloring.

Yield: 4 cups.

	Phenylalanine (mg)	Protein (gm)	Calories
Using Richwhip			
Per recipe	92	4.2	1301
Per ½ cup serving	11	0.5	163
Using Coolwhip			
Per recipe	258	7.4	1165
Per ½ cup serving	32	0.9	146

Lemonade Sherbet

Replace orange juice with 1½ tablespoons of frozen lemonade concentrate and add ½ cup water. Delete red food coloring and add 3 to 6 drops yellow food coloring.

Yield: 4 cups.

	Phenylalanine (mg)	Protein (gm)	Calories
Using Richwhip			
Per recipe	8	0.2	1233
Per ½ cup serving	1	trace	154
Using Coolwhip			
Per recipe	172	3.2	897
Per ½ cup serving	22	0.4	112

Fruit Ice (Churned)

Basic Recipe

1 cup granulated sugar
3 cups water

1 cup fruit juice or purée (see fruit options below)

In a saucepan over medium to low heat, gently boil sugar and water for 5 minutes (no stirring necessary). Chill thoroughly. Pour into can of a 2-quart ice cream freezer. Mix in chilled fruit juice or fruit purée and coloring indicated. Freeze according to ice cream freezer manufacturer's instructions.

Transfer fruit ice to a plastic freezer container and freeze firm. Remove from freezer about ½ hour before using, serving slightly slushy. You may also remove the fruit ice from freezer 1 to 2 hours in advance of using; break up and beat with electric mixer or food processor until smooth, then return to freezer until serving time.

Yield: 5 cups.

Orange Ice

1 cup orange juice
2 teaspoons grated orange rind

2 drops yellow food coloring
3 drops red food coloring

	Phenylalanine (mg)	Protein (gm)	Calories
Per recipe	30	1.5	884
Per ½ cup serving	3	0.1	88

Peach Ice

1 cup fresh peach purée
1 drop yellow food coloring

1 drop red food coloring

	Phenylalanine (mg)	Protein (gm)	Calories
Per recipe	52	1.7	875
Per ½ cup serving	5	0.2	88

Pineapple Ice

1 cup pineapple purée (purée   2 drops yellow food coloring
    canned or fresh pineapple)

	Phenylalanine (mg)	Protein (gm)	Calories
Per recipe	17	0.7	1028
Per ½ cup serving	2	0.1	103

Raspberry Ice

1 cup raspberry purée (purée
    1 heaping pint raspberries
    and strain seeds)

	Phenylalanine (mg)	Protein (gm)	Calories
Per recipe	70	1.8	871
Per ½ cup serving	7	0.2	87

Fruit Freeze

Colorful and refreshing for summer.

15 oz can apricot halves   15¼ oz can pineapple chunks
1 cup granulated sugar   29 oz can sliced peaches
16 oz pkg frozen strawberries

Drain juice from apricots into a small saucepan. Add sugar and heat a few minutes to dissolve sugar. Combine all fruits and all their juice; pour into a 13 × 9-inch metal baking pan. Freeze firm. After fruit is frozen solid, for convenience, cut into smaller pieces and freeze individually in plastic bags. About 30 minutes before serving allow to thaw slightly and serve rather slushy.

Yield: 9½ cups.

	Phenylalanine (mg)	Protein (gm)	Calories
Per recipe	185	6.8	2258
Per ½ cup serving	10	0.4	119

Frozen Fruit Dessert

½ cup granulated sugar   1 tablespoon lemon juice
½ cup water   ½ cup orange juice
¼ cup (40 gm) mashed banana   8 oz can crushed pineapple,
    (3-inch section), not overly   undrained
    ripe

In a saucepan, heat sugar with water until sugar dissolves. Add remaining ingredients and mix well. Pour into a shallow metal baking dish. Freeze until almost firm, then remove mixture to a bowl and beat with electric mixer for several minutes, until smooth and fluffy. Return to freezer and freeze firm. About 15 to 20 minutes before serving, allow to thaw slightly and serve rather slushy.

Yield: 3 cups.

	Phenylalanine (mg)	Protein (gm)	Calories
Per recipe	43	1.7	653
Per ½ cup serving	7	0.3	109

Fresh Strawberry Frost

Wonderful fresh strawberry flavor in an easy summer dessert for the whole family. Your own fresh-frozen strawberries can also be used at other times of the year.

3 cups (450 gm) fresh
    strawberries
1 cup granulated sugar

¾ cup orange juice
3 tablespoons lemon juice

Place half of the strawberries and remaining ingredients in a blender container or food processor. Cover; blend until smooth. Add remaining strawberries; blend again until smooth. Pour into an 8-inch square or round metal baking pan; freeze until soft-frozen, several hours. Place in a bowl and mix with mixer on low speed until smooth. Pack mixture into a plastic freezer container. Freeze several hours or overnight. To serve, remove from freezer 20 to 30 minutes in advance, or reblend in food processor to soften.

Yield: 3¾ cups.

	Phenylalanine (mg)	Protein (gm)	Calories
Per recipe	60	3.9	992
Per ½ cup serving	8	0.5	132

Vanilla Creampops

1 pkg (4-serving size) Jell-O Instant Pudding and Pie Filling mix (vanilla, french vanilla, banana cream, or butterscotch)

8 oz carton liquid Rich's Richwhip Topping and 1½ cups water, or 1½ cups Rich's Coffee Rich and 1 cup water

Combine pudding mix, Richwhip Topping or Coffee Rich, and water and blend on low speed of a mixer, or by hand, until mixture thickens slightly (about 2 minutes). Fill 12 Tupperware Ice Tup molds, leaving ¼-inch space at top. Freeze.

Yield: 12 creampops.

Note
Four-ounce paper cups and Popsickle sticks may be used in place of ice tups. Fill cups, then freeze partially; insert sticks and freeze firm.

	Phenylalanine (mg)	Protein (gm)	Calories
Using Richwhip			
Per recipe	8	0.2	1000
Per creampop	1	trace	83
Using Coffee Rich			
Per recipe	52	0.9	704
Per creampop	4	0.1	59

Chocolate Creampops

1 pkg (4-serving size) chocolate
Jell-O Instant Pudding and
Pie Filling mix

8 oz carton liquid Rich's
Richwhip Topping and 1½
cups water, or 1½ cups
Rich's Coffee Rich and 1 cup
water

Follow directions for *Vanilla Creampops.*

Yield: 12 creampops.

	Phenylalanine (mg)	Protein (gm)	Calories
Using Richwhip			
Per recipe	56	1.6	1040
Per creampop	5	0.1	87
Using Coffee Rich			
Per recipe	100	2.3	744
Per creampop	8	0.2	62

Banana Pops

two 6-inch bananas
4 Popsicle sticks
⅓ cup (60 gm) Nestlé semisweet chocolate chips

⅜-inch piece (4 gm) of paraffin
   wax

Peel bananas. Cut in half crosswise. Insert Popsicle sticks in cut end. Place bananas in a shallow pan. Freeze firm, 2 to 3 hours. Melt chocolate chips with paraffin in top of double boiler or in microwave oven. The chocolate should be very hot so it will be thin enough to coat bananas. Spoon chocolate over each banana, spreading to coat completely (chocolate will harden soon after coming in contact with the banana, so work quickly). Eat immediately; or refreeze, then thaw slightly before eating.

Yield: 4 pops.

Note
   Calculations assume 2 teaspoons of chocolate are left in the pan, as it is difficult to get all of it onto the bananas.

	Phenylalanine (mg)	Protein (gm)	Calories
Per recipe	207	4.9	531
Per pop	52	1.2	133

Frozen Suckers

The strained fruit gives the suckers a nice flavor as well as texture.

2 small jars Gerber strained
   apricots with tapioca

½ cup orange juice
1 tablespoon granulated sugar

Mix all ingredients together in a bowl. Fill 6 Tupperware Ice Tup molds, leaving ¼-inch space at top. Freeze firm.

Yield: 6 suckers.

	Phenylalanine (mg)	Protein (gm)	Calories
Per recipe	53	1.4	258
Per sucker	9	0.2	43

Orange Pudding Pops

Very similar to commercially made pudding pops.

¾ cup (6 fl oz, ½ of 12 oz can) frozen orange juice concentrate, thawed
1½ cups (12 fl oz) water
3 tablespoons cornstarch

⅓ cup granulated sugar
1 cup (69 gm) Coolwhip or whipped liquid Richwhip Topping

Mix all ingredients together in a saucepan. Cook over medium heat, stirring slowly until mixture thickens and becomes clear. Cover and chill. Fold in whipped topping. Fill 10 Tupperware Ice Tup molds, leaving ¼-inch space at the top. Freeze.

Yield: 10 pops.

	Phenylalanine (mg)	Protein (gm)	Calories
Using Richwhip			
Per recipe	90	4.4	897
Per pop	9	0.4	90
Using Coolwhip			
Per recipe	142	5.4	855
Per pop	14	0.5	85

Variation

Grape Pudding Pops

Replace orange juice with ¾ cup (6 fl oz, ½ of 12 oz can) of frozen grape concentrate.

Yield: 10 pops.

	Phenylalanine (mg)	Protein (gm)	Calories
Using Richwhip			
Per recipe	90	4.2	1029
Per pop	9	0.4	103
Using Coolwhip			
Per recipe	142	5.2	987
Per pop	14	0.5	99

Miscellaneous Desserts

Try any of the recipes in this section when you are looking for extra calories and variety to add to a lunch or supper meal. All are designed to be suitable for the whole family. All but one are fruit-based. All are delicious.

Several of the recipes have very "low" versions, which you make by cutting down on relatively high protein ingredients (for example, reducing the amount of oatmeal in the fruit crisp recipes), or replacing a regular ingredient with a low protein one (using homemade low protein graham crackers in place of regular graham crackers in the *Peppermint Crunch Dessert* recipe).

Cherry Delight

¾ cup (70 gm) Nabisco or
  Keebler vanilla wafer
  crumbs (from 19 cookies)
8 oz container Coolwhip (3½
  cups) or 8 oz carton liquid
  Rich's Richwhip Topping,
  whipped

3½ cups (137 gm) mini
  marshmallows
21 oz can Comstock or
  Wilderness Cherry Pie
  Filling

Distribute ½ cup of the crumbs over bottom of an ungreased 11 ×
7-inch pan. Mix whipped topping with marshmallows. Spread half of
mixture over crumbs. Cover with pie filling. Spread remaining whipped mixture over top of pie filling. Sprinkle with remaining ¼ cup
crumbs. Chill several hours.

Yield: 16 pieces (½ cup, 66 gm each).

	Phenylalanine (mg)	Protein (gm)	Calories
Using Richwhip			
Per recipe	297	7.9	2036
Per ½ cup (66 gm) serving	19	0.5	127
Using Coolwhip			
Per recipe	465	11.1	1900
Per ½ cup (66 gm) serving	29	0.7	119

Blueberry Buckle

Both diet and family recipes can be made out of one heaping pint of blueberries. Diet recipe is as delicious as the family recipe.

Diet Portion

2 tablespoons softened margarine or butter
¼ cup granulated sugar
2 tablespoons Rich's Coffee Rich or water
1 tablespoon water
½ teaspoon vanilla

½ cup (55 gm) Wel-Plan Baking Mix
½ teaspoon baking powder
⅛ teaspoon salt
1 cup (160 gm) fresh or frozen blueberries

Crumb Topping

¼ cup granulated sugar
¼ cup (27 gm) Wel-Plan Baking Mix
⅛ teaspoon nutmeg

¼ teaspoon cinnamon
2 tablespoons softened margarine or butter

Preheat oven to 375°. In a mixing bowl, cream together margarine and sugar. Beat in Coffee Rich, water, and vanilla. Stir together the Baking Mix, baking powder, and salt; add to creamed mixture, mixing well. Scrape batter into a greased 9 × 5-inch loaf pan or other small baking dish. Distribute blueberries evenly over the batter.

For *Crumb Topping*, combine the sugar, Baking Mix, and spices in a small bowl. Cut in the margarine until the mixture resembles coarse meal. Sprinkle over the blueberries and bake for 40 minutes. Serve warm, either plain or with whipped non-dairy creamer.

Yield: 2 cups (375 gm).

Family Portion

¼ cup softened margarine or
  butter
½ cup granulated sugar
1 egg
1 teaspoon vanilla
½ cup plus 2 tablespoons flour

1 teaspoon baking powder
¼ teaspoon salt
⅓ cup milk
2 cups fresh or frozen
  blueberries

Crumb Topping

½ cup granulated sugar
½ cup plus 2 tablespoons flour
¼ teaspoon nutmeg

½ teaspoon cinnamon
¼ cup softened margarine or
  butter

Prepare as for *Diet Portion*, mixing ingredients in the order listed. Use a greased 8- or 9-inch round or square baking pan. Bake for 40 minutes. Serve warm, either plain or with whipped cream. Makes 6 to 9 servings.

	Phenylalanine (mg)	Protein (gm)	Calories
Per diet recipe	162	3.7	1080
Per ½ cup (94 gm) serving	40	0.9	270

Peppermint Crunch Dessert

¾ cup (65 gm) graham cracker crumbs (from 10 squares)
3 tablespoons granulated sugar
¼ cup melted margarine or butter
½ cup (95 gm) crushed peppermint candy
8 oz container Coolwhip (3½ cups) or 8 oz carton liquid Rich's Richwhip Topping, whipped

3 cups (125 gm) mini marshmallows
4 to 6 drops red or green food coloring

Crush graham crackers with a rolling pin. In a bowl, mix graham cracker crumbs with sugar and melted margarine. Press crumbs firmly into an ungreased 8- or 9-inch square or round baking dish. Crush candy (an easy way to do this is to place candy in a heavy plastic bag, then pound it with a rolling pin until finely crushed); mix with whipped topping and marshmallows. Add coloring. Spread this mixture over prepared graham cracker crust. Chill.

Yield: 16 pieces (⅓ cup, 39 gm each).

	Phenylalanine (mg)	Protein (gm)	Calories
Using Richwhip			
Per recipe	259	5.7	2278
Per ⅓ cup (39 gm) serving	16	0.4	142
Using Coolwhip			
Per recipe	427	9.0	2142
Per ⅓ cup (39 gm) serving	27	0.6	134

Variation

Low Peppermint Crunch Dessert

Prepare crust, using ¼ cup (35 gm) *Cinnamon Graham Cracker* crumbs, 1 tablespoon sugar and 1½ tablespoon melted margarine. Press into small dish or bottom of a 4-inch pie pan. Prepare whipped mixture as for *Peppermint Crunch Dessert*. Spread 1 cup of the whipped mixture over crust.

Family Portion
Use remaining filling mixture and spread on regular graham cracker crust.

Yield: 3 diet pieces (⅓ cup, 39 gm each).

	Phenylalanine (mg)	Protein (gm)	Calories
Using Richwhip			
Per diet recipe	16	0.3	471
Per ⅓ cup (39 gm) serving	5	0.1	157
Using Coolwhip			
Per diet recipe	48	0.9	447
Per ⅓ cup (39 gm) serving	16	0.3	149

Apple Crisp

1½ cups (180 gm) sliced tart
  apples
2 tablespoons granulated sugar

¼ teaspoon cinnamon
1 tablespoon water

Topping

¼ cup (28 gm) Wel-Plan Baking
  Mix
¼ cup packed brown sugar
2 tablespoons (10 gm) oatmeal

¼ teaspoon cinnamon
2 tablespoons softened
  margarine or butter

Preheat oven to 350°. Mix sliced apples with sugar and cinnamon in a small baking dish or 7 × 4-inch loaf pan. Sprinkle with the 1 tablespoon water.

For *Topping*, in a small bowl stir together Baking Mix, brown sugar, oatmeal, and cinnamon. Mix in margarine with a fork, pastry blender, or your fingertips until mixture is crumbly; sprinkle evenly over apples. Bake for 30 minutes.

Yield: 1¼ cups (295 gm).

Family Portion

Make a double recipe of apple mixture. Put into an 8-inch square pan or other baking dish. Make a double recipe of *Topping*, substituting flour for Baking Mix and adding more oatmeal if desired (up to ½ cup). Bake for 35 to 40 minutes.

	Phenylalanine (mg)	Protein (gm)	Calories
Per diet recipe	141	3.0	765
Per ¼ cup (59 gm) serving	28	0.6	153

Variation

Low Apple Crisp

Replace oatmeal in *Topping* with 2 additional tablespoons of Baking Mix.

Yield: 1¼ cups (295 gm).

	Phenylalanine (mg)	Protein (gm)	Calories
Per recipe	22	0.8	766
Per ¼ cup (59 gm) serving	4	0.2	153

Peach Crisp

1½ cups (300 gm) sliced
  peaches
2 tablespoons granulated sugar
1 teaspoon cornstarch (for very
  juicy peaches only)

¼ teaspoon cinnamon
1 tablespoon water

Topping

¼ cup (28 gm) Wel-Plan Baking
  Mix
¼ cup packed brown sugar
2 tablespoons oatmeal

¼ teaspoon cinnamon
2 tablespoons softened
  margarine or butter

Preheat oven to 350°. Mix sliced peaches with sugar and cinnamon in a small baking dish or 7 × 4-inch loaf pan. Sprinkle with the 1 tablespoon water.

For *Topping*, in a small bowl stir together Baking Mix, brown sugar, oatmeal, and cinnamon. Mix in margarine with a fork, pastry blender, or your fingertips until mixture is crumbly; sprinkle evenly over peaches. Bake for 30 minutes.

Yield: 1½ cups (399 gm).

Family Portion

Make a double recipe of peach mixture. Put into an 8-inch square pan or other baking dish. Make a double recipe of *Topping*, substituting flour for Baking Mix and adding more oatmeal if desired (up to ½ cup). Bake for 35 to 40 minutes.

	Phenylalanine (mg)	Protein (gm)	Calories
Per diet recipe	185	4.4	700
Per ¼ cup (67 gm) serving	31	0.7	117

Variation

Low Peach Crisp

Replace oatmeal in *Topping* with 2 additional tablespoons of Baking Mix.

Yield: 1½ cups (399 gm).

	Phenylalanine (mg)	Protein (gm)	Calories
Per recipe	67	2.2	701
Per ¼ cup (67 gm) serving	11	0.4	117

Rhubarb Crisp

1½ cups (180 gm) sliced
   rhubarb
¼ cup granulated sugar

¼ teaspoon cinnamon
1 tablespoon water

Topping

¼ cup (28 gm) Wel-Plan Baking
   Mix
¼ cup packed brown sugar
2 tablespoons (10 gm) oatmeal

¼ teaspoon cinnamon
2 tablespoons softened
   margarine or butter

Preheat oven to 350°. Mix sliced rhubarb with sugar and cinnamon in a small baking dish or 7 × 4-inch loaf pan. Sprinkle with 1 tablespoon water.

For *Topping,* in a small bowl stir together Baking Mix, brown sugar, oatmeal, and cinnamon. Mix in margarine with a fork, pastry blender, or your fingertips until mixture is crumbly; sprinkle evenly over rhubarb. Bake for 30 minutes.

Yield: 1¼ cups (315 gm).

Family Portion

Make a double recipe of rhubarb mixture. Put into an 8-inch square pan or other baking dish. Make a double recipe of *Topping,* substituting flour for Baking Mix, and adding more oatmeal if desired (up to ½ cup). Bake for 35 to 40 minutes.

	Phenylalanine (mg)	Protein (gm)	Calories
Per diet recipe	183	3.9	707
Per ¼ cup (63 gm) serving	37	0.8	141

Variation

Low Rhubarb Crisp

Replace oatmeal in *Topping* with 2 additional tablespoons of Baking Mix.

Yield: 1¼ cups (315 gm).

	Phenylalanine (mg)	Protein (gm)	Calories
Per recipe	64	1.7	707
Per ¼ cup (63 gm) serving	13	0.3	141

Maple Baked Apples

4 medium, tart apples (about 130 gm each after coring)
½ cup (80 gm) raisins
¼ teaspoon cinnamon

¾ cup maple or maple flavored syrup
¼ cup water
¼ cup margarine or butter

Preheat oven to 350°. Pare top two-thirds of each apple, then core to within ½ inch of bottom. Place in a baking dish. Combine raisins with cinnamon; fill apple cavities with this mixture. Pour 1 tablespoon maple syrup into and over each apple. Pour 1 cup water into bottom of pan; cover apples with foil. Bake for 30 to 40 minutes or until apples are tender but still hold their shape. Combine remaining ½ cup syrup, margarine, and a dash of cinnamon in a small saucepan. Bring mixture to a boil, return heat to low and simmer 5 minutes. Place baked apples in individual dishes; pour some of hot maple mixture over each apple.

For Microwave Oven

Prepare apples as above. Place in microwave-proof dish; cover with plastic wrap. Microwave on High for 5 to 6 minutes or until apples are barely tender. Combine remaining syrup, margarine, and dash of cinnamon in microwave-proof 2-cup bowl. Cover with plastic wrap and microwave on High 5 minutes. Pour some hot maple mixture over each apple.

Yield: 4 apples.

	Phenylalanine (mg)	Protein (gm)	Calories
Per recipe	103	4.2	1695
Per apple with 2 tablespoons sauce	26	1.1	424

487

Fried Apples

2½ cups (300 gm) thickly
    sliced, unpeeled tart apples
¼ cup packed brown sugar

¼ teaspoon cinnamon
3 tablespoons margarine or
    butter

Prepare apples. Blend brown sugar with cinnamon and mix with apples. Heat margarine in a large skillet; fry apple slices in a single layer until tender (about 10 minutes), stirring occasionally. Apple slices should become glazed as they fry.

Yield: 1½ cups (290 gm).

	Phenylalanine (mg)	Protein (gm)	Calories
Per recipe	33	1.0	689
Per ½ cup (97 gm) serving	11	0.3	230

Hot Curried Fruit

Especially good in the winter, since it is served warm. Curry can be omitted but adds an excellent flavor.

1⅔ cups (215 gm) sliced
    bananas
15 oz can apricot halves,
    drained
16 oz can sliced peaches,
    drained

16 oz can sliced pears, drained
    (juice reserved)
15 halved maraschino cherries
⅓ cup juice from pears
½ cup packed brown sugar
1 teaspoon curry powder

Layer bananas in the bottom of a shallow baking dish. Combine the remainder of the fruits and arrange over bananas. Mix juice from pears, brown sugar, and curry powder in a saucepan and heat to a boil, stirring. Pour sauce over fruit. Bake at 300° for 1 hour, or microwave on High for 8 minutes, stirring once.

Yield: 3¾ cups (700 gm drained).

	Phenylalanine (mg)	Protein (gm)	Calories
Per recipe	213	6.3	971
Per ¼ cup (47 gm) serving	14	0.4	65

HELPFUL HINTS

Attitudes and Perspectives

Try to view your child first as a normal child, and only second as a child who happens to have PKU. In your concern about PKU, don't lose track of the most important goal—for him or her to develop into a happy, independent child and adult.

Take one day at a time. Don't project too far into the future, worrying about how you will cope with the diet. You will learn, day by day.

It is important to remember that there is nothing you could have done to prevent PKU or to have known about it. Early after the diagnosis, try to deal with your feelings of anger, pity, embarrassment, or guilt, talking with other parents if possible when you are ready. It usually takes many months to come to terms with the diagnosis and your responsibility as a parent.

When your child is still very young, examine your own attitudes about food and those of your family. Do you eat to live, or live to eat? Do you enjoy cooking, baking? Could you learn, if not? What kind of meal planning strategies do you use? How much food variety? What about snacking? In order to facilitate optimal diet management, you may need to make some changes, many of them subtle rather than dramatic. Start trying to expand your family's diet—add more fruits, vegetables, maybe cut down on meats. Experiment with low protein cooking, baking, and new menu ideas.

Develop confidence in yourself. Convince yourself that you *do* possess all of the skills necessary to cope with the diet. Parents of a child with PKU are responsible for their child's intelligence in a way most parents are not. While it is a heavy responsibility, you *can* manage, as many others have. Rely on love for your child, common sense, and accurate information about the diet to see you through.

Dedicate yourself to strictly adhering to the diet, which is absolutely necessary. Admit that the diet will be difficult at times, but certainly *not* impossible. If you thoroughly accept the need for the diet, your child will too, and confrontation with others over being "different" will melt away.

Don't attribute your child's undesirable behaviors or illnesses to PKU. Your child should *not* have any effects of PKU when well controlled on the diet.

Encourage your child to develop interests in a variety of activities and to develop special skills—sports, music, or whatever. If he or she has something outside of school to focus on, something that is really enjoyable, food will become less important.

Instead of talking about the small amount of food your child can eat or the things he or she cannot have, try to emphasize all that he or she *can* have and that because of the diet he or she does well physically and in school. Emphasize the similarities rather than the differences.

Try not to feel sorry for your child. Train yourself to think positively about the diet (for example, think of the good fortune that there is a diet which can so effectively prevent mental retardation). Accepting the diet as much as possible as a normal part of life will shape your child's attitude toward the diet in a positive way. Have, feel, and express sympathy: "No, I agree; it's not fair that you have PKU." Never express pity; while sympathy puts the child on the same basis as you and eases the hurt, pity subjugates the child to your feelings.

Try to encourage a partnership with your child in working with the diet, not a master-slave relationship, or the slaves will eventually rebel!

Be careful not to compensate for the lack of "fairness" by becoming overprotective or overindulgent. There is a fine line between accommodating the child on-diet and spoiling him or her. Each family needs to evaluate its behavior towards the child with this in mind.

Develop a positive attitude about PKU and diet. This will help build high self-esteem for the child with PKU and for the rest of the family. Your good attitude will influence others. There are many positive benefits for you and your family in dealing with PKU—think about these:

- Increases your organizational skills.
- Facilitates consideration of family members for each other.
- Develops a caring attitude about the handicapped and others with special problems and needs.
- Increases self-esteem of everyone involved in diet management (yes, you *can* succeed).
- Facilitates flexibility in changing lifestyle if necessary.
- Gives you a chance to be creative.
- Increases appreciation for aspects of life that many people take for granted.
- Teaches discipline and self-control for the child from an early age.
- Can facilitate change in family eating patterns towards more nutritious and healthy habits.

Family Involvement

Fathers

While mothers typically have more responsibility for child care than fathers, mothers should not have sole responsibility for diet management. Father's involvement is also very important—to take over diet in an emergency, to share the responsibility for blood levels, to be supportive when problems arise. Fathers should learn simple things about the diet when the child is an infant—formula preparation, how many exchanges are allowed, etc. Fathers should take the opportunity to spend a day alone with the child every once in a while to learn to manage the diet.

Discuss your approach to the diet—your attitudes and any "rules" you both wish to maintain. When both parents present a unified front and tell the child the same things about the diet, it is more likely that the diet will be successfully managed and that the child will accept it well.

Siblings

Teach non-PKU siblings as much about PKU and diet as is appropriate for their age.

Involve older siblings in diet management, eventually teaching them to calculate the diet. If a big sister or brother gets involved, it may seem a more desirable thing for the child on-diet to learn.

Don't penalize normal siblings for not having PKU. Encouraging them to have limits similar to those imposed on the PKU child is good (such as snacking at predetermined times), but don't constantly remind them that they can eat anything, so the child with PKU deserves all of the treats. The non-PKU children need special treats too.

Certain foods can and should be denied to siblings, within reason—foods that may cause undue jealousy for the child on-diet. These foods can be enjoyed when the child on-diet is not present.

You may find that the best way to keep your child happy about the diet is by having food "special" from that of the rest of the family, especially when there are non-PKU brothers and sisters. One approach is to allow the child on-diet to have foods not allowed for siblings, such as Tang or Popsicles, or other "low" treats. While all of the children may love these things, the child on-diet can be given the opportunity to share these items with others *if* he or she chooses.

Provide at least some snacks to other children in the family that are on the diet. Train other children to ask before eating anything, as you should train your child with PKU.

Stress to siblings that what is on their diet is just as important for growth as the PKU diet is for their sister or brother. For a sibling who does not enjoy meat or other high protein foods, explain that he or she gets the necessary vitamins and minerals from those foods while the child with PKU gets them from the special milk.

Grandparents or Close Relatives

Consider individual personalities and abilities to accept and understand PKU, giving reassurance and emphasis where most needed. Emphasize good results of treatment and the child's potential for a normal life and good health. Give more explanation about diet to those who will be caring for your child regularly.

Talk to relatives, especially grandparents, about the kind of attitudes that you think are important for good diet management and your child's healthy outlook on the diet.

Ask your clinic if they provide counseling for extended family members, or if they are allowed to visit the clinic.

Encourage a grandmother who lives nearby to periodically participate in low protein baking, if she enjoys baking. Grandfathers may enjoy this too.

Education

From a Young Age . . .

Encourage your child's independence in managing his or her own diet as early as possbile. The age at which you can begin teaching your child will depend on your child's individual readiness, but might begin as early as age 2. The right age can be as soon as the child learns "yes" and "no"—especially "no!" You can begin to show him or her foods and ask, "Is this a 'yes' food or a 'no' food?"

Your child's ability to make appropriate food choices in unfamiliar situations, and in general to accept food restrictions, can be promoted in the following ways:

Always be consistent with diet restrictions. Absolute consistency in allowing only foods permitted on your child's diet from the very beginning is crucial not only to the child's development, but to his or her learning the 'rules' of the diet and to learning to accept them as well.

Talk about measuring or weighing food at home. Show your child that you are measuring (or weighing) and counting everything that he or she eats, except "free" foods. Frequently measure (or weigh) and count foods together with your child, especially when he or she has learned to count to 5 or 10 or has some concept of numbers. As you become more adept at the diet you may be able to "eyeball" quantities fairly accurately. But it is important to *always* measure or weigh not only to ensure accuracy, but to show your child that nothing is eaten, except "free foods," without first determining quantity.

Talk openly about PKU and the diet at home and elsewhere, without making it a major focus of everyday conversation. This will help your child to become open about it with friends, defusing the diet as a subject for taunts. Respond to your child's questions as honestly and simply as you can and take advantage of opportunities to explain why you are doing certain things (for example, why you take blood, why you measure and count foods) even before you feel your child can fully understand. He or she will at least become familiar with certain words related to PKU and the diet and know that there *is* a reason for what you are doing.

Use teaching materials written especially for children (such as *You and PKU**) when your child seems ready to sit still and listen. Read the book yourself before you think your child is ready, so that you can begin using similar vocabulary related to PKU and the diet and perhaps use some of the ideas presented.

Teach your child from a very young age that he or she must ask you before eating any foods. This will promote your child's learning of what is on the diet and what is not. As your child grows older, he

*Schuett, V., and Taylor, M., *You and PKU,* second edition, 1998. Available from Dietary Specialties, 865 Piscataway, NJ 08854. Telephone: 1-888-MENU123 or 732-980-6700.

or she should have learned to discriminate allowed from not allowed foods and can be encouraged to use his or her own judgment rather than depending solely on yours. Encourage your child to continue asking you when he or she is unsure of the phenylalanine content of any food.

Observe your child in away-from-home situations where food is available and you are still there to supervise. Allow your child to make decisions on his or her own. Praise your child when he or she refuses not allowed food that is offered. When a correct decision is not made, explain what was not correct and why. Better yet, get a friend or a neighbor to do it for you and report. This takes pressure off the child and lets you get a better feeling for what the child will really do when you are not there. Use the information gained as background information to improve your teaching, not to confront the child with the choices he made.

As Your Child Grows Older . . .

Teach your child that some foods are "high" and other foods are "low" or "free." Reinforce this concept by frequently offering the child choices of different foods with different phenylalanine/protein values at snacktime or mealtime. Let the child know that choosing one food (that is, the "low" food) means that he or she can have more of that food than the other food, or more of a different kind of food at a later time; likewise, choosing another food (that is, the "high" food) means that less of that food can be eaten than of the other choice, or that less food will be allowed later.

At home, give your child the opportunity to be responsible for the diet when you are there. For example, consider giving the child a package of crackers or potato chips and tell him or her how many are allowed, letting the child count them. He or she should know that if too many are eaten, the difference will be made up at the next meal. Letting the child make the choice (from age 4 or 5) makes him or her feel responsible, and grown up too.

Encourage your child to help with simple food preparation at home, especially with low protein products. Talk about how low protein foods are different than regular foods that may look just the same (for example, special foods that you make don't usually have eggs and use a different kind of flour). This will help your child to become aware that some baked goods that look the same as the special kinds made at home are not the same, and may be very "high" instead of very "low."

Supervise your child serving himself or herself from the family meal on a frequent or regular basis, when you feel that he or she is ready to begin making some independent choices. As your child becomes sensitive to the idea of measuring and counting foods, to the idea of "high" and "low" foods, and has some knowledge of appropriate portion sizes of commonly eaten foods, you should be able to rely on him or her to report to you what was eaten when you are not present. Encourage your child to describe to you what he or she ate at school or in other situations, and to show you how much was eaten (until your child is able to do this reliably, you may need to depend on the child's teacher or an adult to report to you).

You may need to enforce certain "rules" that will facilitate diet management (for example, "If you are not sure, don't take it" or "Potatoes only once a day").

Help your child learn that it is important to ask if something is sweetened with NutraSweet or aspartame (see page 29 for description of general food items which may contain NutraSweet or aspartame). Praise your child for having the boldness to do that on his or her own.

Remember that your relationship with your child is *the* most important factor in helping your child to accept and learn about his or her diet. More than your child's specific knowledge of PKU, your attitude toward the diet and openness in talking about it with your child from a very young age will help to foster the responsible behavior that he or she will need to have in situations away from your guidance. The fear of allowing your child independence, after the years of control required to maintain the diet, will be much less if you have prepared him or her for such growing-up times by taking advantage of the suggestions presented here.

Teaching Your Child to Keep Track of Diet

There are a number of ways that can be used for teaching your child to keep track of his or her own diet from a preschool age, gradually teaching the child to internalize the information and techniques needed for eventual self-management.
- *Purchase color-coded measuring cups and spoons* (or make them with colored tape) and make a chart indicating measurement size of the color-coded cups and spoons. Let the child practice measuring. "Hands-on" experience teaches best.
- *Create a picture book.* Teach your child to recognize portion sizes appropriate for his or her diet, for foods commonly eaten. Make a

book of pictures of these foods, cut out of a magazine or hand-drawn by child or parent, indicating the portion size for a given amount of phenylalanine or protein (or for a given number of exchanges).

- *Use a "token" system.* When your child has some basic concept of numbers, give him or her some responsibility for keeping track of phenylalanine or protein, through use of a token system. Give the child poker chips or other convenient and fun "tokens," with various colors or shapes representing numbers to indicate exchanges or milligrams of phenylalanine (or grams of protein). At the beginning of the day, give the child his or her phenylalanine or protein allowance in "tokens" and let him or her "buy" food from you using the tokens. This could be done on a daily basis or, after the "game" is learned, at certain intervals. In place of tokens, a corkboard with colored tacks, a peg board and pegs, or an abacus with colored beads could also be used. (To teach your child why high protein foods are not allowed, show him or her how many tokens, pegs, tacks, or beads would be used up for one egg, a piece of cheese, etc.).
- *Design a food chart.* Make a colorful chart for the child to use, recording exchanges with small colored stickers from an office supply store. Give your child the number of stickers to correspond to the allowed number of exchanges or milligrams of phenylalanine (or

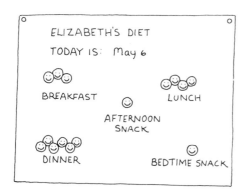

grams of protein). After each meal, have the child put stickers on the chart to show exchanges or milligrams as they are used. This system teaches simple math skills and the visual representation allows the child to see the consequences of his or her food choices, as reflected by a diminishing supply of stickers.

Example:

For a base, use corrugated cardboard covered with shiny gift wrap and decorated with Sesame Street characters cut from a maga-

498

zine or with fanciful stickers. Use transfer type for child's name and meals/snacks. Place clear contact paper over the chart, allowing stickers to be added and replaced daily.

For older children, a small portable log for keeping track of phenylalanine could be devised, so the child can keep a running total by subtracting phenylalanine after each meal.
Example:

Type or print out the form, several on a page; Xerox, cut apart, then put small pages in a tiny notebook with rings.

- *Encourage older children to keep their own food records for PKU clinic use.* Children as young as 8 years of age can learn to write down what they have eaten (including amounts) for routine monitoring done by your clinic. This may be done for only one of the days required at first; later the whole record can be done. This facilitates communication between clinic staff and the child, as well as teaching the child responsibility.

Holidays and Special Occasions

General Tips

Food is an important part of everyone's holidays. While other aspects of the holiday can be emphasized, let your child on-diet get excited about special low protein treats made just for the occasion. Have several recipes which you use only for special days. Let your child choose which one to make.

Don't overestimate the importance of eating to a young child; small children are often too excited to eat much at a party and will often settle for a snack before and/or after the event.

For all family holidays bring food along not only for the child on-diet but bring something he or she can share with other children present, for example a Jell-O salad or relish tray.

When a younger child has been invited to any function where food will be served, call ahead to the adult in charge. If your child can't have the food, you may be able to duplicate it very nearly; or volunteer to send something all children can eat (such as *Rice Krispie Marshmallow Treats*).

For dinner at friends' houses, call ahead of time to the hostess and ask what is being served. People will usually offer to have something on hand that your child can eat. Sometimes you may have to talk the hostess out of buying too much food for your child; many times people don't realize that your child won't eat a very large amount. Or they may want to prepare something "special." Usually, the best way to handle this is to have the hostess supply the drink, relishes, or vegetable and for you to bring the rest. On occasion the best-laid plans won't work out, so it is best to be prepared for any eventuality. It is a good idea to keep your child's phenylalanine or protein intake for the day as low as possible before a party because it is usually the higher protein foods that will be available.

Potluck dinners can be a problem because often there will be nothing the child on-diet can eat. Volunteer to bring a plain fresh fruit salad or relish tray (something that is not often included in the contributions), or take a low pro macaroni salad for everyone—it's good enough! In addition, take some other foods along for your child so that he or she will have some variety also. This may be one of the times when your child will be envious of the choices open to other people.

For young children, don't leave the house without taking foods for the diet; if you are attending parties, weddings, etc., and there are only off-limits foods, these will give you an important back-up.

At the holiday or social gathering do not specifically talk about your child's diet in his or her presence unless the child is included in the discussion. Do not feel sorry for your child or encourage any other adult to feel sorry for the child and how little he or she can eat.

Talk to an older child before attending a dinner that will have all kinds and an abundance of food. Discuss what will be served there, what he or she can have and how much; then let the child manage alone as much as possible.

Let a young child role-play what he or she will say to an adult who offers him or her something not on the diet; there's nothing like rehearsing so that the child has a ready answer rather than accepting food because he or she feels awkward not knowing what to say.

For holidays, start a special project (for example, build a Christmas Creche), or read about non-food aspects of the holiday (for example, learn about the Pilgrims before Thanksgiving). Stress religious aspects of the holiday, or family togetherness.

Whatever the occasion, relax and enjoy yourself!

Valentine's Day

This holiday is one of the easiest to contend with, since many of the Valentine candies are of the "free" variety—candy hearts, cinnamon candies, etc.

- Buy a heart-shaped box at the store, take out the candy and refill with things the child on-diet can have—save and reuse the box for several years.
- Make *Basic Cut-Out Cookies* in heart shapes. Decorate with frosting. Adapt cookie decorating ideas which appear annually in women's magazines.
- Make *Rice Krispie Marshmallow Treats*, cut out in heart shapes; frost and decorate with red candy sprinkles.

Easter

- Start an Easter project. Make an elaborate Easter basket. Let your child decorate eggs with sequins, fancy braids or trims, etc. and decorate a sturdy basket. Make the Easter basket for use year after year so that your child looks forward to seeing the basket, not the contents. It's another constant in his or her world, and will make it feel more like Easter than all of the chocolate bunnies would.
- Make your own Easter baskets by buying the appropriate candy, covering the basket with cellophane. Make the largest item in the

501

basket a toy of some kind to eliminate the need for the traditional large chocolate bunny or chocolate egg.

- Consider giving a "spring-summer" gift—for example, a wagon, wading pool, basketball, books, or small toys, and giving less candy.
- Instead of hiding boiled eggs, use plastic eggs and place 5, 10, or 25 cents inside—the more money, the more difficult the hiding place—or fill plastic eggs with jelly beans or other "free" candies, or a few M&M's.
- Even at very young ages, make sure the child knows the exchange value (or number of milligrams) for the candy he or she is allowed (include this information in the basket) and understands that the candy must be rationed out one at a time if it contains protein.
- Use chocolate molds to press *Rice Krispie Marshmallow Treats* into Easter shapes and decorate with "free" icing. Use *Jiffy Fudge* or *Easy Fudge* to cut out a chocolate or colored Easter rabbit, using a small cookie cutter.
- Press *Rice Krispie Marshmallow Treats* into muffin tins, making an indentation in the top. Color coconut green with food coloring and sprinkle a little in each nest, along with candy eggs or small gumdrops. Set a yellow marshmallow chick on top (estimate phenylalanine/protein content based on size or weight in relation to a large marshmallow).
- Make chocolate or colored Easter eggs using the *Chocolate Bon-Bons* or *Pastel Bon-Bons* recipes.
- Decorate low protein cupcakes baked in tart-sized muffin pans with white "free" icing (see *Cakes* section), green colored coconut, and a jelly bean.

Halloween

- Consider asking close neighbors to have a special treat on hand for your child. Neighbors can be wonderful. View it as giving them a chance to help your child; most respond very well.
- When the child is old enough to "trick or treat" by himself or herself, let the child collect whatever he or she is given and then bring

it home to be sorted out—the things that can't be eaten can be in turn given out at your door, recycled to other children in the family, or collected and given to your local hospital's children's ward.

- Use a family "barter" system if there are other siblings (or neighbor children who are playmates). Let the child on-diet "trade" a chocolate candy bar for gum, etc., until all high protein items are eliminated. Other children are usually willing participants, since they will likely feel they are getting the better part of the deal. Children will also learn to "help" in this way, and to be considerate of the child on-diet.

Thanksgiving

- If you are eating away from home, many low protein foods can be made ahead of time and reheated.
- For the immediate family, consider having a non-traditional meal such as a Chinese "hot-pot"—heat oil in an electric wok (or fondue pot) in the center of the table and place individual servings of a specially prepared deep-frying batter at each person's plate (for diet serving use *French Fried Veggies* or *Master Mix Pancakes* for batter). Let each person dip a variety of sliced vegetables such as mushrooms, cucumber, cauliflower, green pepper, or zucchini into his or her batter and deep fry his or her own in the hot oil—serve this with hot rolls and a salad; it is very filling because of the batter. Include chunks of raw chicken or turkey breast, shrimp, or thin sliced beef for other family members.

Suggested Recipes from "Low Protein Cookery" and Other Food Ideas

(See *The Low Protein Food List for PKU* for nutrient content of non-recipe items.)

Main Dishes and Vegetables

Apple and Raisin Dressing
Apple-Filled Sweet Potatoes
Baked Apples and Carrots
Candied Sweet Potatoes
Candied Sweets
Green Beans Supreme
Savory Dressing
Spicy Candied Yams
Stuffed Mushrooms
The Great Stuffed Pumpkin

Breads

Cranberry Bread
dinner rolls (any of the recipes in this book)
muffins (any of the recipes in this book)
Pumpkin Bread

Salads

Blushing Apple Cranberry Salad
fruit salad (any of the recipes in this book)
Holiday Cranberry Salad
Waldorf Salad

Desserts

Apple Pie
Pumpkin Pie
Pumpkin Pudding

Other Food Ideas

apple cider
cranberry relish or sauce
cranberry applesauce (commercially available)
mashed potatoes and gravy
relish tray with carrot and celery sticks, olives, spiced apple rings, and pickles

Christmas

- Have a "Sweets Exchange" with other families who have children with PKU. Your clinic may be willing to sponsor such an event, drawing families from a distance as well as locally. This is done annually at the Waisman Center. Families bring several dozen low protein treats and return home with an equal number of a great diversity of cookies and candies.
- When decorating your tree, put candy canes on the tree (put them on last!). Give one to all "helpers" as well as to children who come to visit during the holidays.

***Suggested Recipes from "Low Protein Cookery"
and Other Food Ideas***

Any of the recipes or food ideas suggested for Thanksgiving would also be very appropriate for Christmas dinner. In addition, the following special treats, salads, and other ideas are especially festive for the holiday season.

Desserts/Treats

Basic Cut-Out Cookies, decorated
Brownies, with green mint icing
candy—any, but especially easy and nice:
    Candy Pretzels
    Chocolate or *Pastel Bon-Bons*
    fudge (any of the recipes in this book)
    Marshmallow Rice Krispie Candy
    Marshmallow Treats
    Never-Fail Toffee
    No-Peanuts Brittle
    Peppermint Bark
Chocolate and Cherry Christmas Cakes

Chocolate-Covered Cherries
Crispy Date Bars
Gingerbread Cookies
Holiday Steamed Pudding
Neapolitan Cookies
Party Fudge Bars
Spritz Cookies

Salads

Frozen Strawberry Banana Salad
Strawberry Salad
Yum Yum Salad using red or green Jell-O or Prono

Other

Christmas Biscuits
snack mixes—*Cinnamon Munch* or *Low Pro Snack Mix*

Birthday Parties

Birthday Parties for the Child On-Diet

If there are other families with children on-diet of an age similar to your child who live within a reasonable driving distance, you might invite them to your child's party routinely. Your children will grow to realize that they are not alone on the diet.

- Plan a party that won't include serving a meal, such as a beach party, tobogganing, roller skating, or a special theater event.
- Stress games rather than food. Your child may also find it more fun to plan or help make decorations or invitations than to concentrate on food planning.
- Provide snacks that all children can eat—mints, popcorn, chips.
- Bake a low protein cake and have it decorated by a bakery. Many bakeries are happy to do this. Bake a regular cake for others at the party, or serve the low protein cake to everyone.
- Make one of the recipes using cake flour rather than wheat starch (*Sunshine Cake* or *Banana Cake*) or a 1-egg box cake (*Quick-Mix Cake*). Allow your child to save phenylalanine/protein for a normal-sized piece.
- For a young child, make a low protein cake in "doll-size" pans so the child can eat the whole thing if he or she wants. Consider making several of these small cakes and freezing them, to be used when your child is invited to other birthday parties.
- Make a "train" cake—make the engine from *Tastes-Like-Devil's-*

Food Cake in a doll-size loaf pan; then make regular cake cut in rectangles, for the other cars—frost and use candy Lifesavers for wheels and write the children's names on each car.

- Make a Raggedy Ann cake, baking a low protein cake for Raggedy Ann's heart. The child on-diet will have a decorated heart on his or her plate, while others will have to settle for parts of head, feet, etc.
- Make *Rice Krispie Marshmallow Treats* and press into a greased round bowl. Let harden, then tip out of bowl. Frost with a "free" frosting and decorate.
- *Chocolate Pinwheels* with a candle in the center are very attractive and *all* of the children will love them.
- Instead of a cake, fill a Tupperware Jel-N-Serve mold with a favorite Jell-O flavor; "frost" with Coolwhip or whipped Rich's Richwhip Topping tinted with a little food coloring.
- Make *Vanilla Creampops* or *Chocolate Creampops* in party cups rather than Tupperware molds. Freeze until soft, then set a candle in the midde and freeze firm.
- Serve ice cream clowns made out of grape ice (purchased from a Baskin-Robbins ice cream store).
- Make any of the low protein ice cream or sherbet recipes in the book and serve to everyone.
- Serve a main dish which can be adapted to accommodate all of the children, such as a macaroni casserole, or make-your-own pizza (*Kids-Love-It-Pizza;* or use *Traditional Pizza Crust, Quick Pizza Crust,* or *Thick Crust Pizza* for the child on-diet).

- You may want to avoid food-related games, but several are fun for young children at a party. Have a treasure hunt. Put small toys and candy that your child on-diet can eat into small bags and hide them. Or have a "marshmallow bob." Have children bob for regular-sized marshmallows hung from a string (attached to a low ceiling), with hands behind their back.

Birthday Parties for Another Child

- Call the child's mother in advance—if you call early enough she may offer to work around what suits your child best. Send a low protein alternative along, especially cake, and homemade low protein ice cream if ice cream will be served; or offer to provide part of the meal, such as a Jell-O salad.
- For a birthday party at a pizza place, call and find out the menu. Talk to your child and explain what he or she can eat and what other children will be eating and let the child decide whether he or she wishes to attend under circumstances where there may be very little to eat. Or bring along (or take in advance) a low protein pizza. If you explain your child's needs, most pizza parlors will be happy to bake your pizza in their own oven and serve it along with the rest.

Birthday Parties for Other Family Members

- Serve a low protein cupcake for the child on-diet.
- Make one of the recipes using cake flour rather than wheat starch (*Sunshine Cake* or *Banana Cake*), or a 1-egg box cake (*Quick-Mix Cake*) and serve to the whole family, allowing your child to "save" phenylalanine/protein for a normal-sized piece or ½ of a piece.

508

Picnics and Cookouts

Plan ahead. If you can, check to see what types of food people are bringing; have a similar menu for your child if foods are not suitable.

Plan your child's other meals for the day in order to allow for any picnic treats and extras.

Have any special foods you bring premeasured so you can keep track of your child's intake with minimum bother.

If there will be a cook-out, grill vegetables in foil or make *Shish kabob* for your child.

Bring plenty of fresh fruit—eating fruit is a good thing to encourage at an early age anyway.

Have your child drink formula before going to the picnic.

If a picnic will last all day, bring along a small cooler filled with ice for formula—put the formula in a thermos or insulated container to keep it maximally cold.

Suggested Recipes from "Low Protein Cookery"
and Other Food Ideas

(See the *Low Protein Food List* for nutrient content of non-recipe items.)

Main Dishes

Burger Bun with relishes
Garden Fresh Casserole
Mexican Rice
Mock Baked Beans
Mushroom Burgers
Mushroom Soup and Rice
Quick Asparagus Casserole
Rice and Mushrooms
Spanish Rice

Salads

Brown Rice Salad
Coleslaw

Cucumber Salad
Curried Fruit and Rice Salad
Five-Cup Salad
Fruit Delight
German Coleslaw
German Hot Potato Salad
Golden Coins
Marinated Mushrooms
Mixed Vegetables and Pasta Salad
Orange Tapioca Salad
Pistachio Fluff Salad
Potato Green Bean Salad
Potato Salad
Watermelon Boat Salad
Yum Yum Salad

Desserts

Cherry Delight
cookies (any recipe in this book)
Peppermint Crunch Dessert
pies (any of the "dream" pies with graham cracker or cookie crust)

Other Ideas

fresh fruit platter
Kool-Aid
marinated fresh vegetables
potato chips or pretzels
relish tray
watermelon

Eating Out

First and foremost, never be embarrassed by the fact that your child on-diet cannot have everything the rest of the family is eating. Ignore unfriendly stares from other people in the restaurant who may think that you are depriving your child. If explanations seem to be in order, say merely that "He (or she) is on a special diet."

If you do not know the restaurant menu in advance, call ahead and find out if there are specific items served. If there is nothing for the diet, take food along or find another restaurant.

Allow your older child to order his or her own food, even if you know the choice will always be french fries. Give your child that independence—and that responsibility.

Do not hesitate to ask for simple modification of food items on the menu—for example, macaroni with margarine or butter rather than a sauce, vegetables without sauce or breading, etc.

Introduce salads at an early age, and eat them regularly as a family. Salad bars are widely available at restaurants and can provide a varied and interesting meal out for the child on-diet.

For a more balanced meal at a fast-food restaurant, consider taking along a green salad and piece of fruit. This will diminish hunger for french fries and provide a more satisfying meal. (Fortunately, many fast-food restaurants now offer salads or a salad bar.)

For sit-down restaurant eating, take a low protein pasta casserole and/or a vegetable dish or low protein dinner roll for bulk (restaurants are almost always willing to warm up the food when told there is a special diet need) and fill in with available vegetables and fruit from the restaurant.

Freeze unbaked low protein pizza, complete with sauce and toppings, using the *Traditional Pizza Crust* or *Thick Pizza Crust* recipes. Many pizza restaurants will be happy to bake a low protein pizza for you (for an individual pizza, bake about 10 to 12 minutes in their very hot oven). Call ahead to make sure this service is available. If not, call ahead to order the family's pizza so it is ready when you arrive; bring a preheated low protein pizza wrapped in foil or a plastic container to keep hot.

A smorgasbord or cafeteria-style restaurant usually has a good variety of lower protein foods to choose from.

Try to choose a restaurant with a salad bar. A variety of fruits, vegetables, and crackers will be available.

Sunday brunches usually have a wide selection of acceptable foods on a vegetable and salad bar.

- Breakfast ideas:
  toast (if allowed)
  hash brown potatoes (beware, some have a coating on them)
  dry cereal (most restaurants have the small individual cereal boxes)
  orange juice
  fruit cup or any fresh fruits in season
  hot herb tea
- Lunch and dinner ideas:
  french fries
  baked potato
  side dish of vegetables (for example, mushrooms, green beans, or carrots)
  crackers or bread sticks
  part of a dinner roll (if allowed)
  salad bar
  fruit
  sherbet
- Mexican restaurants: rice, guacamole, part of a tortilla, salad or salad bar. Take in your own *Taco Chips* and use with the house salsa.
- Chinese restaurants: rice, vegetable dishes. Since many of the dishes are vegetarian or mainly vegetables, the child can eat from the same dishes as the rest of the family, eliminating "high" items such as chow mein noodles and bean sprouts as well as meat and other high protein ingredients.
- Steak houses: french fries, baked potato, salad bar.
- Fairs and carnivals: cotton candy, snow cones.

Tips for Young Children

When your child is a baby, feed him or her before you go out to eat, and take along a bottle of formula.

Bring a supply of finger-sized cereals and small toys, books, crayons, etc. to keep the child occupied.

Feed your toddler at least a small amount before going to the restaurant to diminish his or her appetite.

Take formula with you in a covered Tupperware glass or have the child drink formula before you go to the restaurant.

Beware of restaurants that provide highchairs already set up with hand puppets and crackers. Make sure you remove the crackers or any other treat before your child sees them.

For a preschool child, buy a lunchbox. Your child will love to take it "out to dinner." At the restaurant order something from the menu, augmented by formula and other "low" foods from the lunchbox.

Babysitters

For a sitter who will become a "regular," when he or she first starts watching your child, a good booklet to give him or her to read is "Living with PKU" (Mead Johnson, 1995).

Always plan ahead and leave enough of your child's daily phenylalanine or protein allowance to permit leaving more than enough food for the babysitter to give him or her. Nothing is worse than a hungry child who can't be fed.

Try to feed your children any main meal before the sitter gets there, so all he or she does is clean up. If that's not possible, make up the plates and put them in the refrigerator with instructions on how to reheat in the oven or microwave. The sitter usually can add a simple green salad. If the sitter will be there for a meal, make up a plate for him or her, too.

For a babysitter you know well, leave *The Low Protein Food List for PKU* to use, showing him or her what to do.

If your child will be allowed choices, depending on the child's age you may want to explain diet options to both the child and the sitter at the same time, putting at least some responsibility on the child.

If you want to give the sitter only limited choices, because many sitters may not easily understand an exchange system, write out a list of foods and the amount the child can have, allowing the sitter or child to choose from a select number of items in specific quantities for snacks. Have the sitter check off which items were eaten, as well as indicating amounts.

If you are not comfortable with the sitter making food choices and calculating your child's intake, have all food prepared and measured (and written down for yourself). Instruct the sitter not to throw away uneaten food. When you return, recalculate your child's intake if necessary.

Leave a "free food" bag for snacks.

Warn the sitter about NutraSweet and other foods that contain aspartame.

For Day Care or All-Day Care

Giving your daycare sitter a complete sample menu for a day with calculations will give the sitter an idea of how your child's food is calculated and measured each day, enhancing understanding of the importance of keeping track of everything eaten by your child (this can be done for a sitter who is a "regular" but only spends a few hours with your child).

If your child goes to a sitter regularly while you work, take groceries to the sitter's house once a week. Each morning take formula and a notebook. In the notebook, record breakfast. Have the sitter record lunch and snacks eaten. When you get home, simply add up phenylalanine/protein eaten for the day, then plan supper accordingly. Supply sitter with *The Low Protein Food List for PKU* or your own condensed list and quantities to feed. Also recommend which foods shouldn't be served together (such as two "higher" vegetables) and provide a variety of "low" or "free" candies, cookies, or other snacks.

If the sitter will be providing a meal, you may want to write your planned menu out completely for the sitter—what and how much. For snacks, it may work out best to leave a list of several choices of foods with amounts that all have approximately the same amount of phenylalanine/protein.

If your sitter has several children to care for, it may work out most conveniently to send lunch with your child as you would for school—lunch pail, including a thermos of formula.

For daycare, label "snacks" and "lunch" in child's lunchbox. Instruct the sitter to give the child nothing but what you have sent or approved.

If you plan to be away for a whole day, place foods in separate plastic bags marked "Breakfast," "Lunch," "Dinner," and "Snacks," with any special preparation instructions noted.

Send along more formula than you think will be needed, to compensate for any spills or a larger intake than you anticipate. Send it premixed, or in powder form with special instructions for preparation.

When You Are Gone Longer than a Day

If you feel the sitter is able to make wise food choices based on the child's diet allowance, have a card stuck on the refrigerator door or kitchen wall with a list of commonly eaten foods and phenylalanine/protein content.

If you do not want to rely on the sitter's judgement, plan menus in advance, with perhaps several alternate choices for certain food items.

If you will be gone for an extended time, plan 3 or 4 days of menus that could be used repeatedly.

For children whose food likes and dislikes are predictable, prepare foods in advance and package according to meals (for example, a bag for Monday breakfast, Monday lunch, etc.). Refrigerate or freeze as appropriate. If items will need reheating, label with instructions.

For formula, prepackage the measured or weighed amount of dry formula in plastic bags for each day you will be gone, indicating how much water (or milk, when necessary for infants) should be added to the formula. Make up a few extra bags.

Travel

Food

Don't stay at home just because it's easier to manage the diet at home! The diet should never be an excuse to say "no" to an activity or travel—anywhere!

Take *The Low Protein Food List for PKU* with you, especially if your child is young and occasions may arise where a new food is available.

- Hotel rooms with kitchenettes are very handy.
- Try to limit restaurant eating to once a day. Eat other meals in the car, motel, or picnic grounds.
- Make up small plastic bags filled with "low" or "free" treats, one for each day of the trip. Or take a small tin filled with "free" candies of different sizes, shapes, flavors.
- Tupperware cups, bowls with lids, and the hamburger stacker are great for traveling—in the hamburger stacker put different cereals, raisins, oatmeal/low protein porridge, minute rice, low protein pasta, popcorn, etc. and carry in your suitcase if you are flying. The Tupperware Velveeta cheese holder is perfect for storing a mini loaf of low protein bread. It also has a cutting board inside. The Tupperware loaf keeper stores a large loaf of bread.
- Try to have many of the same snacks available for all of your children.
- If you will be staying in a room with a kitchenette or will be camping, it may be convenient to cook vegetables in advance, then put in diet serving sizes in plastic bags and freeze. Keep them on ice when you travel.
- Drink boxes (individual sizes), dried fruit, and fruit roll-ups are great for traveling.
- Take snack-pack cold cereals for variety breakfasts and snacks while traveling or camping. Those not on diet can pick out the "high" cereals. Mark on the box top the number of exchanges or mg of phenylalanine in each one.

- Lipton Cup-of-Soup is handy. Some motel hot water taps are hot enough, without heating, for preparing soup.
- If you are planning to visit close relatives or friends, consider sending a few special recipes ahead of time (along with any special ingredients), and special foods and formula.
- Airlines are good about preparing fruit or fruit/raw vegetable plates if you let them know your needs at least several days ahead of time. Specify that you do not want cheese, meat, or eggs. Even so, not everything may be suitable for the diet, but your child will have the fun of getting a meal on the plane. Have some extras ready to fill out the meal if necessary.

Foods for Camping

When camping, remember that being out of doors increases appetites, so take along plenty of low protein foods, especially breads and pastas which are filling.

- Use low protein bread and Ragu sauce and heat over an open fire.
- Take along low protein *Burger Buns* and serve with condiments when others have wieners or hamburgers.
- Take frozen low protein waffles and reheat in a skillet over a fire or stove.
- Plan vegetables wrapped in foil and cooked on a grill.
- Campbell's Vegetable Soup makes a hearty camp "stew."
- Two vanilla wafers and "free" vanilla Pillsbury Frosting (or another "free" flavor) makes a carefree dessert.

- Make "s'mores" using chocolate chips instead of chocolate bars and put on low protein graham crackers.
- Make up small baggies of dry ingredients for pancakes (using *Master Mix Pancakes* recipe); take vegetable oil to add later.

Formula

- Always take formula for several extra days than the number of days you think you will need. Then you will be ready for emergencies (spilled container, extended stay, snowed in, etc.).
- If you are flying, put 3 to 4 days' worth of premeasured formula powder in your carry-on bag in case your luggage is delayed.
- For infants who may be adversely affected by changes in water, purchase distilled water for formula preparation.
- For infants, divide daily formula powder allotment by the expected number of feedings per day. Put powder in the bottle and add warm water, then shake.
- For a 1-day trip, the Tupperware Gravy Shaker holds 18 oz and fits perfectly into a 2-quart thermos (freeze water in bottom of thermos).

For Trips of More than One Day

- Premeasure daily amounts of formula and put in little plastic containers or bags. Then when needed, pour into measured amount of water in a Tupperware Gravy Shaker or other tightly covered plastic container and mix.
- Ice is usually available at hotels/motels for daily mixing of premeasured formula powder.
- For car traveling, if you do not want to mix formula en route, freeze prepared formula in 1-day amounts. Put formula in its own ice chest, opening the chest only to use the formula. Frozen formula will keep well-frozen for about 5 days, as long as the weather is not extremely hot. Freeze formula in the Tupperware tall slim juice containers, which you can then use for juice and other beverages once each day's supply has been consumed.
- Another suggestion for longer trips: carry 1 wire whisk, 1 Tupperware container for mixing, premeasured baggies of formula powder, and 2 flip-top thermoses. Make up the formula each night in the 2 thermoses. Freeze one thermos in the motel manager's freezer and put one in the refrigerator (people are very generous if you explain your child's need to them). Use the refrigerated formula for breakfast. Pack the other in an insulated bag. If you use a little Blue Ice (or similar product), the frozen formula will be thawed but still cold for lunch and supper.

School Lunch

Food

Bag Lunch

Let your child help you plan lunch, offering choices he or she can make. As your child grows older, allow him or her more choices in what to pack for lunch or allow the child to pack the lunch alone, depending on age and skill. This reinforces what he or she has learned about the diet and allows more control of choices, very important for developing self-esteem.

- As first-graders learn to read, special notes tucked into the bottom of a lunch box can brighten your child's day.
- The child-size Tupperware lunchbox set has the perfect size containers for small appetites and lots of variety.
- A wide-mouth, short thermos is good for vegetables or soup. Teachers may be cooperative about a quick reheat in a microwave oven if necessary and one is available.
- Freeze small juice cans or juice-pack drinks, or fresh fruit in season (peach slices and berries do well) in small sealable containers. Slip into lunch box frozen. By lunchtime the fruit or juice will be thawed but still cold.
- If your child is used to eating raw vegetables and fresh fruit at room temperature rather than straight from the refrigerator, he or she may accept these items in a school lunch more easily.
- If most other children take hot lunches, try to get a menu in advance and pack a few things in your child's lunch box that are the same as (or close to) the hot lunch.

Hot Lunch

Depending on the age of your child and the extent of general participation in the school's program, occasional participation by your child can be important to him or her. Arrangements might be made with the cafeteria staff to put only allowable foods on the child's plate (based on your instructions); or if your child is trustworthy and knowledgeable enough about the diet, he or she may be able to select foods from the entire plate that are acceptable and report to you what was eaten, giving away or leaving unacceptable foods.

You may wish to choose days when the menu offers at least two items on the diet—usually fruit and a vegetable. You may want to pack an added item to round out the lunch. Depending on the particular school situation, the teacher may appreciate a note on the days your child chooses to take hot lunch, indicating which food items your child will be eating. A special reduced rate for the lunch may be available if you inquire.

Formula

- Freeze a Tupperware glass or flip-top thermos with half or two-thirds the amount you want to send. In the morning, add the remainder. The frozen formula will keep the fresh formula cold, but will be thawed by lunchtime.
- Send formula to school in a plastic thermos. Put the thermos in the freezer at night, without formula in it, then add fresh formula in the morning. Formula should remain cold until lunchtime.
- For children who are uncomfortable with friends smelling or seeing their formula, send a straw and let the child drink right from the thermos.
- For older children, purchase a plain thermos, without a picture. A child in 4th or 5th grade will not want to carry pictures of cute cartoon characters, etc.
- As children get older, some may not enjoy taking formula to school. Although formula should ideally be consumed mid-day as well as morning and evening, don't necessarily insist that formula must be consumed at school if the child is willing to drink it before and right after school and for supper or in the evening. Send fruit juice or fruit drink for lunch.
- For a child who resists drinking formula in front of other children, consider exploring the possibility of keeping formula in a refrigerator in the cafeteria or teachers' lounge and allowing the child to drink it in private before or after lunch.

School Lunch Ideas

(See *The Low Protein Food List for PKU* for nutrient content of non-recipe items.)

Bread/Crackers

sandwich with low protein bread (see pages 523–24 for ideas)
low protein dinner roll/margarine
low protein or regular crackers (plain or with dip)
muffin (any recipe in this book)
slice of low protein bread or quick bread with butter

Vegetables/Fruits

raw vegetables cut decoratively, plain or with dip (carrot sticks, celery sticks, radish roses, cauliflower flowerets, green pepper slices, mushrooms).

marinated mixed vegetables (any of the above marinated in Italian dressing)

pickles, olives

lettuce salad with seasoned croutons made from low protein bread

potato salad

coleslaw

low protein pasta salad

soup (homemade or canned)

fresh fruit (banana, apple, orange, fresh cherries, grapes, nectarine, peach, pear, tangerine, cubes or slice of melon, berries)

fruit salad

canned fruit

Prono gelled dessert

snack pack canned fruit or frozen fruit cups

6 oz can of juice (apple, grapefruit, orange, pineapple)

juice drink box with a straw

dried fruit (dates, small raisin box, banana chips, apricots, apples)

raw sliced apples sprinkled with lemon juice, then cinnamon and sugar

Weight Watcher's Apple Snacks

dried fruit roll-ups

fruit bars

Snack Items/Desserts

popcorn or caramel corn

pretzel sticks

snack-size bag of potato chips

Taco Chips

Pringles potato chips

mini M&M's packet

"fun-size" candy bar

Million Dollar Candy Bar

Hunt's lemon snack pack pudding

pudding made with non-dairy creamer (see page 399)

Junket Danish Dessert

cookies (any recipe in this book, or low protein commercially available varieties)

cupcakes or mini cupcakes baked in a tartlet pan (any recipe in this book)

"free" candy
vanilla wafers filled with "free" frosting
Cinnamon Graham Crackers filled with "free" frosting
Chocolate- or Fruit-Filled Turnovers
Chocolate Pinwheels or *Vanilla Pinwheels*
Donuts
Garlic Snack Croutons
Low Pro Snack Mix
Rock 'N Roll Raisin Mix

Sandwich Ideas

Put any of the following ingredients, in amounts desired, on low protein bread (see the *Low Protein Food List* for nutrient content):
apples (chopped), raisins, and a sprinkle of cinnamon
apple butter, cinnamon, and raisins
avocado (sliced or diced), Miracle Whip Salad Dressing,
and tomato
banana (thin sliced) and Miracle Whip Salad Dressing
brown sugar and "free" margarine
catsup and onions or pickle relish
carrots (shredded), raisins, and Miracle Whip
Salad Dressing
carrots (shredded), black olives, and Miracle Whip
Salad Dressing
celery (diced), raisins, and Miracle Whip
Salad Dressing
cucumbers (sliced or chopped), and chopped
onions or tomato
green peppers and onions (chopped), fried
green pepper (chopped) and apple (chopped)
with a little lemon juice
honey-butter, plain or with raisins
jam with a few Rice Krispies sprinkled
over it for crunch

523

jam or jelly and margarine

lettuce, sliced onion, tomato, and Miracle Whip
    Salad Dressing

mushrooms (canned, sliced, or chopped)
    and chopped olives

pickle relish (or pickle slices) and mustard

pineapple (slices or cut-up tidbits) and Miracle Whip
    Salad Dressing

potato chips (crushed) and Miracle Whip
    Salad Dressing

radishes (thin sliced), and Miracle Whip
    Salad Dressing

tomato (sliced), onion, and Miracle Whip
    Salad Dressing

School Snacks and Parties

For preschool and kindergarten snacks, you may be able to arrange with the school to have orange juice or fruit drink delivered along with milk that the other children will drink. Or send a supply of juice or juice drink boxes each week or month; or send Kool-Aid or Tang in a thermos. Tang could also be prepared right in the classroom by a willing teacher.

Very "low" preschool snacks to consider suggesting to the teacher:

½ banana

½ cored apple

½ graham cracker, or low protein *Cinnamon Graham Crackers*

mini box of raisins

individual cup of Prono low protein gelled dessert

At the beginning of the school year, deliver to the child's teacher a large supply of individual baggies filled with "free" candy, gum, or treats tied in a bright ribbon. When birthdays arise, the child may choose what to have.

Keep in touch with your child's teacher. Find out who the room mothers for parties are. If you contact them ahead of time, they will usually be more than happy to work around the diet, or can let you know what will be served so you can make a similar treat.

For an unexpected party, the teacher may be happy to keep frosted low protein cake or cupcakes in the school freezer. *Tastes-Like-Devil's-Food Cake* as cupcakes or *Chocolate Pinwheels* are great keepers. These are even good frozen, so defrosting ahead of time isn't necessary. Or give your child's teacher a Tupperware container with a box of graham crackers (or container of low protein *Cinnamon Graham Crackers*) and a can of "free" vanilla Pillsbury Frosting Supreme, or a box of Wel-Plan low protein cookies. You might also consider giving the teacher a supply of small bags of M&M's, always a favorite, for a ready treat. The children in the class may even learn to bring an identifiable treat like the M&M's, along with their birthday treats, especially for your child.

Give the teacher a list of snack-type foods that are allowed on the diet and appropriate portion sizes for unexpected treats or "food experiences," etc., in the classroom.

If either the teacher or your child is not sure whether a certain food is allowed on the diet, instruct the teacher to call you or have the child bring the treat home.

For times when your child can eat what is being served at snacktime, teach your child to report to you what he or she had and how much. You can check on your child's accuracy by periodically contacting the teacher to verify what your child has told you. Contacting your child's teacher periodically (or perhaps talking with the teacher at a regularly scheduled parent conference), to find out how responsible your child is in general about the diet in the classroom is highly encouraged.

The child's teacher must be told about aspartame and cautioned about the myriad of products that contain it. Be careful which list you give the teacher; old food lists may not contain information about products that have been reformulated to contain aspartame. In addition to or in place of a list, advise the teacher about *types* of foods/drinks that typically contain aspartame (see page 29).

Hospitalizations

Arrange through your child's admitting physician to meet with the hospital dietitian. The dietary staff may not be knowledgeable about the diet, but will probably allow you to special-order menu items appropriate for your child.

Even though you may have the full cooperation of the hospital dietitian, be prepared to provide most of the child's food yourself. If the stay will be longer than a day or two, before you go to the hospital it would be wise to pack a variety of non-perishable foods, such as your child's favorite cereals, canned soups, low protein crackers or cookies, etc., to have available.

Remember that your child is being treated for an illness—not PKU. A few days "off" the prescribed diet is not going to have disastrous results. Your primary concern should be to make a sick child well, following the advice of the physician, and then to re-establish the diet.

UNIVERSITY HOSPITALS
MENU

Breakfast

☐ orange juice
☑ apple juice
☐ grapefruit half

☑ cold cereal *Rice Krispies please!*
☐ hot cereal

☐ fried eggs
☐ pancakes
☐ French toast

☐ milk *We will provide PKU formula— Ann Smith*
☐ coffee
☐ tea

GOOD MORNING!

EVERYDAY TIPS

General Food Storage and Labeling Tips

Tupperware sells handy labels for anything you want to identify. These are great for babysitters, your freezer or refrigerator, or for travel. You may also purchase plain white or colored labels from any office supply store.

For infants, label each baby food jar after purchasing it and before putting it away, with portion size and phenylalanine or protein content so you can easily identify those with a "high" or "low" content when needed.

Label all of your home-baked items with the name of the recipe, portion size, and phenylalanine or protein:

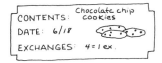

When you buy cereal, use stick-on labels in bright colors (which stand out from package labels) to identify serving size and phenylalanine or protein content. Put the labels in a consistent place (e.g. upper right-hand corner). If it's a product you use continuously, use the removable labels; you can just peel it off and stick it on the next box.

For snacks and for any occasion, premeasure all types of foods—from carrots to cereal. Keep them in airtight containers or plastic bags and store appropriately. Label as above.

Especially during the summer and early fall when you may be freezing the season's harvest, measure out appropriate servings, put into small empty margarine tubs and label. It is then handy to use premeasured fruits and vegetables from the freezer as needed.

Tupperware products are excellent for storage of all kids of low protein foods—for refrigerator or freezer.

Consider storing wheat starch in a Tupperware cereal container. The opening is about the size of a ¼ cup measuring cup and allows you to spoon out the starch without the "fly away" problems of working with wheat starch directly from the bag. It is also convenient to put Wel-Plan Baking Mix in a cannister or other larger container.

Food Freezing Tips

Want to avoid the what's-for-the-diet-blues forever? Make use of your freezer to stockpile an assortment of ready-to-eat dishes and a variety of foods. Then cash in on your assets whenever you need them. Think of your freezer as a creative tool, not merely a storehouse for leftovers. The key is knowing what to freeze, how to package it, how to keep track of it, and how to use it.

Planning

Develop a plan based on your child's favorite foods, keeping the inventory changing.

Freeze meal-sized quantities.

Keep a running inventory. It will help you to plan menus and ensure that no foods stay frozen too long. The inventory should have name of recipe, date, portion size, and amount of phenylalanine or protein. Cross off items when they are used.

As part of your record-keeping, label every package you put in the freezer, to match your inventory information, using stick-on labels. You might want to add "reheat at 350° for 10 minutes" or some other brief instructions.

Packaging

Adequate wrapping is the key to successful freezing. All foods should have an airtight seal, and the wraps and bags used for freezing foods must be strong enough to withstand the jostling that invariably occurs while you search for items.

Choose a freezer wrap that retains the moisture-vapor in foods. Moisture is the most significant factor affecting a food's freshness. If moisture-vapor escapes, your food can also suffer from freezer burn—drying out of food through loss of moisture. In tests of freezer wraps, Saran Wrap has been found to be the best. The common plastic-coated paper types of freezer wraps also work well but are more expensive then Saran Wrap. Ziploc freezer bags, with food wrapped in Saran Wrap first, provide excellent moisture-proof storage. Seal-A-Meal bags also work very well for vegetables, soups, etc.

Aluminum foil retains moisture but is expensive and crinkling up the foil creates tiny holes that can let moisture out.

Plastic containers with tight snap-on lids will also work well. If the lid is not very snug, put several layers of Saran Wrap over the top of the container, then put the lid on. Square and rectangular containers use space most efficiently. Select those that stack nicely when in use and nest together when empty.

Save little plastic margarine tubs and use for freezing vegetable dishes and casseroles. The tubs can be heated in a microwave oven and the food served directly in the tub for convenience.

If you are short of casserole containers, let the food freeze in the baking dish, then remove it when frozen hard and wrap it in plastic wrap or freezer paper. When you're ready to reheat it, slip it back into the dish.

Freezing and Defrosting

It is important that food freezes quickly. When freezing fresh or freshly prepared foods, don't stack the containers. Leave an inch or so of room between them so that cold air can circulate and remove heat. Then stack them once they are frozen. Placing the containers in direct contact with the freezer surface also speeds freezing and minimizes flavor loss.

When you are preparing dishes specifically for freezing, undercook slightly. Reheating will bring them to their optimum state.

Do not refreeze food that has been cooked, frozen, and reheated unless it is a baked item like bread, cookies, etc. A second reheating may overcook. In addition, as the food sits in the serving dish for a second time, and then cools to go back to the freezer, bacteria may flourish.

Food that has been defrosted in the refrigerator and has not reached more than 40°F (ordinary refrigerator temperature) for a short period of time *can* be safely refrozen as long as color, odor, and texture seem acceptable to you.

To reheat frozen foods, you can thaw first, or cook straight from the freezer.

It is best to thaw frozen foods in the refrigerator. If you need to speed the process, run lukewarm water over the package, or thaw in a microwave oven according to manufacturer's instructions. When you haven't time to thaw, you can cook food that is still frozen. If oven-heating, use freezer-to-oven-ware and allow about 50% more baking time. Top of the oven heating will require only a little more time than the recipe says.

Do not keep frozen items for longer than 3 to 4 months; in time, the quality of even properly packaged food will diminish.

Foods to Freeze

- Homemade soups.
- Vegetable dishes/main dishes (but be aware that freezing can leave potatoes somewhat mealy and pastas softer). Low protein pizza and/ or pizza crusts are a "must." Low protein pot pies and turnovers and filled or unfilled crepes are also appealing, "low," and freeze well.
- Freeze items such as pizza sauce in ice cube trays, premeasuring amounts. When frozen, place in a plastic freezer bag, and remove as needed.

- Onions. Chop coarsely in blender or food processor, drain well, spread out in a single layer on a cookie sheet, and freeze, then put in a freezer container. Use frozen onions to speed preparation for a variety of vegetable/main dish recipes as needed.
- Low protein bread, rolls, muffins, quick breads, crackers, tortillas, and waffles (freeze tortilla and waffles on a paper plate for support, with waxed paper or plastic wrap between each), frosted or unfrosted cakes and cupcakes, pie crust, cookies.
- Frozen bread dough is also ideal for making fresh dinner rolls. Freeze dough in small balls; thaw, shape as desired, let rise and bake as for any of the dinner roll recipes in the book. (The rolls may not rise as much as rolls from unfrozen dough, however.)
- Cookie dough. Freeze in bulk, small portions, or as *Freezer Cookies.*
- Pie dough either in bulk or made into small pie shells.
- Bread crumbs or croutons (crusts and stale bread make great crumbs or croutons). For crumbs, if necessary, dry bread in oven. Crumble as fine as desired in food processor or blender. For croutons, cut in small pieces, pour melted margarine over them, and toast in oven, or make *Garlic Snack Croutons* or *Low Pro Snack Mix.* Both can be frozen in a bag or other small container.
- Non-dairy creamer. Rich's Coffee Rich and Richwhip Topping keep well in the freezer for months. Freeze small portions in an ice cube tray, then remove to a plastic freezer bag for convenient use.
- Crumbs from *Cinnamon Graham Crackers* for a later pie crust or topping.
- Small measured containers of fruit (such as blueberries in portion sizes to be added to pancakes or muffins, strawberries for *Instant Strawberry Ice Cream,* various fruits for *Banana Smoothies* and fruit smoothie variations, etc.).

Food Ideas

If you run out of wheat starch, you can try substituting cornstarch. The quality of the item *may* be very similar, though you cannot be sure of this. Do *not* substitute cornstarch for Wel-Plan Baking Mix, as the recipe will probably not be successful.

For a new flavor, add a little Nestlé Chocolate Quik to a mixture of one part hot cooked cereal and low protein porridge or add chilled applesauce, cinnamon, and a few raisins.

As a handy substitute for low protein porridge, grind low protein pasta in a blender or food processor until fine. Mix with regular hot cooked cereal to lower phenylalanine content.

When preparing hot cereal using a mixture of regular cereal and low protein porridge, add them to the water *first*, then cook, and you will not get lumps.

Some commercial low protein cookies can be quite hard; soften and freshen them by putting in a microwave oven for a few seconds, or store in an airtight container with a piece of apple or bread.

Use Wel-Plan Sweet Cookies for making an ice cream sandwich, using low protein ice cream. Or frost the cookies and decorate with candy sprinkles.

Take any crumbs from low protein cookies and continue accumulating in a container that you keep frozen over a period of time. Add to the container any special baked items which your child dislikes or is bored with and grind in a blender. Your "crumbs" can be used to make crumb pie crusts, sprinkled on pudding, or used as toppings for fruit crisps. Do the same for low protein bread crumbs and use for casserole toppings. Low protein bread crusts can also be saved and made into croutons, for making *Garlic Snack Croutons* or *Low Pro Snack Mix*. Stale bread also makes excellent croutons.

Rather than baking a cake (unless for a birthday party), make cupcakes. Freeze with or without icing. Wrap individually in plastic wrap if unfrosted. It takes only a little while for the cupcakes to thaw, and if stored in airtight containers in the freezer they keep well for 3 to 4 months without losing their good taste or texture.

For low protein *Vanilla Creampops* or *Chocolate Creampops*, or other frozen pops use regular wooden Popsicle sticks in Tupperware Ice Tups instead of the plastic ones provided so they look more like the commercial kind eaten by siblings or friends.

Add either catsup or steak sauce to plain white rice for a change.

"Stretch" rice by mixing with equal amounts of cooked Aproten Anellini or Wel-Plan Spaghetti Ring Style.

To make mashed potatoes the whole family can enjoy, mash them with margarine and hot potato water; or use Rich's Coffee Rich diluted 1 : 1 with water.

Weigh a corn cob before and after your child is finished eating. Or choose a small cob and weigh or measure it before and after cutting off the corn. Do this several times so you have a rough idea of the proper size of cob to give the child for a given amount of phenylalanine.

Formula Tips

If you dislike making formula every day and have freezer space, try preparing formula for a few days or up to one week and freeze in individual covered containers. Each night before you go to bed take out a container for the next day to thaw in the refrigerator. Or premeasure daily formula powder into jars or plastic bags for quick and easy use.

Prepare formula in the Tupperware Gravy Shaker rather than a blender; generally it works just as well. If you need more than the amount it holds, put in all of the formula powder, mix with some of the water needed, then pour into a larger pitcher and add cold water to equal the total volume desired.

As an "emergency back-up," consider leaving a can of formula at a nearby relative's or friend's house.

Try using formula rather than non-dairy creamer on any cereals; as the child grows, continue using formula on cereal.

Try using formula rather than non-dairy creamer for making Jell-O instant pudding, using 2 tablespoons plus 2 teaspoons pudding mix with ½ cup formula (texture will be thin but many children don't mind).

For variety, add Nestlé Strawberry Quik, or almond, orange, or mint extract to formula. A few drops of your black coffee with a little sugar, a few drops of vanilla with a little sugar, Tang, or other protein-free drink powders are also good for masking the taste of formula.

Mix formula with any of the low protein ice creams or sherbets for a "shake."

Some children prefer formula that is icy cold, so you might try freezing it and serving it slightly slushy, or putting an ice cube or crushed ice in it. This is especially nice for hot summer days.

If you have trouble with your child's drinking enough formula, a positive approach will always work better than threats. Motivation for a child as young as preschool age can be enhanced by giving the child pleasant experiences to associate with drinking formula. A reward of a special activity, food, or anything your child enjoys could get you over a formula "slump" and avoid future battles.

A special glass or a straw may help formula go down better. Formula that won't go down any other way just may taste wonderful out of a shot glass, or a little liqueur glass, instead of in a large (overwhelming) glass.

For children who are not fond of formula, adding it to other foods to increase intake is usually not successful, though it could be tried (puddings, ice cream, baked goods).

For older children, reinforcement by PKU clinic professionals of the importance of formula for growing and being healthy may be helpful in fostering a positive attitude.

Remember that your child's appetite and interest in drinking formula will vary from day to day. As with any child, such variations are normal and you should not expect your child to get exactly the same volume of formula every day. If the clinic has prescribed a certain volume of formula, you should try to attain this as an *average* over about a *one-week* period, with some days less and some days more than the prescribed amount.

Consult your PKU clinic nutritionist for advice on appropriate changes in formula density or composition, to suit your child's individual needs, as well as taste and volume preferences.

Eating Habits and Mealtime

Your child needs to learn to accept the diet from a young age, observing what is on the diet and what is not. You should not dramatically alter your diet to accommodate the child's diet (i.e., eliminating meat) but you may want to avoid regularly eating foods that are especially child-appealing in his or her presence. "Closet-eating" may be appropriate for you at times.

In general, don't use food as a pacifier or a reward, or withhold it as a punishment.

Set a good example. Children copy their parents' likes and dislikes.

Try new foods and recipes. You cannot expect your child to do so if you do not.

Taste-test your child's low protein foods. This will promote a positive attitude towards these foods, for both you and your child. Avoid showing distaste for any of the foods.

Introducing a wide variety of vegetables and fruits at the earliest age possible will help avoid the "picky eater" syndrome. Make a special point of letting your child try foods you do not necessarily like. Don't ignore the more unusual fruits and vegetables. Remember that a young child's taste for foods is just developing and the wider his or her taste experience, the more likely it is that he or she will come to enjoy many different foods, and the easier diet management will be.

Toddlers can be encouraged to eat vegetables by serving them in unfamiliar forms, such as in matchstick pieces. Serve raw vegetables at the start of the meal, when the child is most apt to be hungry.

Don't force your child to eat a food he or she dislikes, but do insist that the child eat or at least taste two different foods at each meal.

Try new foods for your young child at lunch time. If the food is refused or less than the expected portion is eaten, the diet can easily be adjusted at dinner time.

Limit the amount of "undesirable" foods you keep in the house. Have on hand plenty of fresh fruit, fresh vegetables, and low protein items. Avoid having tempting snack foods such as chips in the house.

Don't be afraid to set limits. Say no to "unhealthy" foods and explain why the child should eat low protein foods.

Try to eat meals on a regular schedule. When a meal is overdue, there is a tendency to snack, leaving fewer exchanges for mealtime.

Consider establishing a general rule (with some exceptions allowed) that no single meal can contain more than ⅓ (or ½) of the child's total daily phenylalanine or protein allowance. Give your child a range of food choices for meals to encourage consideration of phenylalanine/protein intake and to change the emphasis from the foods that are forbidden to foods that are allowed.

Don't dwell on the diet at mealtime. A little discussion about exchanges may be needed, but plan ahead with your older child so that he or she knows what to expect by the time the family sits down.

Have a positive attitude at mealtime. This should be a relaxed time for sharing and for happy conversation—not a time for reprimanding.

Don't rave about meat. *Do* comment on the goodness of foods the child is able to eat along with everyone else.

Encourage conversation at mealtime. The child on-diet will typically have less to eat than others, so use conversation to fill the extra time. Have everyone remain at the table until *all* are finished.

Consider having periodic "special event" meals at home. For example, have all family members make their own salad, pizza, or ice cream sundaes, using appropriate low protein ingredients for the child on-diet. Or try table-top cooking with a fondue pot or wok, using vegetables for everyone and adding meat for those not on-diet, or have a cookout and grill vegetable shish kabobs.

Have the whole family participate in occasional "meatless" meals, or meals when everyone eats a special low protein item.

The child on-diet (beyond toddler age) should be served just as everyone else is served, either "family style" or with prefilled plates, after you have considered the advantages of both methods. The method you use can be varied, depending on time and on what is being served.

Family Style

All food is on the table in plain view. The child on-diet learns to choose proper food, measure and/or count and pass up what is not allowed. With a young child you can take the opportunity to explain what is included in his or her diet and what is included in your diet and others' diets. In this method, measuring devices or a gram scale become part of the child's place setting. The child should be told how much to serve. Tupperware has a ⅛ cup (2 tablespoons) measure that works well for smaller portions.

Prefilled Plates

Weigh and/or measure diet portions as you dish up appropriate serving portions for others in the family. If diet food gets too cool by the time this is done, it is convenient to briefly reheat it in a microwave oven. This method allows more precise control of phenylalanine intake and avoids commotion if the child wants foods not allowed.

Meal Planning

When possible, prepare meals for your child as much like those for the rest of the family as possible. Take advantage of the many recipes adaptable for diet *and* family, or make your own simple adaptations (for example, when eating bacon, lettuce, and tomato sandwiches give your child the same, omitting bacon and using low protein bread).

Try to plan dinner meals so that the child can share at least one part of the meal that everyone else will eat.

In general, if the whole family eats simple, unadorned foods it will be easier for the child to partake in the meal.

Sometimes it may not work out for the child on-diet to have something similar to what others will be eating. Don't be overly concerned. The child needs to become accustomed to the differences and may not mind or even notice. Here's an opportunity to encourage individuality by not being "just like everybody else." Children on-diet do it *their* way!

Try to make your child's plate as colorful and attractive as possible. This is very important! Consider buying your child special dishes designed for children; they are colorful and add much to mealtimes. Children look forward almost as much to seeing "their" dishes as they do to the food on them. Colorful plates and placemats can be found in many discount stores, department stores, or specialty stores. Beginning when your child is a toddler, try to arrange food attractively on the plate, as you would find it in a fine restaurant. Look at this as a creative challenge. Naturally, you won't do this for every meal, but a bit of garnish and an eye to colorful foods do much to make most meals more inviting. An example of adding color: With the wide variety of vegetables the children on-diet can eat, pastas can be made especially appealing by using chopped red and green bell peppers, black olives, red tomatoes, green herbs, a little paprika and even curry powder.

As children get older, the *number* of items on their plate becomes important—perhaps even more important than *what* is on the plate for children of certain ages. Be conscious of equalizing the number of items on the child's plate so it is the same as those that others have, or at least the same as siblings have. Even one olive or a pickle may be enough in the child's view to "count" for one item.

Food Ideas for Breakfast, Lunch, and Supper

Breakfast

Banana Breakfast Toast
Best White Bread or *Best Homestyle Bread*, toasted, buttered, and
    sprinkled with cinnamon and sugar
Broiled Pineapple Toast
Caramel Rolls

Cinnamon Raisin Bread toasted, with apple butter or honey butter
Cinnamon Rolls
Donuts
French Toast
Filled Coffee Braid
Frosted Orange Creme, using formula
Hot Cross Buns
muffins (any recipe in this book)
Orange Freeze, using formula
pancakes (any recipe in this book)
Peach Toast
Waffles
Beverages:
   fruit juice (any)
   Tang or Start
Cereal:
   cold cereal with or without fruit
   hot cereal with added low protein porridge
Fruits:
   banana
   fresh berries
   fresh peach or nectarine slices
   grapefruit slices
   melon wedge or chunks
   orange slices
   tangerine

Lunch

sandwich using low protein bread (see pages 523–24)
School Lunch Ideas (pages 521–24)

Supper

Any of the soups, salads, main dishes and vegetables, bread or dessert recipes are suitable. Especially note the Quick-to-Fix Food Ideas in the Quick and Easy section of the book (pages 292–294.)

Food Ideas for Special Theme Meals

Chinese

   Chinese Fried Rice
   Chinese Sweet-Sour Vegetables
   Chop Suey
   Chow Mein
   Mock Egg Rolls

Sweet and Sour Sauce
Vegetable Stir-Frying
mixture of rice and Aproten Anellini or
    Wel-Plan Spaghetti Ring Style with a dash of soy sauce
rice with a dash of soy sauce
Wel-Plan Short-Cut Spaghetti cooked
    firm-tender (to resemble Chinese noodles)

French

Broccoli Crepes or *Asparagus Crepes*
Crescent Roll
fresh fruit ice (any recipe in this book)
green salad

Italian

Breadsticks
green salad with marinated vegetables
    and Italian dressing
low protein garlic bread
marinated vegetable plate
spaghetti sauce on low protein noodles
Veggie Spaghetti

Mexican

Burritos
Guacamole
Mexican Rice
Salsa Fresca
Taco
Taco Chips with taco sauce, salsa,
    or guacamole
Taco Salad

Middle Eastern

Mediterranean Vegetable Casserole
Low Pro Tabouleh

Snacks

Establishing a regular time for snacking is advantageous for maintaining best control of diet. Non-stop or unscheduled nibbling can be avoided if your child is taught from a young age that snacks are limited to several defined times (afternoon/after-school and evening, or for preschool children perhaps also mid-morning).

Analyze family snacking habits and work on making adjustments in the whole family's patterns if necessary.

Educate your child on-diet that nibbles can quicky add 1 to 3 exchanges per day, much the same as they add calories for someone on a reducing diet; it all counts, measured or not, since the quantities of phenylalanine or protein allowed are so small in the first place. Parents with chronic nibblers should take quantities equal to the amount nibbled and put them in measuring cups to show the child how much extra he or she is getting in the diet by nibbling. This, more than outright cheating, is the source of "going over" the diet allowance for most older children.

If possible, snacks should be eaten away from the television set, unless "free" items are being eaten. It is easy for the child to "forget" that he or she has just consumed something, asking for more within a short time. Snacks should be savored and appreciated, away from distractions.

Realize that requests for snacks by young children are many times a request for mom's or dad's attention.

When other children in the family have snacks, encourage the use of foods which the child on-diet can also have, at least part of the time.

For young children, put premeasured treats or "free" foods in plastic bags. Attach to your refrigerator with a cute kitchen magnet. When your child wants a snack, he or she knows this is available without asking, at allowed times. Or put low protein items on a special shelf or in a drawer marked with the child's name.

Gently steer your child away from snacks or foods that are "higher" than you think desirable. "Let's have some _____, it's better for you."

When you take your young child to visit playmates, take along extra snack foods to offer the others if your child can't eat what they have (e.g., raisins, pretzels, etc.).

Snack Ideas

Suggested Recipes from "Low Protein Cookery" and Other Food Ideas

Banana Pops
Breadsticks/Soft Pretzels
Chocolate or *Vanilla Creampops*
Chocolate or *Vanilla Pinwheels*
Chocolate Turnovers

Fruit-Filled Turnovers
Cinnamon Graham Crackers
Cinnamon Munch
cookies (any recipe in this book)
cupcakes (any recipe in this book)
Donuts (or donut holes)
Finger Gelatin
Frosted Orange Creme
Frozen Suckers
Fruit Smoothies
Garlic Snack Croutons
Grammys
Grape or Orange Pudding Pops
Ice Cream Sandwiches
Low Pro Snack Mix
Mini S'More Snacks
Mock Angel Food
muffins (any recipe in this book)
Orange Freeze
quick breads (any recipe in this book)
Rock 'N Roll Raisin Mix
Snack Crackers

Strawberry Shake
Taco Chips plain, with dip, or with taco sauce or salsa
Toasted Cinnamon Sticks
Toasted Honey Sticks

Other Ideas

carrot or celery sticks
dried fruit (apples, apricots, banana chips, pineapple rings, pears,
    raisins)
fresh fruit
dried fruit roll-ups
fruit bars
olives, pickles
rice cakes, either plain or spread with margarine, jam, or honey
    (plain ones made only of puffed rice, available in grocery stores
    and natural food stores; one cake equals 30 mg of phenylalanine,
    8 gm protein, 34 calories)
Wel-Plan crackers
any of the snack items listed on pages 522–23.

Diet Management Tips for Older Children and Teens

For school lunches, expect considerable peer pressure for food to *be* like (not just look like) what others are eating. Small bags of chips, mini candy bars, etc., will become important "junk food" which can still be supplemented with fruits, low protein sandwiches, etc.

Often "blending in" is more important to older children than what is eaten in situations away from home. Do not make "waves" for your child to accommodate diet (unless he or she wants this). The child may choose not to eat at all rather than bother someone to make or to have available an allowable food substitute.

Try to refrain from "oversupervising" your child's food weighing/measuring/counting activities. With appropriate earlier teaching, the child should be allowed responsibility to handle the diet as much as possible, without parents constantly looking over his or her shoulder.

"Cheating" may be inevitable to some extent for most older children/teens. Absolute adherence to the diet at all times, with perfect counting/measuring and keeping track is probably an unreal expectation for anyone. Occasional indiscretions should be handled calmly, or ignored in some circumstances, especially if it is a matter of the child eating *more* of allowable foods rather than eating forbidden foods. It is important to strike a balance between absolute rigidity and overindulgence. However, high blood levels over prolonged periods should be avoided and the child should take responsibility for keeping levels low.

It may occasionally be important to allow an older child/teen a food for which the phenylalanine content is not precisely known, making an estimate based on knowledge of phenylalanine content for a similar food (for example, a dinner roll at a restaurant or a plain cookie at a potluck dinner). In such instances, it will be wise to estimate "high" rather than underestimating.

Allow the child/teen to make decisions about how many exchanges to use for each meal, based on his or her knowledge of the total number allowed. Some guidelines may be provided. Be sure to forewarn the child ahead of time if a meal out or a relatively "high" food is planned for dinner so that exchanges can be planned accordingly.

Diet should never be an excuse to say "no" to an activity or travel. Opportunities will arise for school trips, camping with scouts, traveling with a marching band, etc. It *will* be extra work to plan for diet, but saying "yes" to such activities will promote a positive self-image and prepare the child for "solo" diet management. Coolers, hot plates/toaster ovens, etc., can be used for accommodating diet needs.

Teenagers should be taught what to ask to have eliminated when ordering a "vegetarian" meal on their own in a restaurant. Many good restaurants do have vegetarian alternatives, but some may include high protein foods, such as cheese. The eliminated items will typically be replaced by additional vegetables and/or fruits.

Plan dates around activities rather than food. When eating is part of the date, fast-food restaurants can be suggested, where french fries and cold drinks are always available, or a restaurant that serves a salad bar, baked potato, or fruit. Your child/teen may not really mind eating fries and salad while others eat pizza, etc.

INDEX

Index

M

Q

R

S